Shahriar Shahir's life turning point was Shana's birth in 2011. His main characteristics are being patriotic and a philomath and having a great passion for learning. His motto is love, courage, effort, and faith.

He has dedicated his life to work and striving for success, growth, and development. Although he faced obstacles during his path, he gained valuable achievements.

He got a scholarship from Emirates Flying School and obtained a pilot's license. He had the incredible privilege of having many careers. However, his passion has always been business and he believes he grew up in it.

He implemented the dream of establishing a business with global standards in the franchise industry. At the same time, he created the Hoopoe brand, which is the fruit of many years of experience in the business world. In parallel, he published nine books about the standardization of the franchise industry which contain more than 1,000 pages and are registered and certified by the UAE.

With the birth of his second child, Michael, in 2024, he has found even greater inspiration to continue his journey as a writer, creating timeless works.

To those who have inspired me to explore the depths of human nature.

To the thinkers and dreamers who dare to question the norms.

To all who seek understanding in the complexities of life—this work is dedicated to you.

Your influence, guidance, and curiosity have fueled my journey.

Shahriar Shahir Barzegar

SEX

A Look at Human Alienation in the World of Sex

AUSTIN MACAULEY PUBLISHERS®
LONDON * CAMBRIDGE * NEW YORK * SHARJAH

Copyright © Shahriar Shahir Barzegar 2025

All rights reserved. No part of this publication may be reproduced, distributed, or transmitted in any form or by any means, including photocopying, recording, or other electronic or mechanical methods, without the prior written permission of the publisher, except in the case of brief quotations embodied in critical reviews and certain other non-commercial uses permitted by copyright law. For permission requests, write to the publisher.

Any person who commits any unauthorized act in relation to this publication may be liable to criminal prosecution and civil claims for damages.

Ordering Information
Quantity sales: Special discounts are available on quantity purchases by corporations, associations, and others. For details, contact the publisher at the address below.

Publisher's Cataloging-in-Publication data
Barzegar, Shahriar Shahir
Sex

ISBN 9798895433188 (Paperback)
ISBN 9798895433195 (Hardback)
ISBN 9798895433218 (ePub e-book)
ISBN 9798895433201 (Audiobook)

Library of Congress Control Number: 2025902491

www.austinmacauley.com/us

First Published 2025
Austin Macauley Publishers LLC
40 Wall Street, 33rd Floor, Suite 3302
New York, NY 10005
USA

mail-usa@austinmacauley.com
+1 (646) 5125767

Table of Contents

An Introduction to an Introduction   13

Chapter One: Sad Human in the World of Sexuality   25

    What Is the Relationship Between Love and Sex?   29

    Is Sex Biological or Mystical and Emotional?   31

    The Gap Between Sex and Virtue   33

    The "Bipolarity" Between Sex Is a Product of Creation Consciousness   37

    Sexual Satisfaction Is a Window to Spiritual Evolution   42

    The Short World of Inversion of Feeling   49

    Would the World Be a Better Place Without Lust?   51

Chapter Two: The Lost Half of Humanity   55

    Finding the Right Partner or the Right Way to Relate to Him   55

    Matching Is a Superficial Work or a Work Related to the Inner Human Being   57

    The Role of Human Childhood in Mating Aesthetics   60

    From Dating to Flirting, from Greetings to Sex   62

    Holding Hands Is the Beginning of the Trust Stage   64

    A Kiss, the Beginning of Contact Between the Insides and the Exit from Loneliness   65

    Getting Naked, the Beginning of the Deep Symbiosis of Cells   66

    Departure from Normal Behavior, the Beginning of the

Fusion of Souls	*71*
Orgasm Is the Peak of Oneness of Souls	*75*
Reject Requests for Sex and Relationship	*79*
Chapter Three: The Glory of the Sacrifice of Bodies	**82**
Late Sex, Its Causes and Consequences	*82*
Coldness of Temper, Impasse of Sensual Affections	*87*
Poetic Feast of Sex	*89*
Sacrifice of Bodies in Ideal Sex	*90*
Refreshing Sex Requires Creativity	*93*
Can Sexual Playfulness Be Permanent?	*94*
Rejuvenation of Sexual Attraction	*96*
A Night in a Hotel or Anywhere Other Than Home	*98*
Defamiliarization in Sex	*99*
Artistic Sex, an Opening out of the Dead End	*104*
The Philosophy of the Originality of the Body and the Issues Surrounding It	*107*
Leave the Habit and Discover Another	*113*
Removing the Imposed Masks	*117*
Escape from the Archetype of the Holy Woman	*118*
Mankind and Its Masks	*128*
Chapter Four: Sexually Defective Activism	**134**
Kamasutra, Understanding Sexually Defective Activism	*134*
Relationship Management; See a Therapist	*138*
Sexual Impotence and Premature Ejaculation	*141*
Female Abilities and Male Disabilities	*143*
Multiple Ejaculations Versus Single Ejaculation	*144*
Sense Organs—Sexual Organs	*145*

Inequality of Women in Sex	146
The First Factor: Male Impotence	146
The Second Factor: Cultural Crises	147
The Third Factor: Religious Restrictions	148
The Fourth Factor: Social Taboos	149
Man's Physiological Weakness, the Reasons for an Enmity	150
The Fifth Chapter: A Bridge to Transcend Oneself	**156**
Love Is the Astrolabe of God's Secrets	156
Bridges to Cross Oneself	158
The Two-Way Nature of Love	159
Love Is Plurality but Unity	160
Love and Spiritual Refinement of Society	163
Love Can Be Learned	167
Relationship Between Marriage and Love	168
Marriage and Love; Two Mismatches or Two Pieces of a Puzzle	174
Love, Sex, Marriage, Free Relationship	189
Love and Betrayal: Two Sides of the Same Coin	194
Chapter Six The History of Male Tyranny	**197**
Humans of Every Gender Are Organs of One Body	197
Should the Female Soul Be Loved Only?	201
Suppression of Women, Instead of Competition and Opportunity	204
The Role of Religions in Marginalizing Women	212
The Exclusive Advantages of Men and Women	216
A Sign of Women's Freedom in the Process of Sex	220
A Window to the Future	222

Humiliation of Women in Linguistics	*226*
Male Deception	*231*
Literary Texts Are Tools of Male Propaganda	*232*
Eastern Burned Mother, Archetype of the Flaming Candle	*238*
The Fundamental Rights of a Natural Sinner	*241*
Sexual Power Is the Criterion for Evaluating a Woman	*243*
A New Era and the Beginning of New Relationships	*244*
Motherhood—Femininity	*251*
Children, Mothers, Fathers and Educational System	*252*
The Third Type of Mother-Child Relationship	*255*
Family Without a Center of Authority	*258*
Family Incompatibility with Women's Freedom	*260*
Sex for Reproduction, That's It and Nothing Else	*261*
Women Flourish in the Absence of Traditional Relationships	*265*
Democracy and Women's Revolutionary Movement	*267*
Is Mankind Doomed to Be Alone?	*273*
What Is the Problem of Being a Man or a Woman?	*282*
Chapter Seven: Free Relationship, Pornography, Homosexuality, and Other Cases	**288**
Free Relationship, Why and How?	*288*
What Is Sexual Fetishism?	*293*
Pornography, Requirements of the Modern Age	*298*
The Relationship Between Pornography and Art	*303*
Animals and the Conventional Limits of Sexual Morality	*306*
Female Homosexuality Is More Logical than Male Homosexuality	*308*
Legal Violation	*313*

Female Circumcision, a Brutal Russian Way to Suppress Female Sexuality — *316*

The Purpose of Female Circumcision — *317*

Other Factors Affecting Female Circumcision — *318*

Menstruation Is Aimed at Creation, Not Opinion — *319*

Chapter Eight: Marriage, Reproduction and the Philosophy of Absurdity — **326**

Marriage Is Not the Same as Having Children — *326*

Marriage, a Pattern of Communication Between Men and Women; Buts and Ifs — *329*

Marriage and to Educate Children — *330*

Marriage and Mental Betrayal — *348*

Procreation and the Philosophy of Emptiness — *351*

The Solution to Birth Opponents — *356*

A Child Is Not an Imitation Machine — *357*

An Introduction to an Introduction

Sex or sexual intercourse is one of the most fundamental components of the human biological system. If we want to demonstrate several important factors in the formation of human life and its continuity to this day, sex, or "sexual force," is one of them. Sexual force not only ensures the continuity of the human race systematically but has also been a powerful driving force in regulating human relationships in social realms, beliefs, and personal relationships, moving them forward.

The evolutionary history of humans is just one of the results of the functioning of sexual force in life. Not only does evolutionary psychology attribute a significant role to the impact of sexual activity on human mental health, but one of the most fundamental theories related to evolution, known as the Darwinian-evolutionary theory, is based on human sexual behavior.

We will explain that according to the Darwinian biological evolution perspective, humans naturally strive for the highest probability of success in reproduction and ensuring the health of the offspring through sexual selection, based on the genetic data recorded in the genetic map.

The self-regulating sexual behavior has ensured the evolutionary process of human evolution through sexual mechanisms for centuries. However, this is not the only thing that highlights the issue of sex in human life.

Throughout history, regulatory or religious institutions have made extensive efforts to channelize the element of sexuality. In the face of these constant challenges, humans have always viewed sex as a significant "issue" and witnessed conflicting forces waging war to control it. This continuous experience has gradually sedimented in the human subconscious and in their DNA system, turning into a historical complex.

The intervening forces have been so powerful that they have extended their areas of influence and control to even the bedroom and the intimate space of men and women. A look at religious books dedicated to teaching the principles of procreation is indicative of the fact that the religious institution in its controlling nature has no limits and does not recognize personal boundaries.

If the actors of these institutions were to focus on finding effective keywords for understanding and optimizing sexuality instead of concentrating on defining the social boundaries of sex, this social issue would have gained an acceptable order and structure, and humans would have experienced a more peaceful life alongside sex.

Limitations in resources and scientific channels, lack of information and effective education about the general and combined functions of sex (based on science rather than religion), lead to any effort (including the small effort you see in this book) to serve as an introduction to books that should be written in a deeper and more thoughtful manner and provide impartial and unbiased guidance to humanity. Therefore, we have titled these lines "An Introduction to an Introduction" to indicate how much the field of sex lacks comprehensive scientific research from various perspectives.

Areas such as psychology, sociology, evolutionary biology, philosophy, theology, criticism, medicine, aesthetics, ethnography, history, and the like should responsibly and deeply focus on this fundamental human subject and, through their different lenses of knowledge and awareness, shed light and insight on it.

If this is the case, it can be expected that in the decades to come, humanity will, through the achievements of these studies, come to a proper understanding of sexual matters, the principles and standards of romantic relationships. This can shed broad light on the dark paths of ignorance and misunderstanding and, in the first place, reduce the various deviations, distortions, and misinterpretations that dominate sexual matters.

The orbit of the discussion on the issue of sex or lust is that to enter this field, one must set aside prejudices and critically examine its review and reconsideration. This means that a person, as a 'whole' with a set of existential elements, should be subject to scrutiny and not minus some of them.

Humans are multidimensional beings. The attempt to eliminate some of its dimensions, especially when speaking of the sublime human, is unscientific and unrealistic. Desire is an inseparable part of human existence, and if it has been misunderstood and misused in social interactions so far, it is not because of the nature of sensual matters, but because of the nature of human action in dealing with sensual matters.

If sex was a reprehensible matter, it would not have been entrusted by the all-knowing essence of existence to the human being. A look at the mechanisms and functions of this natural and divine force shows that this force has been manifested with biological purposes and a spiritual and profound approach.

Separating nature of humanity in terms of lust, especially in domains such as mysticism, Sufism, and sacred matters, contradicts the process of human evolution and opposes divine command. When religion aims to eliminate this influential and motivating force, it implies a perceived flaw in the creation of the Creator, and religion seeks to rectify it and optimize the work of God.

Regardless of the accuracy and validity of religious institutions or realms such as mysticism and Sufism, ignoring inner desires in the path to reaching spiritual and meaningful realms indicates the weakness of the practitioner's actions and their inability to confront their own desire.

To clarify the issue, it is sufficient to look at the lives of real prophets. It does not seem that any of them have imposed restrictions on sex. They not only did not imagine such restrictions for their followers, but even for themselves, they did not envision such limitations and even excelled more than others.

One of the major problems, which exists in the human encounter with sex, is the presence of a constant conflict between the power of sex and ideological structures that through controlling institutions; Like religion, politics, ethics, etc., it has been going on. Throughout human social history, the forces and colonies of power, including ideological, educational, political and social, have always tried to confiscate the act of sex in the field of personal and public relations. It is clear that such a confrontation is not an attempt in line with a kind of social tact and thinking to discover its existential dimensions. However, this effort could lead to dressing up human disorders and neuroses and freeing him from his challenging position in the field of sex.

Human nature is averse to suffering. The desire of a person to reach his lover and have sex with him should be in a natural and easy way without suffering and hardship. Therefore, the art of loving, whether in the form of marriage (which we will talk about its strengths and weaknesses in this book), or in other forms, is a fundamental and desirable thing and not a side issue or reprehensible.

A spiritual person is not a person who ignores or isolates a part of his being; rather, he is a human being who, with all his existential identity, takes a step in a path that he believes to be correct. Now, whether this path is religion or mysticism, economics or law, art or philosophy and the like, it does not make a difference in the story.

But the matter is not that simple. The element of sensuality has been the cause of countless perversions throughout human history. Sex has become a reason for the sad exploitation and exploitation of a group of people against another group and a vehicle for the exercise of sovereignty and the expansion of authority and the promotion of selfishness. Sexuality has become a conduit for enslaving fellow human beings and a vehicle for exercising sovereign or male and even corporate authority. Sexual power has become an opportunity to hunt for desires and obtain reprehensible goals that some people have been looking for in their lives. It is not a secret to anyone that in these powerful equations, women are an exploited type, to what extent they are passive and have been embezzled.

All this is due to the fact that, since the beginning of history, the erotic matter and generally the subject called woman has been a train that is based on the rails of a huge misunderstanding and at different historical moments, some people have greased the wheels of this train and set fire to it. They have added fuel to it.

In the thousands of years of human history, wrong motives have been involved in the movements that have been made to condemn sex, sensuality, and an entity called woman, and this dominant trend has continued almost uninterruptedly until now.

Of course, in the contemporary period, we are witnessing important changes. New science and the contemporary elite population have examined sex as an obligatory knowledge and provided guidelines that the activities and ideas of these thinkers have faced many resistances and obstacles.

Osho, an Indian philosopher and theorist, was among those whose challenging perspectives and ideas on sex hold great importance. His views on promoting joyful sex as a fundamental human principle have been met not only with acceptance in Indian society and Eastern communities but also at times with hostile reactions in developing countries.

However, it should not be overlooked that the enlightenment brought about by those who illuminated the dark world of ignorance has had a significant impact on the dominant thought of humanity, and at the very least, has instilled a "doubtful spirit" among the educated classes of founding societies.

The fundamental theory of Osho is based on the premise that sex is considered a natural phenomenon and as a factor upon which the formation of the human race relies. It should be examined from various perspectives and requires criticism and scrutiny of the positions of religions, clerics, and patriarchal society.

Many books by Western theorists have been written on the nature and identity of sex. However, these texts often inherently contain a form of institutionalized self-identification with the quality of sex in human society. It can be observed that in some cases, a certain acceptance and self-identification with male dominance can be noticed in the theories of Osho. Later, we will see to what extent some of the most prominent scholars have presented disgusting and inhumane views on women and gender equality.

In his writings, Alain de Botton portrays romantic relationships as a circular system, with the man seemingly positioned at its center, despite presenting different perspectives compared to the conventional view of sex. Let's take a closer look at Alain de Botton's theories in certain sections of this book.

The most challenging aspect of sex in personal and human relationships has always been how and to what extent to involve the issue of sex in the upbringing of children. Introducing sex as a taboo in educational systems has led children to quickly face a wide range of conflicts and contradictions in higher stages of their cognitive and personality development, which educational systems have remained silent about. This contradiction within the heterogeneous and inconsistent nature of sex is like a deep-rooted hidden matter. A hidden matter is that without speaking about it openly in all social and biological aspects, there is no possibility of achieving a fundamental explanation.

It can be said that if we consider human life as a full-fledged war in various fields, sex, the fire of desire, is the main source of all these apparent and hidden conflicts and struggles. To the extent that it should be placed at the top among the pyramid of human needs such as food, nourishment, shelter, clothing, dignity, and the like.

An examination of Maslow's hierarchy of needs reveals that sex, sexual desire, a sense of belonging, and acceptance, alongside a significant portion of other biological needs, directly or indirectly influence all levels of this hierarchical system.

Based on Maslow's hierarchy of needs, humans rely on the following needs to sustain a healthy and fulfilling life:

1. Biological needs
2. Safety needs
3. Social needs such as belongingness and affection
4. Esteem needs including respect, self-esteem, values, and the like
5. Self-actualization and self-motivation

With a little attention, the presence of sexual desire can be felt through its various variables in all stages and aspects of human needs. In some of these stages, such as the fourth stage needs, successful sex is one of the main ingredients in creating a "sense of satisfaction." A successful romantic relationship, flawless and sublime sex, "real liking," a sense of belonging and being belonged are among the major items that complete human needs.

An emotionally reactive and unaccepted individual, or someone who has failed in having a genuine intimate relationship, will generally perceive their social needs as neglected. The compounded issue arises where the failure to meet human needs at this stage can simply and directly impact needs and important factors of subsequent stages.

Self-esteem and self-motivation, feeling respected and valued, feeling benefited from biological needs, and ultimately "feeling insecure in the chaotic systems of life" are emotions that a person experiences during the vacuums caused by sex and physical affection.

Therefore, what theorists, activists, writers, and promoters of sexual excellence introduce in the lexicon of a social counselor and reformer is the same sequence of cause and effect that will ultimately lead to the creation of a healthy and dynamic society.

The issue does not end here. When sex is placed on the table as a psychological, sociological, biological, physiological, and even spiritual and philosophical act for a comprehensive and precise evaluation, the outcome will be a roadmap. Based on this roadmap, humanity can identify the dark aspects of individual and social life rooted in the crisis of sex and seek appropriate solutions for its restoration. Without having a roadmap and without going through a process of identifying causes, one cannot definitely pursue causality and treatment.

Without giving in to a structural change, humans must traverse through the same furnace of ignorance where some of the custodians of ethics and spirituality have paved the way before them, facing unknown and unfamiliar pains and problems. Such a process can strike at the roots of social vitality in communities. Humans must keep the sick body of life alive with dirty breaths like various deviations and sexual perversions, and consequences such as pornography and the like.

While this field requires extensive scientific research and refinement, even at this stage, with the available scattered information, signs of an advanced cancer development crisis called "sex crisis" can easily be observed. Some of the crisis indicators can be seen in these statistics:

- High divorce rates, which are said to affect up to one-third of marriages and up to two-thirds in some societies.
- High statistics of unconventional sexual entertainment, including the success of the ten-billion-dollar pornography industry worldwide.
- High rates of profanity, sexual assault, child marriages, abortion, "child marriage," honor killings, and the like.
- The increasing spread of sexual deviations such as homosexuality and the like.
- The increasing proliferation of cultural and social movements that continuously demand civil liberties and other human rights for women, reflecting an accumulation of social demands.
- High statistics of orphaned and undocumented children, child trafficking, resulting from the lack of control over births and the lack of optimal control over the relationship between women and men in underdeveloped societies.

All of these have their roots in the "sex crisis." A phenomenon that continues to exist beneath the surface of practical beliefs, ancient patterns, and educational systems. Dominant systems of belief—religious, political—implicitly accept that this field has a long way to go; however, admitting to the inability to manage this crisis is tantamount to ignoring the benefits that come from this passage. As Parvin Etesami said: "This thieving crow has become soap—despite all the cunning and intelligence!"

The failure of humans in sexual satisfaction and the disarray in managing it has various reasons. For instance, sex, as a personal matter, has less room for discussion and elaboration in public spheres. Consequently, its deficiencies and shortcomings are less countable and studied.

A person who has been plagued by a lifetime of sexual failure due to premature ejaculation carries this affliction with their spouse until the end of their life, unable to articulate it. The initial challenge that such an individual faces involves issues like pride, feelings of inferiority, and the agony of revealing a situation that dominates one of the most private aspects of this couple's life. An improper childhood upbringing system does not allow them to address a simple biological problem as an issue and work toward resolving it.

The behavioral contradiction of humans and the prevailing polarity among different generations is just a part of the great deception that humans grapple with. The same individual can easily access the most intimate sexual qualities of one or more actors through a simple visit to adult content in the digital world; however, when it comes to describing and expanding on their own personal issues, the realm of sex becomes a forbidden zone, and the secrets of their illness turn into unspoken secrets of their life.

While this issue can be addressed through fields such as behavioral psychology, biological achievements, medical services, and pharmacology, not only is it not simple, but her simple inadequacy, like an advanced cancer, engulfs the marital life of the couple. If we revisit the topic related to Maslow's hierarchy of needs, the existing inference is that social failure stems directly from sexual failure. Considering the aforementioned points, in this brief text, we endeavor to shed a fresh light on the dark aspects of the issue of sex. A light that, undoubtedly and by nature of the subject, must be explicit, simple, and unbiased, including solutions and suggestions.

However, considering that in the issue of sex, the female gender is not just a partner and half of the equation, but much more than a mere one-third of the equation, a significant portion of the book revolves around women, their innate and natural essence, their position as a male sexual partner, and their historical foundation. It will be clarified that the historical approach of men toward women, in the equation of a unidirectional life, has generally been dominant, possessive, and oppressive. We will also address the issue of acts of ownership and subjugation, not inherently, but toward goals that at least some part of masculine history has pursued their development.

We will delve into the private domains of men and women to see the implications of sexual failures in the first place and then, in an urgent and companionate approach, identify the resources available to enhance the quality of relationships. We will explore love to determine if it is solely manifested in sexual acts or if it extends beyond the bedroom.

It needs to be clarified how our encounter with love should be and how humanity's current perspective on the concept of love stands. We will briefly examine the historical and mythological roots of love to identify the sources that nourish love and where women stand in this battlefield. We will attempt to pinpoint where misunderstandings regarding love and the functioning of the heart and emotions originate.

This text will mainly focus on the "macro-axis" in most cases; however, in various discussions, we will not overlook data mining based on specific historical contexts. We will critique the statements of scholars and intellectuals to understand where the course of this historical river, which had the discourse of love/sex/sexual matters flowing in it, has deviated or when interruptions have occurred in its movement.

We will not ignore the behavioral and educational perspectives and the evident and hidden contradictions that humanity has faced in the challenge with sex, and we will seek traces in all these cases to demonstrate why women, as half of human society, have always been labeled as the weak, sinful, and guilty gender. We will also seek reflections of this social narrow-mindedness in areas such as mythology, art, literature, religion, philosophy, history, and civilization.

Concepts such as love, marriage, social interactions, and prevailing taboos will be brought to light to shed some light on the darkness of the human mind as much as possible. Topics like sex will be discussed in relation to matters such as virtue, human dignity, social respect, economic relationships, customs, cultural differences between the East and the West, and feminist civil movements seeking to change inappropriate relationships.

The challenges and dysfunctions that humans face in the realm of sex are among the issues we strive to understand and seek better alternatives for. However, enduring issues like challenging old patterns will remain influential in shaping individual and social behaviors in the realm of sex and intimacy.

In order to achieve vitality in social life, the continuation of stable relationships in forms such as marriage, we are looking for the answer to the question of whether sexual ethics and increasing the abilities of men and women in the issue of "sex as technique" and "sex as art" are what potentials and tools. There is more to improve performance and productivity.

The problem called sex in the history of human relations is so complicated that no one claims to have a definitive and radical solution. Most of those who have spoken or written a book in this field admit that the efforts made to correct human attitudes and actions toward the category of sex are to reduce the amount of human misfortunes when faced with sexual force, and it is not so easy to completely eliminate this difficulty.

Sex can be considered as one of the few common languages of mankind. A common language that has formed a kind of social discourse in almost the same way in all parts of the world and throughout history, and since humans have been sloppy in their dialogue with this language, it has caused human distress. The area that Alain de Botton calls "the poverty of human misery."

Alain de Botton has considerable studies on sex as a human dilemma. His writings are not unfamiliar to Iranians who are fond of reading. When this writer talks about finding a common human language to talk about the "sorrowful poverty of man in the world of sex," he certainly did not pay special attention to the more painful poverty of Eastern man. If we consider that the painful alienation of the Western man in the field of sex is so severe, how big can the crisis of the Eastern man be? This comparison makes us understand the necessity of such studies more.

The cultural diversity of societies cannot be hidden from view. If in Western societies the need to review the category of sex and the necessity of new studies is felt, then in the first way, in Eastern societies this issue is much more necessary. This is despite the fact that the restrictions of Eastern societies have made such activity much more difficult.

This book does not have a claim in any of the mentioned topics. Rather, it acts as a "problem plan" and as a "nudge" to remind us why humanity is so desperate and troubled in the issue of sex. For this reason, we welcome the path-breaking views, criticism and compassionate opinions and conflict of possible opinions that the perceptive readers of this article will benefit from Sir Ment, the owner of this pen, with great pleasure and gratitude.

Chapter One
Sad Human in the World of Sexuality

Among the types of mental disturbances and impressions that humans have been dealing with throughout their lives, mental and emotional disturbances caused by sexual power have been one of the most important and deep-rooted mental disorders. Man receives a major part of his emotional waves, emotional pains and lasting sadness from the mouth of his sensual power and his sexual needs and events.

Endless sexual fantasies, numerous images of erotic events, sexual success or deprivation, can form a major part of any person's mental images. Happiness, feelings of success or failure, feelings of sadness and similar sufferings are directly rooted in his mental history, and dependent on the images he has archived from his sensual moments throughout his life.

When a person is alone and thinks about the past in the sad and silent evening of a summer day or in long moments of chronic insomnia, usually the most important mental images are sexual experiences. Each person is different from others in terms of personality and individuality as much as their sexual experiences are different from others.

Internal resentments and sins and destructive thoughts that weigh on a person's conscience are the source of humiliation, jealousy, hatred, pulls and motivations that are hidden inside. Conflicting feelings, which are often not shared, are part of these internal forces that are directly rooted in sensual desires.

Every person, in moments of solitude and solitude, and in the unattainable labyrinth of his mind, also has ideas of the situation of others. Sometimes he imagines that maybe he has a different status in his sex record. He probably thinks that others have been much more successful in this respect. But there is no possibility of any kind of comparison.

Social taboos draw bright red lines between people's private worlds, their imaginations and their erotic repertoire with others. So he'll never know if he's the only one wading through the deep valleys of his own sexual taboos, or if others are in the same situation. It seems that most of the people around us are in the same situation as we are. That is, man is a prisoner in his "sorrowful poverty" in the field of sex and lust, and apparently there is no way to escape from this prison.

The point is that in few books and resources, there is a useful guide for drawing the ideal world of sex and its belongings, so that a person can, without referring to others and without talking to people, be able to measure his deviation, failure, health, or success with a simple comparison. Measure and know whether he has received a passing grade in his sexual performance. In fact, man has been abandoned in his inner world in the worst possible way. A world where at the same time the strictest controls and restrictions are applied to it.

Perhaps the famous example of "elephant in the dark" can be cited about the sensual world of people. In the dark and lonely world of the room of sensual desires and requests, sex is the elephant that we have to identify the general dimensions and the condition of its organs by relying only on our limited experiences. Meanwhile, there is no light that sheds light of knowledge on the dark world of our limited knowledge and imagination.

The reason for these complexities and the nested network of human ignorance regarding sexual behavior is that this issue rarely becomes an issue in the public spheres of life. The category of sex in human social life is the same as "present and absent existence." Sex is present in all the moments and daily relationships of life, and it is one of the most important needs of the biological system, along with important needs such as bread, water, air, housing and clothing. But at the same time, talking about it is limited and forbidden.

The sexual identity of each person is highly personalized and contains many hidden secrets that are impossible to talk about in public. If we go a little deeper and look at this personalization in the imaginations and mental worlds of sexual partners, we will see that even sexual partners who have successful sexual relationships often refuse to admit their sexual interests and fantasies. Fear of humiliation, ridicule, or fear of disgust are just a few of the reasons sexual partners can't reveal their inner passions for sexual fantasies.

All this is regardless of the external limitations that have been imposed on humans in history with varying degrees of severity. The first limiting factors that make talking about sex a difficult taboo are the causes of religious culture and social rules.

Religions have tried to make the masses stupid by instilling superstitious beliefs and have deepened this indoctrination during different centuries, and the sorrowful sojourn of mankind in the valley of sex is more or less the achievement of the authority of religions and taboos. A look at the inscriptions and signs left from the past periods, from the age of stone and metal and hunting to the industrial age, does not give any signs of human happiness in sex. The obvious point is that in all these periods, talking about sex has been taboo. The issue that has continued to this day and the failure of mankind to face the category of sex also comes back to this.

Of course, the entry of man into the industrial age and the start of the next rapid developments caused changes in this equation. A person who has managed to step into other planets and reveal many of his ignorance in scientific and philosophical fields, now thinks of making changes in the field of hidden secrets of the inner world and challenges with sensuality. Although this challenge actually occurs; but the obtained results show that solving human problems in the field of sex is far more difficult than his scientific successes in challenging the problems of physics, chemistry and astronomy.

Man's achievement in facing the challenge of sex in the era of modernity is only limited to the change in some of his beliefs and behaviors and nothing more. The fact that humans in a part of this planet decide to wear bikinis and not consider masturbation to be ugly and act more carelessly in sexual behavior does not mean the root solution of the problem. For this reason, we observe the same psychoses and frustrations in the era of modernity.

Still, sex for humans is accompanied by feelings such as guilt, heartbreak, lack of self-confidence and crises that are rooted in the psychological depth of his problems. Now, due to the requirements of the modern era, sex has become a means of entertainment more than in the past. Group sex, pornography, fetishism and the display of sex images have been the superficial and perverted changes of mankind in his attempt to solve his problems with sex. This is despite the fact that in the depths of his heart, the same "painful poverty" in the challenge with sex still remains. By explaining that his stresses and frustrations, which are the consequences of the age of modernity, have been added to the previous problems.

On the other hand, modern mankind has not only been unable to solve this age-old problem with all its calculation and intelligence, but other variables that have governed the issue of sensuality have remained almost as strong. Strict religious rules, social taboos, restrictions and repression have always been present and now they are confronting modern thought with all their might, and it seems that it has been successful in some cases.

What is the reason why man has not been able to create a logical and reasonable relationship with sex and tame this unpredictable horse in order to optimize his life? Is this powerful and unruly internal force deposited as evil and the origin of evil in the human body? If so, why does the survival of the human race depend on this sinister phenomenon? In principle, is it possible for humans to integrate sex with reasonable and calculated life and the requirements of modern society and curb it?

All these are questions that humanity has asked itself many times. We and you have asked ourselves such questions many times. In response, it should be said that man never seems to be able to limit this strange phenomenon, which basically contradicts things like boundary breaking, de-normalization, and distance from the principles and standards of society, in a specific path and framework.

What Is the Relationship Between Love and Sex?

Even sex in the face of love will not do that. It is because one of the most difficult definitions that can be given is to specify the regularity of love and sex on an objective and quantifiable scale. Regardless of the fact that these two phenomena are neither definable nor structured, their juxtaposition adds to this distress and disorder.

Where exactly is the clear demarcation between love and sex? How are love and sex defined together and in connection with each other? When does love end and sex begin? When does sex end and love begin? When is sex the symbol and climax of love? When does sex indicate the absence of love and the presence of animalistic and predatory traits? When can love turn into sex? When can sex be the gateway to love?

These and dozens of other questions show well how dark and undefined the border between love and sex and the definition between sex and universal concepts such as humanity, civility, dignity, moral virtues, predatoriness, self-control and the like are. These conflicts and contradictions are sometimes so complicated that the legal and moral system and even the power of conscience, which is institutionalized within humans, gets confused in defining the limits and criteria of an event.

But perhaps the biggest unsolvable question is, where is the interaction border between sex and sensuality and human values? At the very beginning, it should be said that the type of encounter of religious leaders in interaction and enjoying the pleasure of sex cannot be considered as a criterion to answer this question. When faced with sex, if not they behaved more mundanely than other people, at least it can be said that they did not act differently. Philosophy and ethics have not provided answers to these questions.

The answer of religion is quite stable and at the same time has fundamental conflicts. The method of religion is to suppress it to the maximum, as a blatant phenomenon, in public spheres and a kind of unrestrainedness in private spheres. Religion's view of women is mainly from the perspective of ownership and sexual slavery. Of course, sexual slavery has also been used against men; but regarding women, the issue is more sensitive. The concept of "slave," which is mainly a semantic unit with religious roots, means exactly sexual slavery and nothing else. Legitimacy of this slavery and different types of sexual slavery, which most of the time even reaches the relationship between couples and in the family center, is provided by religious institutions and laws.

According to all the data that we have from the experience of long human life and according to the philosophical, logical and biological signs and the data that other sciences have provided us so far, it is almost certain that the possibility of a peaceful coexistence with the phenomenon. It is not possible to have sex in such a way that all the aforementioned criteria remain valid and at the same time, sex as a natural thing and with pleasure, does its job well.

Therefore, the ultimate goal of mankind should be focused on how to deal with the phenomenon of sex in a way that brings the least possible damage to us in various fields, has the least conflict with the teachings of religions, and at the same time can benefit from it. It was used as an effective lever for the continuation of family relationships of couples in the form of marriage.

By optimizing traditional views, it is possible to use the gift of sex as a driving engine for the survival of the generation and at the same time in the field of population control and reduction and elimination of phenomena such as marginalization, poverty, homeless children, prostitution and all social problems that are rooted in the lack of population control and the lack of control of pregnancy and pregnancy in an animal way, he took corrective steps. Also, when it comes to a successful harmony, couples should be able to make the most of this natural gift.

Of course, human concerns when faced with sex do not end there. In the end, he has to create balance and logical order between sensual acts and various issues. Things like:

- Caring and educating children and managing their knowledge in the field of sex at different ages.

- Solving problems with sexual partners and resolving life and family affairs without any of them having a negative impact on the other.
- Preventing the penetration of social vices centered on sex into the family and relationship with the spouse.
- Managing a romantic relationship with a considerable amount of sexual benefit while continuing the relationship, not cooling it, not reducing the sexual attractiveness of the parties and preventing the collapse of the relationship and maximum compliance with the expectations of the parties.
- Facing sexual deceptions from those around you and not damaging the two-way relationship because of these poisonous waves.
- Preventing sex without charm and a car that is devoid of any happiness and diversity.
- Avoiding the feeling that by agreeing to marriage or a stable relationship, we have created a world full of sexual deprivation.

These and other cases are among the adversities that a person has to deal with regardless of whether he is in a stable relationship or not, and it seems that no solution has been introduced so far.

Is Sex Biological or Mystical and Emotional?

Maybe the answer to this question can help us find a solution to understand "sorrowful poverty." Or even in the face of the hardships that humanity is dealing with in the valley of sex, it is somehow consoling.

Is sex, as evolutionary biology says, a reward for the human race that humans, like other animals, are persuaded to reproduce in order to perpetuate the generation? In this assumption, sexual pleasure is a reward that nature has prepared for humans so that in pursuit of this pleasure, they will continuously seek the action of sex, and in this way, reproduction and the continuation of the generation with all its troubles will seem acceptable.

If, according to this theory, being lustful is just a trap of nature for humans to ensure the continuation of the species, then what happens to things like love, liking, loyalty, attraction and romantic actions of humans with their sexual partners? Are these in line with the great deception of nature?

If we are captive to nature's beautiful trap to reward and ensure the continuity of the generation, then are the mind games we have made for ourselves all toys taken too seriously? What do toys like love, loyalty, passion, infatuation, mystical trance and the like have to do with sex?

That is, in all these cases, it is the male or female hormones that are guiding our behavior and managing our actions during sexual life, and the above are actually the colors and accessories that we give to this sweet toy? In this sense, beauty is at the service of health and with an intermediary guaranteeing a good delivery and producing a copy of a human being that has perfect health standards.

This process has been prepared by nature in such a way that the process of sex through every channel that passes from the beginning of the acquaintance of two people until its completion at the moment of ejaculation, is clearly and in the most correct way possible in the way of continuity of generation and reproduction. Now, if he encounters various obstacles such as contraceptives or infertility, it doesn't matter. All people have sex and pleasure under the influence of a prevailing current, now if the result is the production of another human being, how much better! If not, nature is the winner of this field based on the law of probabilities. The eight billion people living on the planet is undoubtedly a convincing example of how true this hypothesis is.

If we accept this principle, there are other benefits associated with this process. Benefits such as escape from loneliness, regulation of social and family relationships, escape from isolation, and health benefits that are said to exist in sex, and of course, as mentioned, pleasure from sex (as a reward), can itself be a product of this process.

Sexual act + reward (pleasure) = result (continuity of generation + regulation of affairs and functioning of collective systems)

A look at the process of human life, from the beginning of birth to the time of death, shows that sex is the most fundamental, multiple concepts and the most penetrating phenomenon of his life. Sex should be considered both practically and mentally as an element of every person's life on the planet. This dominance can perhaps be shown in a specific course like this:

- The existence and creation of man and the formation of his life are dependent on the act of sex. Two people perform the act of sex and another person finds life capacity.
- The main mental concern of a person during adolescence and youth is sex. Under the influence of the phenomenon of sex, he deals with prohibitions and restrictions, which are perhaps the most painful experiences of his life.
- A person gets married or experiences a stable relationship or repeated relationships. In his relationships, he is constantly analyzing his situation and struggling with his mental world and his imagination.
- He finishes his period of sex and now in his old age he is busy analyzing his previous experiences and depending on the successes and failures he has had, he evaluates his life as a success or a failure.
- And this process, which is repeated in the case of him and his parents, is also repeated in the case of his children.

The Gap Between Sex and Virtue

Humanity will continue to be stuck in the deep contradictions with which it is challenged until it cannot in a reasonable way fill the gap between sex and virtue, sex and spirituality, sex and dignity, sex and decency, sex and humanity, sex and respect. Mother is not a sex symbol, but it is clear that she brought us into this world in a sensual ecstasy. We try to censor his sensual side.

On the other hand, the wife is supposed to live a sensual and flirtatious life with us, but all the man tries to do is to censor this aspect of his wife's nature and presence. He cannot respect a woman who is sensual and exposes all her desires deeply; but at the same time, he expects that this woman can lead him to the pure ecstasies of a pleasurable embrace. In other words, the sum between virtue and sex is now the sum of opposites.

To solve this challenge, a man usually categorizes the women around him and, in his opinion, sees each of these opposites in the dictionary of one of the types of women he knows. He respects the mother who is the symbol of "sexlessness." Now he should respect his wife in the same way, while his wife is a sex symbol. This conflict is the main cause of many disorders that lead to the collapse of the family institution and the increase in divorces.

This conflict does not exist by itself; but mankind, especially in the Middle East, has established this in the institution of society, and now it is struggling with the deep consequences of this structural and archetypal conflict. If this structural conflict is removed, sexual arousal can give new life to life.

The conflict we talked about is so wide that it calls into question the educational indicators of mankind. The "man-wife" is told at the beginning of life and in childhood that lust is an impolite and shameful act. He grows with this education and gradually opens the doors of awareness to the real world. In the first encounter with the truth, he realizes that this ugly thing was and is going on regularly between his parents. The first blow of this structural conflict has come and it turns out that the ugly thing is one of the obvious events in the relationship between father and mother.

Over time, he realizes that basically sex is the most important issue in human life. Teenagers with open ears chatter about it. In girls, he discovers strange charms that, according to the educational literature of his childhood, seem ugly.

Over time, the philosopher in the child becomes evident. He goes deep into the nature of creation and realizes that he himself is the fruit of one of the same ugly things that happened between his mother and father. He reads literature, art and history and finds that it is full of stories whose main theme is sensuality and sexual attraction.

After some time, he gets a wife. Now his other nasal conflicts are raging. How to resolve the conflict between the ugly thing and respect? This is where the man's crazy behavior begins. He is left alone in the impasse of a systematic conflict.

Sex has stages and ranks, reaching the highest and most beautiful aspects of it requires that the man and woman in flirting leave all the components that indicate respect. They have to do things that don't seem respectful at all.

This conflict causes biological and mental reactions in men. He prefers to leave his wife still respected and untouched and to reach those exciting peaks, which he has been fantasizing about for a lifetime, touch the skirts of other women.

The educational systems of progressive societies have now put enlightenment on sexual concepts on the agenda from the very beginning.

Germany and Japan are among the leading countries in the world in teaching sexual concepts to children. Other countries have also paid attention to this essential education. Countries like America, Canada, Australia, Iceland, Holland and even Islamic countries; Like Lebanon, Turkey and Bahrain, they have implemented such programs either on a trial basis or in the form of programs to prevent AIDS.

In addition to creating the necessary knowledge about sexual organs and their functions, these educational programs teach children issues such as sexual hygiene, the requirements of sexual intercourse, the necessity of postponing sexual activities, and legal and social issues related to sexual activity. The ultimate goal of these training sessions is to increase a person's ability to protect themselves and learn about legal restrictions, and manage sex for a better life.

The Catholic Church and other religions are among the opponents of these programs. Misunderstanding the nature of sex education for children, religious leaders present any talk of sex skills and education to children as promoting sex. They prefer children to grow like weeds without any education and guidance, and by themselves receive incorrect information from the surrounding environment and eventually experience failure and frustration in managing sexual and even marital affairs; but during adolescence, they do not get acquainted with these concepts in the form of formal and controlled education.

The religion's response to controversial issues like these is "non-reaction" and ignoring the issue. Religion, in most fields, in response to difficult questions that require tact and thoughtfulness, tries to ignore it by removing the face of the problem. In other words, religion's response to the important issue of children's sex education is like sweeping dirt under the carpet.

All this while the achievements of progressive educational systems such as the Japanese educational system, show how effective modern education is in promoting social ethics and health. We cite only one example of these educational conflicts in order to clarify what achievements may be achieved by the traditional and backward society in the absence of a modern and developed educational system and the lack of attention to the education of sexual skills as an essential part of education.

A psychoanalyst friend recounted: "Once during my professional career I came across a case that was surprising. The issue was related to a 30-year-old young man who was married; but after several days of marriage, he did not have any relationship or flirtation with his wife. Surprised and disappointed, the man's wife asks the man after a few days, why don't you approach me and nothing happens between us? The man answers in complete astonishment and anger: Do you want me to touch my wife?"

This case shows that in the absence of a modern education system, when children and teenagers are left to their own devices at the discretion of reactionary religions and grow up like weeds in cars, in the absence of sexual skills and the principles of cohabitation, what miracles and virtues are possible. The result of this conservative thinking. A thought that many educational systems of Eastern societies agree with.

It seems that marriage in the form of this method of education has reached a dead end. Or at least, the ideals and adventures of men are not achievable within its framework. He is caught between a mother statue, a respected wife, and the passionate woman of his sexual fantasies. He prefers to leave this field full of fallacies and conflicting forces and slowly pass by it and go to other women for more carefree perspectives. This factor may be the main reason why today's young generation does not welcome marriage.

The "Bipolarity" Between Sex Is a Product of Creation Consciousness

If we accept that the existence of two opposite poles is in line with a balanced structure to advance the goals of creation, then imagining any kind of conflict or enmity between the male and female sexes will be completely pointless. The truth is that men and women are not only not enemies, but they are not even in conflict with each other.

The "evolving" situation between a man and a woman is because, basically, in creating a feeling of attraction and desire, the purpose of which is the continuation of generation and pleasure, the existence of two poles, positive and negative, is inevitable. If there was no "bipolarity" between men and women, the world would be devoid of concepts such as love and belonging. The pleasure that exists in the intimacy between a woman and a man, the pleasure that these two take in harmonizing and caressing each other is due to these two polarities.

When the male soul touches the female soul, it feels that it has regained its lost half or unfinished part. Therefore, if everything goes well, the result of this closeness is the feeling of completeness. If the feeling of completeness prevails, it is obvious that other feelings such as: the feeling of ownership, the feeling of exploitation, the feeling of superiority, the feeling of majesty and servitude fade. Now, if we see that such concepts are widely seen in the history of male-female relations, there is no doubt that man has made a huge mistake in dealing with his other half.

A real man achieves the highest sense of fulfillment and satisfaction in intercourse with a perfect woman. Movements and lines of thought that pursue statuses such as monosex or even equality between women and men are oblivious to the fact that in the deliberate elimination of these differences, the "element of attraction" will be lost. In the absence of such an element, human society will be very dull and life will be devoid of romantic motives, and the human soul will be devoid of intrinsic pleasures.

Naturally, no man wants to hug another man and go to bed. If all the mechanisms of creation are perfect, such an image will also be accompanied by disgust. It is the intelligence of creation that does not allow the world to be devoid of great attraction between men and women. Women who think they have to adopt masculine qualities are neglecting this vital issue.

There is no grace or pleasure in the meeting between a mortal man and a mortal woman.

Sex, in its most sublime form, is the product and result of the ideal state briefly described above. If it is observed that the bio-social record and emotional life of human beings was not like this, it only means that human civilization and culture, until today, has suffered from a great nervousness and abnormality.

By not understanding the category of gender, human beings have not only denied women the gift of an ideal life, but also deprived themselves of the gift of an optimal partnership in order to enjoy life with women.

If such an ideal dominates the emotional life of men and women, then we will see that sex will not only appear in the dictionary of religions and social beliefs and rootless taboos, as a reprehensible and sinful act, but as a sublime behavior and a product of obedience to the guidelines of creation will emerge.

It is obvious that in order to change the "existing situation" to the "desired situation," the first step must be taken by men in thought and action. The first step is a serious revision of the traditional male thinking that wants the woman as a being at his service.

If the man considers the woman as his sexual servant, it is natural that the woman will, at best, only perform the duty. In such a situation, the woman will not use all her capacities and creativity to have a romantic relationship with the man.

The Eastern woman (at least in the traditional and uninformed layers) is now caught in the same situation. The position of the oriental woman in the sexual interaction with her spouse is completely one-sided. He censors himself to accomplish this task with minimum cost and minimum energy. He has lost his natural gifts. Creation in his body includes creative qualities for sex; but she has to ignore them, in the shadow of her partner's sexual tyranny, to the fact that she is a means of immediate and superficial male gratification.

On the other hand, the man (especially the oriental man, at least in its traditional and undeveloped layers) has a free hand to satisfy his sense of sexual diversity. Monogamy imposed on women and polygamy granted to men is one of these cases. While the man is not able to give the experience of a sublime sex to his woman, he reduces the quality of the work and constantly seeks the issue of quantity.

Such behavior is completely against nature's goals. We have strangely witnessed a major error in the intelligent workings of creation. Creation, in the issue of pregnancy and the continuity of the generation, using the female reproductive system, has not taken into account any prerequisites regarding the necessity of transcendental sex. The mere arrival of sperm in the female reproductive system is enough to start the reproductive process. This is a gross error, or at least a negligence in the working of creation, which has ended to the detriment of the woman. Religions and ideological institutions have taken the utmost advantage of this negligence of creation.

The man does not want to release the sexual potential in the woman's body by setting off the primary explosive device. Because he is not able to respond to this latent force, nor is he interested in it. The man's inability to have a deep, long and quality sex has caused him to come out of denial and deny and suppress the woman's capabilities in this regard.

Concepts that have been mentioned throughout history with titles such as "female decency" or "maternal noble spirit" have actually been tricks to perpetuate this oppression.

Activating multiple ejaculations in a woman is actually a disaster for a man. A long relationship with multiple ejaculations is not something a man has the tools to cope with. A man's power in a quick and short sex is limited in the sexual organs and leads to a low-quality ejaculation. For this reason, in some parts of the world, we see a lot of women who have not experienced ejaculation even once.

More than 90% of women in some underdeveloped societies do not experience the peak of sexual pleasure, and the issue of sexual satisfaction does not make sense to them. A woman's historical experience is full of sexual intercourse with men who use her body for a moment in an inappropriate situation and after a quick ejaculation, their grunts fill the room. The man is done with him. Now he is the one who has to deal with this feeling of humiliation.

For this reason, during the millions of years of human life, millions and millions of women have lived and gone in this world, without even knowing about the natural gift hidden in their bodies. Although this issue is a form of self-protection for men; but for women, it has meant severe deprivation.

Natural and ideal sex for a woman starts with the first sparks of feeling and then with caressing and kissing and flirting. Then it moves on to caressing other parts of the body and in a slow process, it leads to the operative stage of sex. This slow process, after several experiences of temporary ejaculation, ends with the final ejaculation in the woman. But this is still not the end point for the process of female sex.

After the orgasm, the moments of caressing and cuddling come. The pleasant feeling of becoming one and touching the soul of the other party and allowing the other to touch one's own soul is part of the levels of sex in women. This special pleasant and slow feeling is what a woman tends to experience during intercourse. But does a man have the ability to manage and implement such a process? The answer is clear. No! Especially, the best and most ideal possible state in sex is that the last ejaculation of the woman is exactly the same time as the ejaculation of the man.

Such a trance-like experience is so far-fetched that it should be viewed as an alchemical phenomenon. The truth is that women, unlike men, are either not stimulated by their genitals, or if they are, their importance is very insignificant. In other words, as much as sex in men is a matter related to the sexual organ and temporary, for women it is a phenomenon mixed with soul and emotion.

A woman's satisfaction is not through the channel of the nervous system of the reproductive system, but through the channel of deep romantic feeling and understanding of her essence. The more successful such a process is, the more naked and unmistakable he will be during sex. Otherwise, it will do what it has done in its historical experience. Remaining on the surface of the body and even without touching the sensory arteries of the body. Becoming a sex machine that can be used at the push of a few buttons without his participation in this matter. Even worse, she turns into a lifeless corpse, which gives the man a priceless opportunity to exploit her sexual organs in a very superficial way. It means flirting with a corpse.

This is a problem that the history of women's sexual experience, mostly, testifies to. In fact, throughout history, millions of men have made love to millions of female bodies, not knowing that their sexual partners are actually nothing more than bodies. The transformation of women into flirtatious corpses, in the first place, was caused by the inferential and strategic error of men throughout history.

The serious problem that has caused men to take the authority to act while suppressing the potential of women in their own way is that if women are fully aware of their capacities, then the sexual ability of men will seem worthless. Therefore, the easiest way that men have taken in the direction of the initiative leading to sexual pleasure is to turn the woman into a passive and receptive creature.

A man starts and ends sex in the easiest and apparently most desirable way possible, without having to undertake the difficult task of satisfying the woman.

Perhaps this is why adventurous women, who see sex as a certain and inalienable gift, mostly avoid marriage and try to find, among their many boyfriends or sexual partners, finally, a man with real and extraordinary capabilities, to choose for a permanent relationship.

On the other hand, when a woman chooses a female partner and engages in a homosexual process, since both have equal and perfect abilities in sex, they are likely to obtain full and perfect pleasure.

From the point of view of homosexual women, a long and maximal love process with the same sex is far better than sexual intercourse with a man whose activity in a two-three-minute process and a quick ejaculation is nothing more than a momentary annoyance.

A woman who is stuck in such a predicament must either give up her right to reach the peak of sexual pleasure or take one of the unconventional ways such as homosexuality. Perhaps it is because Sigmund Freud concluded in his scientific findings that "homosexuality is not considered a mental illness."

Pointing out that men and women are equal and belong to the same species, he says that any theory or philosophy that condemns women is inhumane and due to sexual supremacy. He extends this equality to the field of homosexuality and adds: homosexual people are often distinguished from others by their moral culture and especially high intellectual development. He believes that homosexuality has no advantages, but it is not something to be ashamed of. Because it is neither vice nor degeneration and it cannot be classified as a disease.

Sexual Satisfaction Is a Window to Spiritual Evolution

Sex is one of the serious matters of life, either as a supreme sacred thing in the path of human spiritual evolution, or as a basic need that is done solely for the purpose of the evolution of the generation and pleasure. Based on the emphasis of psychological science, sexual pleasure and satisfaction caused by sex has increased continuously from the earliest decades of human life to the present day. On the one hand, lack of success or lack of desire to have sex can be signs of pathological neurosis, and on the other hand, lack of sexual success in itself can act as a factor in jeopardizing the mental health of a person and society. So happy sex can lead to psychological stability and behavioral control of humans.

Josef Breuer, the great Austrian psychologist and one of Freud's colleagues, believed that every memory carries a certain amount of emotional energy in a person's psyche. Failure to express these memories over time causes the concentration of a large amount of wasteful and disturbing energy in the person's mind, and as a result, disorders and mental illnesses appear in him. Based on this principle, Brewer believed that in order to relieve a person's mental disorder, these energies should be removed. In order to expel these energies, you have to bring the mentioned memories from the unconscious to the conscious and relax yourself by expressing them. It was from here that Freud realized the mechanism of "exhaustion." The discovery of this psychological reality caused psychologists to try to extract hidden and unconscious memories from the patients' unconscious with the help of hypnosis and to reduce the destructive effects of these memories by explaining and expanding them by the patient.

Considering the above fact, it can be concluded that mental knots caused by sexual complexes or memories can be among the most bitter. The ecstasy and solitude of sex is the most appropriate time to express these memories and vent the bitterness caused by them. In this way, we see how important it is to have a healthy sex life and the participation of a sexual partner in a person's mental health and refinement.

The psychological ecstasy caused by ejaculation and the experience of oneness in sex are completely similar to human experiences in meditation, discovery and intuition, and in every way. Perhaps the first sparks that made mankind think of doing activities like meditation was the experience of sexual ecstasy. A person with the experience of sexual ecstasy seeks to develop this experience and tries to get this feeling in a deeper and more intense way. All efforts based on spiritual and emotional transformation follow the path that man has taken in the experience of sex. Orgasm is the sublime point of these spiritual bays. A phenomenon that humans always seek to repeat and improve its quality and quantity.

Relying on the achievements of psychology, it should be said that perhaps the limited success of women in Sufi, mystical experiences, and even meditation and spiritual matters, is because they have been widely denied throughout history to reach the peak of spiritual bliss through orgasm.

Throughout history, women have consistently given men a taste of this feeling without being involved in the spiritual experience themselves. The man followed this experience and resorted to other methods to repeat it, without taking the woman along with him.

The above equation tells us that most spiritual and even divine experiences have physical and physiological roots. Spiritual growth and experience is based on physical experience. Mystical love and reaching the Alevi world is based on physical love and the experience of understanding the presence of a sexual partner. In fact, in order to climb any height, man must start from his body. Those who have not succeeded in understanding physical experiences will not be able to understand deeper spiritual experiences through the first method.

Throughout history, women have been deprived of discovering their physical horizons, and for this reason, the presence of women is clearly limited in the spiritual experiences caused by life.

In the mystical culture and literature of the East, there is a fundamental sentence that specifically refers to this issue. This mystical rule, which was developed by Abu Ali Sina, is the phrase "Al-Majaz Qantara al-Haqiqah."

According to Bo Ali Sina, the theoretical basis of love is expressed in "love in a beautiful and sweet way." Following this idea, other Islamic and Eastern mystics believe that love for women and beauties can be a gateway to divine and holy love.

Other philosophers like Mulla Sadra, like Ibn Sina and his predecessor; That is, in addition to expanding this idea, Ibn Arabi also followed this practice. Of course, some believers in this belief have extended the subject to love with handsome men and even flirting with them. This issue has been widely expressed in Persian and Islamic mysticism and literature in the form of "witness play," which is not the subject of our discussion.

In an article about the love of young people for the beautiful, Ibn Sina explains in detail the philosophical and intellectual justification of the love for the beautiful.

He says that love for beautiful women can increase goodness, and in this way, he can consider love for beautiful women as a way to reach God.

In the seventh volume of a book called Seven Journeys, Mulla Sadra writes in a chapter entitled "Eighth Place in Divine Providence": "To reach God's love, one must taste the taste of human love and enjoy beautiful women and beautiful teenagers."

He explains that "to love and enjoy someone who has a beautiful face and a fit body is something that all people are inherently interested in, so these things should be praised based on God's wisdom." He believes that there is a difference between the love of beauties and caring about attractive faces and the love that arises between two people when they are officially married. Because the attraction of the second type is present in almost all male and female animals. True love is the love that begins between two people, not based on extreme sexual acts. In true love, usually an attractive face is important along with good and cute manners and charisma and rhythmic movements of the beloved, a humane and spiritual behavior.

According to Mulla Sadra, such love for the beautiful and humorous face of the lover softens the heart and raises the mind.

Mulla Sadra clarifies that: "The philosophy behind the love for beautiful women is that a person gains consciousness by benefiting from this physical beauty, and with the help of the beautiful face and body of a human lover, he awakens the aesthetic feeling in himself and for be prepared to reach spiritual beauty and God's love and eternal life in the other world. In Greek philosophy and theology, love is one of the main foundations of human life."

In a book called *The Symposium*, Plato writes: "Chaos had engulfed the universe until the earth was created. Earth became the center of all things and then love appeared. After that, earth and love replaced the original chaos and formlessness of existence."

It is mentioned in another part of this book that after this change and transformation, love began as the greatest source of humanity for the human race and every human being living on earth. Before love, life had no benefit and no happiness in itself, but now that love exists, there is nothing better than loving someone and they love you back.

In this book, which is written in the form of a discussion, we see an idea that has existed in Eastern theology in the same way, this idea is that "carnal love can be a bridge to divine love."

When it comes to Aristotle's speech, he puts forth the theory of the "ladder of love" with a passionate speech and with a great quote from one of his favorite teachers, a woman named Diotima. This is the mystical theory that is thousands of years old in the culture of the East.

The summary of Diotima's statements is as follows: "The one who, led by love, looks at the earthly beauties and uses them as a staircase that will lead him step by step to his goal and destination, will reach from one beauty to two beauties and from there to the beauty of the body and the body, and in general, from there to the beauty of morals and good behavior, and after that, it reaches the beauty of knowledge and endless wisdom. This is the knowledge that is his aim and purpose." According to the theory proposed by Diotima, love is the center of the universe. Love is like an angel that establishes a connection between earthly man and transcendental wisdom and the Creator of the universe, and man has no choice but to seek help from love to reach his essence. Love is like a ladder that, as Rumi says, can connect a person to his "true roots."

In this theory, traces of the "authenticity of truth" theory, which Attar proposes in the story of Simorgh, can be seen. In the Greek philosophical point of view and as explained by Diotima, the principle of truth is the principle of love, which the seeker must achieve by learning to see, walk and follow the path.

Diotima explains that: "Whoever wants to walk the right path of love must fall in love with a beautiful face in his youth." He continues: "And if his guide has shown him the right path, he will only fall in love with one beauty and that's it." Attachment creates a good and beautiful thought for him, and when this happens, he will realize that the beauty of a body is like the beauty of other bodies, and therefore, in general, he will fall in love with a body...After this stage, he will realize the beauty of the soul will become and he will find it much higher than the beauty of the body, and when he reaches a higher stage, he will understand that the beauty of the soul is higher than the beauty of the body.

Love exists both on earth and in the highest heavens, playing a crucial role in the journey toward perfection. In earthly life, love is a transcendent and spiritual force that not only lacks meaning without physical presence but truly finds its essence in the realm of body and emotions. By embedding love in the mechanism of creation, especially in the creation of man and woman with their complexities and unique moments, creation has blended the essence of humanity with love.

The most significant area where earthly love can be a source of goodness and evolution for humans is the understanding of the presence of others. A woman's presence as a contributor to the evolution of man and as a ladder for progress and excellence.

The historical experience of the relationship between man and woman shows that love has been widely forgotten. The failure of the materialistic human experience in the past, which manifested itself by eliminating love in social life, indicates that in order to return to the original roots and reclaim human identity, one must once again encounter love. The most important meeting point of human and love is manifested in the intersection of man and woman. The result of a romantic life can be the production of generations whose main policy is love in life. However, the problem here is that the process of reproduction occurs without the slightest attention to the feminine essence and without considering the sensitivities of women, even depriving them of their right to love. Human materialism causes women to remain deprived of understanding this gift, as only male ejaculation is deemed sufficient to shape the process of reproduction.

Happiness stemming from physical love is an evolved form of relationship and intimacy, serving as a catalyst for human growth and evolution, much like Diotima described in detailing the stages of romantic evolution. Ideal sex can simulate a state of contemplation for women and even men. This is because women who prioritize their sexual lives based on feminine priorities are generally livelier, more sociable, more vibrant, and healthier. The significant prevalence of social depression among women in underdeveloped societies is primarily due to sexual suppression and deprivation of the blessing of love. Love, enlightenment, spirituality, evolution, and even divinity are all different stations on a specific path that culminates in the experience of "perfection," as witnessed in the stages traversed by the seeker in "The Seven Cities of Love."

The ideal situation in all these cases is for a man and a woman to walk side by side, not as strangers or one without the other. According to Osho, an Indian philosopher, the reason many women have not reached the stage of enlightenment is that they have never tasted the peak of sexual pleasure. A pleasure that can open a door toward the sky. Women have mainly lived, had children, and died. This is because biological processes and masculine behavior have led them to not even know what the peak of sexual pleasure means.

This Indian theorist adds: "I have questioned very intelligent, educated, and cultured women and realized that they have no concept of it. In fact, there is no word in Eastern languages that can translate the word orgasm. There was no need for this word; this issue has never been addressed. Men have taught women that only prostitutes enjoy sex. These prostitutes moan, scream, and almost go crazy during intercourse! To be a respectable lady, you should not do these things! So, the woman remains in tension and feels degraded deep inside because she has been used. Many women have reported to me that after lovemaking, when their husbands fall asleep, they cry."

This is a situation that should be referred to as the lack of "understanding the presence of others." The situation of "two strangers" or "one without the other."

The reality is that a woman's body is a sublime work of art that cannot be viewed as a commodity or a tool for understanding its aesthetic nature. The combination of the body with the soul, heart, and feelings of a woman creates a complete and magnificent set. Any negative attitude or action toward this being is a flaw in purpose and a denial of its existential nature. A nature that stems from the fundamental principles of creation and a humanistic perspective.

If a man understands that, in the interpretation of Diotima, one body is no different from other bodies, then pursuing other bodies will not turn into an endless quest for him. To bring a musical instrument to vibration, one must strike its strings in a professional and precise manner. Any kind of inconsistency and deviation, both in taste and temperament, can lead to producing harsh and disturbing sounds. This is exactly what men are doing. The feminine protest we witness around the world is actually a reproduction of a sound that has been played on the wounds of women unjustly.

A musician who aims to produce the most excellent and emotional melodies from their beloved instrument never views it as a soulless tool or a sound-producing machine. They engage with the source of beauty creation with their spirit and emotions. They caress it. Embrace it. They intertwine their soul with its essence and identity, ultimately resulting in a harmonious and unified process, creating an artistic masterpiece.

The body, soul, heart, and feelings of a woman should also enter the process of empathy and self-awareness with the same feelings and artistic passion. Beautiful words, kisses, caresses, harmony, and ultimately mutual climax are steps that can elevate the process to a sublime level for both sides and create a masterpiece of mutual success.

A man who falls asleep after a short and emotionless sex, leaving his partner without even starting the motivation process, is someone who has not been educated in the art of empathy and creating great musical excitement. He is an unevolved being who is unaware of the existence of a woman. He is an uncivilized and artless individual who, with his ugly behavior, disregards all the elements and criteria of aesthetic beauty hidden in the process. In a place where love should begin as the beginning of the evolutionary path, with such a clear mistake, it turns into a place for the end of the journey.

The Short World of Inversion of Feeling

When a person enters the world of sex, they are completely sure that these moments are passing and immediate moments of satisfaction. This alone can be a source of stress. The mutual feeling given by the sexual partner can be helpful and comforting. Therefore, when sex is limited to those short moments of sexual excitement and is held without foreplay and aftermath, it violates its purpose. In fact, even the highest sexual experiences are short. Psychologically, when a person is in a pleasant situation, time passes quickly, and when in a difficult situation, time passes slowly.

One of the shortcomings of sex in general, particularly for men, is its transient and unstable nature compared to other pleasurable activities. Sex is like a spark of immense energy that is suddenly released and uncontrollable, similar to the immense energy stored in clouds responsible for seasonal rains and storms. A great force gradually builds up in the two opposing and symmetrical natures of the clouds. When the two clouds collide, the roar of thunder and the release of hidden energy lead to the release of immense energy. However, everything comes to an end after a few moments. Even the longest of sex acts, with the help of external factors, do not last much longer than an hour. If we do not consider the prerequisites, preliminaries, and aftermath, this time will be significantly shorter.

This is why it is said (and women appreciate this) that sex should be a slow and fundamental process that begins with loving words, kisses, cuddling, romantic conversations, caresses, body massages, arousal, and intimacy, ultimately culminating in an orgasm.

In ideal sex, even orgasm is not the end point. The buttocks, like foreplay, matter. But lovemaking is important both in determining the level of love and affection, and in terms of human ethics and valuing feminine identity.

The crucial point here is that sex is the main factor in reaching a soft and humane character and creating tenderness and affection. Or to put it better, it should be so.

The gentle sorrow that occurs after orgasm is due to humans getting closer to their nature and human roots. It is a sign of inner grief in humans, which, in the words of Rumi, stems from being cut off from the gardens of nature and deep human roots.

Sex is one of the transformations in human life that can bring individuals closer to these worlds and signs each time. It is evident that all of this is conceivable assuming the realization of an ideal sex. Otherwise, it is clear that when a man turns away from his partner after a superficial, short-lived, and one-sided orgasmic sex and engages in playing with his mobile phone or raises loud animal-like noises, expecting such expressions and worlds from it is entirely futile. Sex is a double-sided coin. It can be a behavior that embodies the abomination and depravity of humanity, as well as a catalyst for human and divine aspects, referring to his deep human roots. Conversely, when sex manifests in its demonic forms such as rape, spousal abuse, obscenity, and the like, it becomes one of the most demonic behaviors.

Sex can be a powerful purifier that refines undesirable aspects of human nature and impurities. Here, we speak of a systematic confrontation embedded in the human institution. The clash between gentleness and violence, boredom and joy, uniformity and freshness, hardness and softness, coldness and warmth, compassion and indifference, strangeness and camaraderie, disconnection and connection, love and otherwise, and generally the confrontation between good and evil. Sex in its ideal form softens these matters.

The behaviors exhibited by men in the process of relationships reveal significant cognitive indicators in the fields of psychology and cultural sociology. Sex is not a simple physical behavior based on an outdated and condemned instinct, but primarily a credible channel for the emergence of love. Therefore, elsewhere in this text, it is mentioned that loves that do not culminate in bodily unity are not only sacred and ideal; they also indicate a form of psychological sickness or are themselves agents of a psychological sickness.

The concept known as platonic love (between a woman and a man) can generally be considered invalid and a kind of word play. The desire for love and the desire for sex are fundamentally definable and distinguishable from each other. These two aspects constitute a significant part of human psychological needs and can serve as a vehicle for mental health, followed by physical well-being, and ultimately social health of individuals.

Would the World Be a Better Place Without Lust?

With all the challenges and hype surrounding sexuality, suddenly the question arises in the inquirer's mind: Would humans truly be happier and more content without sexual desire? Humans have plenty of means and ways to enjoy life. But why should they endure so many challenges and tensions for the sake of an additional possibility? Without desire, humans could have had a more peaceful coexistence. Many competitions and hostilities would have been eliminated. Humans wouldn't have to exhibit ugly and repulsive behaviors driven by their primary motivations in sexual hormones. Without desire, love could have been much more genuine and humane. Establishing a balance between desire and love wouldn't have been obligatory.

Love without sexual exploitation, as seen between a mother and child, could showcase one of the most beautiful social and elevating aspects of humanity. Without lust, human life wouldn't be divided into major stages like childhood, youth, and old age to such an extent. Many of these divisions are driven by sexual impulse.

Eastern cultures hold great respect for the elderly. This respect, often interpreted as wisdom, seems to stem from the fact that in old age, a person is devoid of destructive force and sinful lust. Whatever they exhibit reflects a greater purity and human dignity. They can easily interact with young women without the stigma of sinful behavior or sexual motives.

In old age, sexual attractions do not determine behaviors and decisions. This is because the ancient archetype of "wise elder" is widely present in the Eastern world. There are many proverbs in Eastern languages that highlight the conflict between old age and wisdom and the power of sensual love. For example, there is a proverb that says: "If the love of an elder stirs, disaster will follow." The story of Sheikh San'an and the girl and the parrot is based on this cultural conflict. These and countless other questions have clear answers that nature has responded to. By placing sensual power within humans, nature has ensured the beauty of life even in non-sensual environments and realms. When looking at a painting, a significant portion of the artistic pleasure is due to the activity of sexual hormones.

The beauty of the Mona Lisa painting lies in the hidden sensual energy in the underlying layers of the image. This energy connects with the viewer's inner sensual energy, resulting in an aesthetic enjoyment. A significant portion of literature and art is infused with hidden sexual motivations. Without tapping into this hidden sensual force, humans couldn't even fully appreciate the beauty of a sunset. Human emotional sparks arise from their inner sensuality when facing the phenomena around them.

Human culture has classified almost all phenomena based on sexual criteria and has structured its system accordingly. Language reflects a significant portion of human desires and perceptions, with the female represented as SHE and the male as HE. Most languages adhere to similar sexual requirements in their rules.

Language can be distinctly divided into masculine and feminine components. Poetry without the presence of sexual elements will be devoid of any artistic subtlety and aesthetic capacities.

Even in entirely masculine and religious environments, sexuality and sexual desire persist in a concealed manner. Music without the involvement of sexual elements almost loses its aesthetic appeal.

A significant portion of the world economy is directly or indirectly dependent on the element of sensuality. The beauty and valuation of objects are linked to their connection with feminine beauty and sensuality. Gold is considered beautiful and precious primarily because we associate it with the traditional patterns of feminine beauty. A gold necklace gains value solely by imagining it on the bare chest of a woman.

In silver dishes and grand hotel halls, there is a strong aura of sensuality and sexual attractions in flux. Travel inherently involves a sensual act. Seclusion and intimacy are inherently based on a sensual perception. Creation is entirely based on sexual attraction. Plants, animals, galaxies, stars, and planets are all the same. When we look at a villa in the midst of a garden in the light of the setting sun, there is a sensual feeling intertwined with the explanation of its beauty and authenticity. The sun, symbolizing heat and beauty and serving as a source of energy, has a feminine nature. The moon, as a great ancient symbol of life, holds a sexual identity with an uninterrupted connection between earthly beings and the sensual and feminine beauty aspects of the moon.

The daily life of a human in stock exchanges, factory environments, and company offices holds intrinsic value and is filled with relentless effort and dedication that ultimately leads to the seclusion of a bedroom. Colors generally have a sensual and sexual nature. Colors can divide a person's living space into masculine and feminine environments, with the main factor being sexual behavior. The vast industry of cosmetics and grooming is important because it can provide a small service to enhance human beauty, which in itself serves the element of sensuality.

Sex is a factor in strengthening internal power and a factor of aggression and effort in humans; a great force that shapes humans in the face of worldly events. The relationship between a father and son behind the scenes, based on a sexual act that provides the prerequisites for the birth of a child, is conceivable. In fact, every child is a sign and effect of the sexual power of their parents. Without hidden sexual energy in the audience, the most important literary masterpieces in the world, such as Pride and Prejudice, Wuthering Heights, and famous paintings like The Kiss by Gustav Klimt, Girl with a Pearl Earring by Johannes Vermeer, or The Birth of Venus by Sandro Botticelli, would be devoid of artistic identity and value, lacking current impact.

The sexual force, by incorporating a primary element called sadness, is constantly refining the human soul. Without the sexual factor, humans would become dangerous and merciless beings, turning the Earth into an uninhabitable place. All these factors that give meaning to life constitute a great mission that creation, with its abundant intelligence, has placed on the shoulders of the female gender. The female gender, with a different psyche and immense energy it generates in earthly creation, is tasked with being the driving force of life on Earth, considering its highly influential components.

Chapter Two
The Lost Half of Humanity

Finding the Right Partner or the Right Way to Relate to Him

In the process of mating, humans have focused the utmost attention on finding the "right person." However, a high level of precision in the selection process has led to a strategic error in the continuation of the process. This means that humans concentrate all their efforts on "finding the right person" and then fall short in finding the "appropriate communication method" with that person. Just as finding the right person is important, finding suitable ways to communicate with that person is also crucial. While a considerable amount of love can ensure the prospect of a lasting relationship, love alone cannot thrive in an unsuitable and suboptimal environment without continuous attention to its growth.

Many relationships start with great love but gradually, it is observed with utter disbelief that the flame of love diminishes and eventually, like a flickering candle, it declares its last sparks and suddenly goes out. The unexpected endings of lives lie in these negligence, lack of sufficient experience in managing relationships, and the inability to nurture love. In the words of the poet: when the "relationship lights" are out, continuing the path in darkness, even with the help of love, will not be possible.

In other words, humans today, due to their innate backgrounds, naturally know how to fall in love and experience it. However, in the next phase related to "staying in love" and "making someone fall in love," or better put, "the art of loving," they become vulnerable.

Perhaps this weakness stems from childhood upbringing. Men learn in childhood that love is a one-way street, and to have and maintain love, there is no need for reciprocal action. A mother unilaterally devotes her love to her child, and he continues to draw from this wellspring of affection until he is on her deathbed, and even beyond. For him, love is an endless one-way stream that he can draw from whenever needed. To sustain this situation, there is not much need for reciprocal action.

When men extend this rule to others during adolescence and in times of love, they exhibit rough and thoughtless behavior. They believe that as soon as they fall in love, an endless stream of affection should flow toward them and never be cut off. This misconception leads them to disregard the considerations and obligations of behavior when faced with love.

Many times, due to a man's emotional dependencies, in accordance with the "Oedipus complex" rule, the role and identity of the mother are transferred to the spouse, and he seeks nurturing and motherly behavior from his partner. The combination of these two situations undermines the emotional foundation of the man's relationship with his spouse much sooner than expected.

When we talk about the importance of frequent circular checks by a mental health center, it means that a skilled therapist who is knowledgeable about the masculine nature, emotional dependencies, and fantasies of a narcissist gradually tries to rescue them from this unintended error. A therapist will remind a man that unlike the romantic relationship with the mother, a romantic relationship with a woman is a two-way process that requires consideration and delicacy, neglect of which can lead to the decline of romantic feelings.

Many times, men are the main factor in breaking up relationships; but they are not the main culprits. Because of the same feeling of dependence and the idea they have of a one-sided childhood love, they naturally exhibit behaviors that are not conscious or malicious; but in any case, it causes a break in the relationship.

The woman tries to endure this situation for some time and waits for the situation to improve; but in the absence of an external factor that corrects and educates the man and corrects his behavior and actions, there will be no chance for transformation and improvement. In the absence of a psychotherapist, oftentimes critical relationships will not have a chance to survive.

Matching Is a Superficial Work or a Work Related to the Inner Human Being

To start any relationship, in the first place, the physical body, along with some behavioral and emotional sparks, will be the criterion of action. At this point, we may be faced with a kind of paradox. Based on his natural instinct, man makes sexual attraction a criterion for evaluation and choice. But modern ethics tells him that looking sexually to evaluate a woman's character is against human dignity and possibly insulting. His mind is aware of the sensual aspects, the chiseled nose, the combination of eyes and eyebrows, the extension of the hands and the height of the stature. Even during the conversation, he visualizes the sexual and hidden parts of the woman in his imagination and recreates a scenario of the possibility of embracing the woman. At the same time, another force warns him that: "A beautiful face is nothing in appearance/ O brother, bring a beautiful face."

But nature takes its own course, and the primary criterion for selection, following the intelligence of creation, is external attractiveness, and the function of the inner personality will be determined in the next steps.

When life becomes stable and some time has passed from the relationship, sexual attraction and inner personality reach a balance point and each takes an equal share in strengthening the relationship. The longer the cohabitation, the heavier the balance becomes in favor of spiritual convergence. The priority of sexual attraction decreases and its quality decreases due to the repetition of the act and increasing age. Now men and women are continuing the same life, which at the point of decision, sensual attraction was involved in the beginning of it in a fateful way.

Many people decide to establish a relationship and get married based on sensual judgments before they have the chance to truly know each other. Sensual imaginations and fantasies to spend a pleasant and peaceful night, during a conversation about the basics of manners, usually play an essential role in determining the main lines of destiny. How many people make their final decision even by seeing a photo?

Alain de Botton believes that in understanding the basics of the aesthetics of attraction, the findings of evolutionary biology provide us with important information. Evolutionary biology indirectly determines a man's preferences for being attracted to a woman. Although this criterion is imperceptible, it is decisive and has been institutionalized in man over the centuries.

According to this theory, the hidden measure of sexual attraction is the issue of reproductive health. That is, in the initial meetings, when a man evaluates a woman, the beauty component is a convincing reason that guarantees that his partner is a healthy person and can give birth to healthy children and ensure the evolutionary process of the generation and the family.

In other words, the beautiful appearance of a woman indirectly promises that she is completely healthy in terms of the immune system, has a strong physical structure and strong muscles, and a fit and balanced body, so the prospect of life with her is ideal. Such a woman promises sexual pleasure, happiness, health and great energy that she can share with her man and his children. This knowledge is more than dependent on a man's rational inference, it is an intuitive ability based on the lived experience of generations that has been institutionalized in his existence. The enormous intelligence of life, with the installation of this intelligent filter, makes humans act in such a way that important criteria such as health and beauty, which guarantee the quality of the generation, are always prioritized in choosing a mate.

In explaining the theory of the "Principle of Species," Darwin writes about sexual selection: "As mentioned in the hypothesis of the struggle for survival and its result, i.e., natural selection, new species are formed due to having some privileged and beneficial properties, they transfer their traits and advantages from generation to generation in the form of inheritance to their descendants, and other traits and specialties are gradually depreciated due to the mixing of different individuals of the same type."

Thus, evolutionary biology and Darwinian evolution both state that a woman's beauty inspires that the next generation will be protected from the scourge of ugliness and disease. This survival conflict system is actually the defense mechanism of the human genome to eliminate pests.

By putting together this network of self-control of life and conflict with the issue of human dignity of women, we arrive at the answer to that basic question. That is, based on the intelligence of creation, the sexual view of a man toward a woman and a woman toward a man is in accordance with a huge intelligent system and thus does not conflict with the human dignity of women; rather, it is basically parallel to nature.

In fact, nature has entrusted us with a recognition mechanism based on instinct, and when we evaluate the pair, we actually look at the opposite subject from our human biological aspect. In such situations, nature can automatically make complex and correct decisions and save us from confusion.

The data encoded in the human genome can contain even more precise criteria. In order to find out this, evolutionary biology scientists have started research. These studies have shown that men mainly use the same general criteria to find a woman beautiful.

Researchers randomly showed pictures of men and women from around the world to a group of people. The reference group was asked to categorize the owners of these images in terms of their sexual attractiveness and aesthetic criteria.

The results showed that the aesthetic criteria for sexual attractiveness are surprisingly similar in different regions of the world. Evolutionary biologists determined that the criterion of beauty and attractiveness for people in different parts of the world is the subject of "symmetry." That is, a sensual and beautiful face is one whose left and right parts are physically symmetrical.

The evolutionary logic hidden behind this human taste is completely clear and based on the human experience and his historical memory regarding facing all kinds of diseases and injuries.

Symmetry is the opposite of "difference" and "unalignment." A phenomenon that occurs in various diseases such as mongolism and diseases caused by chromosomal abnormalities. Man's historical sixth sense tells him that symmetry means health and health means beauty. To evaluate himself, he relies on the intelligence that the intelligent system of existence has embedded in him. The intelligent system of existence works in the same way on the whole earth, and therefore the aesthetic standard is exactly the same in all parts of the earth.

Man is not aware of the presence of this innate intelligence in him. Therefore, his choice is more instinctive than logical.

Now, when a man sits facing a woman for the first time and evaluates her sensual and aesthetic capacities, he is using this hidden knowledge without realizing it. The man's inner feeling tells him that this beautiful woman promises a long life for him, and a wide range of happiness for the man and guarantees the production of beautiful and healthy children.

In this way, it can be said that arousal is not inherent in itself and depends on other prerequisites and resources in the whole human existence, of which beauty and health are the most important.

The Role of Human Childhood in Mating Aesthetics

A person's worldview is significantly influenced by his educational mechanism, especially during childhood. Depending on the general and geographical culture of the parents, a person's worldview may be completely different. This is the point that cannot be known at first glance and by evaluating the person's appearance.

Mental deficiencies are one of the most important factors affecting the formation of a person's macro worldview. Failures can create deep holes in character. Vulnerable and unbalanced points of a person's personality are hidden in the lower layers. When two people live under the same roof for a long time, they will reveal their hidden realities whether they like it or not.

In a long relationship, there comes a time when the parties, willingly or unwillingly, put their fingers on the vulnerable points of each other's souls. Sometimes a life after decades suddenly falls apart overnight. This is the time when the unbalanced and weakened part of the soul of one of the parties has been hit.

For this reason, in the correct evaluation of dating days, we should not only emphasize the person's strengths and virtues; it is equally important to know the weaknesses of the character. The greater the scope of these conflicts, the more likely it is that a joint life will not end.

Sex, as one of the most important factors in the continuation of a joint life, is no exception to this rule. Psychological and educational gaps may affect a person's sensuality while creating different sexual tastes. The amount of deprivations and mental complexes caused by the tensions of early educational periods may lead to tensions in the stable sexual relationship of both parties.

There may be conflicting characteristics that complement each other in the case of a correct choice. For example, if a passive and introverted personality is combined with a passionate and extroverted personality, the two can fill each other's mental voids. But if two conflicting souls are placed next to each other, the possibility of reconciliation and the index of repulsion are higher. A pragmatic and passionate personality can complement a thoughtful and introverted personality. However, two thinking and introverted characters double the state of conflict caused by the intensification of introversion, as an example of the mathematical rule "negative in negative is equal to negative."

The element of sensuality may be intensified or reduced based on these psychological relationships. When people find signs of compensatory traits in the other person, they instinctively feel more sensual toward them.

Because of this, sometimes a person may be interested in only one of them when faced with two completely identical people. Because he feels that his ideal person will complement his inner weaknesses.

In one of his works, Alain de Botton mentions an example to explain this issue. He uses Scarlett Johansson and Natalie Portman as two of the most beautiful women currently living on earth to clean up the aesthetic basics of today. He says that the educational system leading to the formation of the psychological personality of each of us plays a role in choosing one of these two faces as an attractive face.

Showing a photo of each of them, he writes: "If we are faced with two people who seem to have the same health, we may, because of our psychological background, feel that only one of them is really irritating to us. If the parents who hurt us were untrustworthy and over-the-top people, we would probably conclude that based on Scarlett's appearance, she is a little too fond of excitement and melodrama.

Scarlett's cheekbones might be thought to indicate her high talent for self-absorption, a quality we have more of than we'd like, and her eyes, though calm, might give the impression they could burst into a volcano of rage. and become roaring, something that we have a talent for and certainly we don't need someone to strengthen it in us."

Alain de Botton continued by posing the question, "Why don't all healthy and attractive people attract us equally?" Or why are our preferences so different? He writes: "If we are to judge based on objective criteria, Natalie is not more beautiful than Scarlett, but we may find her more beautiful in the end, because her eyes give us exactly the same sense of peace that we ourselves have not received and have always longed for. But we may see a steely and pragmatic determination in Mrs. Portman's forehead and be motivated by it, because we cannot expect such qualities from ourselves, we always lose our house keys and we cannot even fill out our insurance forms with common sense."

"His mouth may also be seductive to us, because it suggests a kind of tolerance and self-restraint that balances our painful tendency to recklessness and indolence. In short, we can explain our attraction to Natalie or Scarlett by reviewing our own shortcomings; Just as our attraction to the paintings of Agnes Martin or Caravaggio can be explained by examining the shortcomings that exist in us as adults."

The result is that every human being instinctively seeks a partner who brings out the wholeness and integrity of his personality and helps him by filling his personality holes. This mechanism remains active not only in sex, but also in other areas of life until the end of our life.

From Dating to Flirting, from Greetings to Sex

Regardless of where a person ends his life on this planet and under what educational and family system, it can be said that the process of establishing a relationship with the opposite sex includes a single and uniform pattern. This pattern has worked for thousands of years and is still working today. From the time when the newly matured cave-dweller, on his hunting trail and behind a large elm tree, first looks at a young and elusive girl, until the meetings are repeated and finally he goes to bed with her, until when in the lonely corner of a In the restaurant, the young man's gaze meets a girl's gaze several tables away, and after certain stages, the story of the bed repeats again, the process is the same as it was: the initial meeting, meetings, subsequent dates, meetings and gifts, approaches, and finally Bed: In whatever way the living environment of these two requires, but there is no difference in the essence of the problem.

Getting to know a man and a woman and getting close to each other can be compared to the circles that are created when a stone is thrown in a pond. But to apply this analogy, we have to reverse the process. Always the first introduction and greeting is the biggest circle. The first feeling of interest brings two people into a circle with the greatest possible radius. In the next meetings, the radius of the circle of feelings and relationships becomes narrower until finally, these repeated circles at the central point of the relationship; That is, the bed becomes a "point of unity."

The first meeting may be a good time to exchange the first glances that express feelings by drinking tea or coffee or having dinner in a restaurant in the city. Signs of the presence of sparks of empathy between the two sides, which seem to be gradually testing each other and putting aside the misunderstandings that have always surrounded human relationships.

Telling a short story about a travel experience or a trip by the sea, or telling stories from high school or university can create openings where both parties can get to know the unknown corners of each other's souls. The end of every narrative, the telling of every story, the draining of every glass of drink, the end of every meal together can be the right place for each of the parties to take an effective step toward each other.

Each time such a step is taken, the parties grant the other privileges to get to know the more private parts of the soul and feelings of the other party.

Emotional evaluations continue throughout these stages. A shopper's look at the clothes or a happy shopper's look at the heat flowing in the skin of a woman who is telling a story and a heroic fantasy about the genitals of a man who is listening to a story. These can flow in the heart of this acquaintance and slow and continuous movement toward the bed.

With each step of closeness and intimacy, the physical distance decreases centimeter by centimeter. This process may be accompanied by determination and foresight. Intimacy has not yet grown enough to be able to initiate physical contact without concern. Therefore, slow and centimeter movement toward the first touch can be the best possible policy to evaluate the other party's reaction.

At this critical and sensitive stage, a simple event may come to the aid of the parties. A collision of hands or face while picking something up from the table, or an accidental contact of the leg while moving under the table, and any other similar incident, may lead to a fake apology, followed by laughter and the collapse of the walls of uncertainty. Whether this shortcut exists or not, eventually the time will come when both sides will take a big step by holding each other's hands and try their luck to break down the wall of fear.

Holding Hands Is the Beginning of the Trust Stage

Finally, what makes the decision of two people to become one begins with the contact of hands. Touching hands can have different meanings in different situations. In a normal handshake in the workplace or when introducing two people or a regular routine meeting, hand contact can have no meaning other than normal pleasantries. But when, after several meetings over dinner and coffee and using dozens of tactics to test the other person and looking for different ways to touch each other's soul, the first contact of hands occurs at the dinner table or in any other public setting, it can mean the beginning of a relationship. Deep body.

After holding hands, intimacy reaches a point where men and women can fantasize about the next pleasant events. Perhaps, after joining hands, we will once again see another stage of tactical retreat. In such a situation, the parties retreat to the previous situation and normal words and other conventional conversations are exchanged again. Without forgetting the important step that has been taken, it is not going to be forgotten without any function.

Dinner is over. This meeting is also close to its end. But the emotional meeting of the hands promises the beginning of which it is not clear where the end will lead. Still trying to maintain a layer of indifference. Trust is not fully established yet. Precautionary forecasts must be on the agenda.

A Kiss, the Beginning of Contact Between the Insides and the Exit from Loneliness

When the man and woman of our scenario go out of the restaurant or the meeting place, each of them is having their colorful fantasies about the stages of a sex. But there is still no definite plan to actualize it. In all these stages, each party may have a share in luck and coincidence. The same event that happened in the accidental contact of the hands played an important role in bringing the two parties closer together.

Outside the meeting place, the task of the following hours should be determined. So the man cautiously suggests that they go to his room for tea and to watch a movie they both like. Since the emotional meeting of hands has taken place, we all know that the proposal will be accepted. But the historical experience of the civilized society, which is supposed to consider the woman in a completely equal position with the man, does not allow the explicit "shameless proposal." Therefore, respect and caution still prevail over all statements and suggestions.

With the agreement reached about the destination, the prediction of the next steps still remains in the state of colorful fantasies. Anything can stop this progress. Therefore, the step-by-step process must be followed completely.

The advantage of equal relationships over relationships under the rule of marriage is related to this issue. In the state of marriage, the man is only a beneficiary who is supposed to use the benefits provided by the marriage rule in any possible way. For him, sex is mandatory, and his fantasies are only about the details of the performance, not about whether or not it will happen. But in our scenario, the man does not have a special advantage over the woman. He is in a completely equal and even weaker position. He must observe all the rules of equality and mutual respect and never commit an act that harms a woman's self-esteem.

In the limited light of the house, when the light of the television shines on the woman's cheeks from the front, the man feels significantly closer to this creature that was not present in his life a few days ago. From the angle he's sitting on the couch next to her, he feels the flushed cheeks and soft fur on her cheek are clear signs of acceptance. So he carefully puts his hand on the woman's shoulders and moves a little closer to her and waits for the woman's reaction. As he expected, the woman's reaction is also due to his desire.

The woman puts her hand on the man's hand and moves a little closer to him. But he continues to watch TV. After a while, the man gets up and brings tea to his guest and then returns to the same position as before. He puts his hands on her shoulders again and pulls her toward him with more courage.

The woman rests her head on the man's shoulders, in such a way that her warm brown hair touches the man's face. A warm feeling rises from the depths of the man's being, and a deep desire from the need to hug him is expressed in him. He touches his cheeks to the woman's warm and flushed face with an attitude that comes from avoiding caution. The woman turns and puts her lips close to the man's mouth. Now the first kiss is formed. They have taken another big step toward becoming one.

Getting Naked, the Beginning of the Deep Symbiosis of Cells

Caution still prevails. Words and sentences are still exchanged within conventional limits and respecting all etiquettes. The adventure of a man and a woman is entering an important stage. The man reaches out and opens one of the buttons of the woman's shirt. Without protesting, he reaches out and opens the second button himself. This completely symbolically means that she has allowed the man to discover her most private part.

Until a few days ago, before this relatively long process, if these two saw each other on the street, the idea of such contacts might have been far from mind and even accompanied by disgust. But in these few days when the stories, conversations, laughter, exchange of private information continued, the process of touching the mutual souls has made the touching of the bodies as the last step before sex, seem obvious and even pleasurable.

Even during these exchanges there might come a time when the discovery of hidden traits on either side would lead to a permanent separation. But fortunately, everything indicated that the man and woman of our scenario are close in every way. This closeness has included spiritual and emotional subtleties, shared interests, shared dreams, shared experiences, understandable failures, and understandable life experiences.

In fact, the process that leads to the final stage should be a completely natural and non-deterministic process. The oppression that is imposed on women in underdeveloped societies in line with marriages is related to this key point. In such marriages without prior acquaintance of the souls, the relationship of an animal species that requires the unquestioning obedience of the woman to the sexual desires of the man is both the beginning and the end of it. In this process, the woman is not respected. His desires are ignored.

The spiritual and emotional world is not important in any of the common relationships.

A few days ago, the idea of sex for a man and a woman in our scenario might have been accompanied by disgust and disgust, because they did not know each other. The Eastern woman succumbs to this disgust in the equation of forced marriage. No one has to discover and understand his spiritual and emotional angles and try to align with that unknown world. The tyrannical social system does its work, willingly or unwillingly, and women are passive receivers who are reduced to the level of an exchangeable object.

In a traditional and regulated sexual relationship based on male dominance and the rule of social taboos, women do not enjoy sexual participation much. This is because a major part of sexual desire and pleasure is independent of physical aspects. Physical action actually flows in the outer layers and at the level of the relationship.

In our scenario, non-physical aspects based on the personality and dignity of both parties are very important. Only by touching the other person's naked soul can we come to the conclusion that someone loves us or not? In fact, one of the most difficult things to ensure the definite fulfillment of which is hard work is to love and be loved. The messages we receive from the other party that we think are signs of love can be incredibly misunderstood and even false.

This is the point of reference that men throughout history have been able to deceive the women in their lives. The message we send after buying an expensive gift may have different interpretations. This interpretation will always be accompanied by great misunderstandings. Perhaps best of all, the man sends a message to the woman that he is happy to play the woman's role as an agent of his highest sexual satisfaction.

This message may be spoken or hidden behind meaningful silence. A man may send the message that he is satisfied with his partner's role as an efficient servant and service provider in raising children and running the household. It is even possible that in the eclectic mass culture, this level of attention can be interpreted as the extreme of loving.

What was drawn above clearly shows that the criteria of loving and being loved are very different. It is certain that being loved from the point of view of a woman with common sense and sufficient awareness and a human and sublime spirit will never correspond to one of the above types of interpretations. Even the most sublime form of love for a woman is not a man trying to understand her. A woman does not need to be understood by a man. Understanding must exist by itself. Trying to understand a woman means that a man suffers from a deep deficiency. A shortcoming that has caused him to be far from understanding the general and historical nature of women.

When understanding itself exists, other factors that become necessary in the process of becoming one can be signs of true love. Factors that are increasingly present from the moment of acquaintance to the event of orgasm and after that. All these are reflected in the man's behavior. In order to know such factors and to know the nature of men's behavior, it is necessary to have some kind of general awareness in women.

For this reason, it can be said that the majority of women in human history have not only been deprived of gifts such as orgasm, but also due to the lack of knowledge related to male behavior in combination with female nature, they have not been able to understand whether they are truly loved or not. No, they are also deprived. In fact, these women remain in compound ignorance, which plunges their lives into despairing neglect.

Now is the stage of getting naked. Undressing is the end of customary precautions. But that's not all. According to Sepehri, "the sacrifice of the surfaces" is glorious; but it does not mean absolute meeting of souls. However, nakedness means accepting another, one of the most important pillars of closeness. Man is not only ashamed of nudity; rather, he is clearly afraid of it. One of the punishments Adam Abul Bashar and Eve faced was nudity. Facing the hardness of the earth and the beginning of the life process, as the first activity, to protect themselves, they began to cover their private parts with tree leaves.

Nudity can make a person completely defenseless and desperate in front of others in unwanted and public situations. For this reason, in some of the tortures applied in authoritarian regimes, they torture the criminals with nudity. A naked person completely loses the independence of action and the power to process things and can cooperate with the interrogator and torturer and fulfill his demands.

Voluntary nudity in front of a sexual partner represents a deep type of trust and union and constitutes the granting of permission to enter the most private privacy. This two-way action and reaction is actually a reward for a sensory convergence. As much as this feeling of convergence and mutual acceptance is more complete and deeper, nudity can have more degrees. Couples who have experienced the highest form of convergence and closeness do not shy away from bright spaces.

The lower the depth of this unity, the more the parties tend to darken the flirting environment to a greater degree, so that the possibility of seeing naked details is limited. The greater the distance between two people, nudity can be accompanied by feelings of anxiety and even disgust. Because under normal conditions, looking at another person's naked body will not be a pleasant sight. Of course, it goes without saying that this issue is not unrelated to the aesthetic issue of people's bodies. But the pleasant attraction of sex can hide a major part of this aesthetic problem.

Actually, sex attraction works like two sides of the same coin. Sexual power can make looking at other organs feel disgusting. This problem is well reflected in the repulsion that the body of newly reached adolescents creates for the surrounding people. When this person was a young child and there was no sign of sensuality in him, either naked or clothed, he was a beloved and lovable being to those around him. But as soon as the power of lust appears in him, his body becomes an unpleasant phenomenon.

The same sexual power in the conditions we mentioned may be exceptionally desirable and pleasant for a person's sexual partner. The two parties are not only flirting in complete nudity, but they have also added soul nudity to it. Each is revealing their most complex and personal fantasies and sexual interests. Hobbies, sexual fantasies, desired arousal, past sexual experiences; Like masturbation, the first sexual experience, sexual creativity and tendencies that cannot be expressed under normal conditions, are revealed one by one.

The sentences and the exchange of information are such that it seems that each of the two people has moral and sexual deviations in a strange way. But the fact is that inside each of the healthy people, there is a moral and sexually deviant person hidden, which can only be revealed in the conditions that the people in our scenario are in now.

This situation in itself is a sign of ultimate unity and closeness. The existence of such latent tastes is as natural as, according to psychologists, a dictator, a murderer, a criminal, a masochist, etc. are hidden inside every healthy person.

The existence of such tendencies is not unnatural, what complicates this issue is the degree and power of action of these internal forces. When one of these forces overcomes and prevails over other forces and tendencies (i.e. all human virtues), then we will witness the emergence of an actual criminal at the level of society.

Departure from Normal Behavior, the Beginning of the Fusion of Souls

For sublime sex, you can't stay within the norms and rules of routine. Being normal is what people consistently follow in public and social settings. When the ultimate intercourse is to take place, baring the soul and showing the naked and unmasked manifestations of the soul can be the right path for this.

Therefore, the man and woman in our story begin to say phrases and sentences that bring them to the naked stage of the soul. This is something that does not happen in a routine and traditional marriage. A married man and woman, who have been guided to a common platform based on the traditional guidelines of society, may enter into the process of sex thousands of times without ever gaining knowledge of each other's hidden personality. Because according to the traditional guidelines of the society, a woman should never become uncontrollably intimate. He must endure the process with the highest form of self-restraint and remain passive.

The words that are exchanged between the man and the woman in our story are a sign of departure from the controlled standards of the relationship. They do not utter these words under normal circumstances. Because sexual arousal can cause a departure from soft behavior. They talk about their personal interests in sex, arousal and other personal interests that lie in the darkest private corners of one's personality.

When both parties are revealing their secrets and sharing their experiences from the beginning of puberty to the present, when they reveal their feelings and sinful behaviors, they are actually going through a great loneliness that keeps them away from society. Mutual acceptance and mutual forgiveness is an attempt to get out of the isolation that humans face in all moments of their lives.

The problem is that sexual partners cannot always give each other such feelings. We see millions of couples who have had sex thousands of times and finally passed away without having come out of their cocoon of isolation with such deep spiritual interaction. Sexual relations that are created in the form of traditional marriages have such a feature. Coming out of the cocoon of sinful isolation with the help of a sexual partner requires prerequisites that, if present, will ensure the durability of the relationship.

Admitting one's spiritual infatuations and sinful and non-indulgent sexual tendencies and baring one's soul in front of one's sexual partner is often in conflict with societies and traditions expectations of couples. Such tendencies are not compatible with childhood upbringing, nor with the conservatism that parents have had in post-puberty education.

If a woman wants to behave in the form of a traditional woman and in accordance with the conventional patterns of society, she should never utter such words and desires in front of her sexual partner. What happens in this semi-dark room is another world where neither conventional rules work nor events can be predicted. So when it is said that "love is the other side of madness," it refers to such an irregular situation. But love and unity appear exactly here and nothing else.

The symptoms that appear in sexual organs and behaviors, changing the tone of words, and transforming the lexical field toward silly or impolite words are a practical example of honesty and acceptance, which realizes the state of loving and being loved in an atmosphere free of deceit.

This genuine excitement, which manifests itself in the reticence of words, grabbing, pulling, squeezing and other non-aggressive actions, gives an irreplaceable pleasure to the parties, which are clear indications of the sincerity of the parties. This is a category that cannot be studied in formal intercourse, or even in a prostitution situation. In other words, the quality of sex-love is achieved in a combination of physiological manifestations with emotional and psychological satisfaction along with honesty and spiritual unity.

The sensuality of the behavior is not even directly related to the degree of benefiting from the aesthetic gifts of a woman or a man. This factor can be very transitory and unprofitable in the absence of the aforementioned backgrounds. What happens in such a bed is so pure and genuine compared to the superficial love and false passions and passions that it can bring sexual partners to the peak of sexual pleasure.

Flirting with women who engage in sex as a duty is no different from the act of needing. A routine work without the involvement of the spiritual agent, to remove a physical product that has been created in the body, and to do it, it is enough to do a simple work without concentration and reasoning.

To put it simply, the conflict between love and rationality is always the main obstacle for the manifestation of true love and feeling. When the factor of rationality prevails in the experience of sex, when both parties are constantly adapting their sexual behavior to conventional social, religious, educational patterns, etc. during flirting, they never reach the peak of unity and closeness.

Insolence in verbal and behavioral relationships and going beyond the limits of conventional behavior on the eve of sexual intercourse is a sign of love and permission to enter privacy. These behaviors may sometimes lead to the use of tools that are discussed in the issue of fetishism and will be discussed in their place.

Hair pulling, profanity, grabbing, words that are normally derogatory, and many other indiscretions are among the things that can be signs of excessive love and a sense of complete belonging. In fact, it can be said that in the conditions of purity of sexual act, the concept of respectful sex does not exist externally. The excessive love of the parties has emerged because they have not only been able to break the framework of their isolation with the help of each other in creating this unity, but for a moment they have gone beyond all the norms of behavior and social etiquette and have reached purity in their actions. If the parties continue to wear the usual masks they wear in society during the process, they will actually be violated and will be deprived of deep sex.

Aggressiveness, indiscretions and the uncensored expression of all secret thoughts and emotions, contrary to what social taboos consider as shamelessness or lack of decency, have no meaning for either men or women.

The sex scene is the moment to overcome fears and doubts. When we allow someone to penetrate into the dark depths of our thoughts and souls, we are actually accepting that this person is the closest to us of all the people living on the planet.

No event like sex can be a place to cultivate and refine the filth inside. When we talk with our sexual partner about all the dark corners of our soul and thoughts, we have actually found a way to lighten the soul and get out of the heavy burden of soul filth. This is because after a quality sex, a person feels light and exalted. A person feels that the purulent secretions of his soul have been removed and he has achieved inner lightness and purity. Now, if a person is deprived of this attainable gift, he must deal with this internal filth and carry it with him forever.

Women who are deprived of experiencing such sex in their lives are often depressed and sad. Such people have never had the opportunity to talk about their inner tensions and dark thoughts in their head in a mutual show. This means bearing the pains that have burdened his soul over time and constantly bother him.

Irregularity of behaviors in the act of sex is part of its nature. A man kisses a woman's sexual organ and puts his mouth, which is one of the most excellent parts of the body, which is always visible to others and a vehicle for the manifestation of his personality, on the most mundane part of the woman. This irregular behavior means that he accepted the lover without judging the whole of his body.

From this point of view, the function of sex is not dissimilar to the process of "confession" in the church system. We all know that confession does not absolve one's sins. A person, in the process of confession, reveals all the bitter and sinful thoughts and images loaded on his soul. Images, experiences, biographies, and mental data remain exactly as they were before after confession. But their speech relieves the soul from their heavy burden and the confessor feels liberated and light. Sometimes the importance of this spiritual refinement is so much that the person's life is divided into before and after confession. This great achievement makes him, after the first confession, always eager to enter into another sweet process of confession.

The transcendental sexual experience of the kind we have described is not temporary or transitory. It is a lasting experience that may remain forever in the minds of both parties. They will seek to repeat this experience and the relationship will last. There are many cases that sexual partners refer to after a long time by remembering and describing their pure experience and experiencing a pleasant feeling by reviewing it. They may go back and review the process of their behavior from the beginning to the climax of sexual pleasure and talk about their feelings at each of those moments.

In the intimacy that has developed, they once again share their true feelings during the time of honest dating. Remembering the first sparks of love at the beginning of acquaintance is usually one of the most pleasant emotional manifestations in the lover and the beloved.

The traditional businesslike and conservative indifference of men in the process of sex is more degrading to women than anything else. The paradoxical situation that lies in the nature of traditional marriages makes most of these marriages either lead to failure and divorce or, if they last, provide a poisonous and painful environment for women.

Of course, men are also noble to this failure; but Beh Lataif Al Haili tries to fulfill his emotional needs elsewhere, away from the family environment and away from the eyes of his life partner. But the problem is that these needs will not be fulfilled anywhere other than entering into a genuine relationship with the main life partner.

In order to realize such a genuine relationship, it is necessary to have sex not as a routine task, but as a game and a deliberate choice to strengthen a part of the relationship. Insolent transgressions should not be limited to outside the home and temporary sex partners in the form of prostitution or polygamy. A change in attitude and performance can restore a broken relationship and bring happiness to both parties. It is enough to get over being bound to the dry discipline and sanctimoniousness of futile dealings with your spouse and look at him as a lover who has wonderful capabilities and capacities and let his talents flourish in a strong partnership. This issue depends on continuous creativity.

Orgasm Is the Peak of Oneness of Souls

The men and women of our story are on the verge of ultimate understanding by going through these wonderful and complicated steps and sharing novel data from their inner menus. What happens on the verge of orgasm is not limited and dependent on physical actions and reactions. Sexual organs and other parts of the body mediate the perception of the presence of another. Sensing the presence of another does not always happen in sex. There may be "another" and sex and ejaculation also occur; but understanding the presence of another is a more complex category.

The perception of the other's presence starts from the very beginning of acquaintance and reaches its climax in orgasm. In Attar's interpretation, what happens at the peak of Qaf is the physical truth of the relationship. In this long journey, the lover and the beloved pass through the "seven cities of love" and reach the presence of the soul in the ecstasy of purity without restraint or fainting. As we mentioned with Rumi's statement. where it says:

There is no difference between two friendships
Both sides are nothing but the light of the East

In other words, orgasm (especially true orgasm in women) is the result of the meeting of souls. Although there are methods and techniques to actualize the capacity of orgasm in women who have this disorder; but a major part of the problem of orgasm (especially in women) is psycho-mental and not psycho-physical.

In order to achieve orgasm and in the best conditions, to experience successive orgasms, a woman needs to be approved and accepted first of all. It requires that it is not limited. His motivation is not physical, but it is rooted in circumstances that are not easy to achieve. If we limit a woman's reactions, we have turned off something in her inner self from the very beginning.

If we believe that a woman's decency dictates that she should be quiet while flirting and not make noise, she is aware of our belief. Therefore, the depth of his being reacts to the fact that he is in our mind and does not cooperate with the cells to reach orgasm. Even more simply, if the environment is such that his voice can be heard by others in the next room, his psyche will engage in self-censorship.

Therefore, having the right environment is the first prerequisite to reach the peak of sexual pleasure in women. Men do not have much problem with this issue both physiologically and sociologically; but he has a wife. So, if you love your sexual partner and if, as a civilized and intellectual man, you care about his natural rights to have sex with you, you may need to soundproof your bedroom.

You may need to use measures to make your sexual partner feel safe and calm. You may need to start exercises to awaken his sleeping physical and mental aspects. These exercises should undoubtedly be with his participation and in a continuous and accurate conversation. Attracting a feeling of trust depends on convincing him of the fact that; He and you are moving on the same rail and you are not a careless and selfish man and you are not indifferent to his smallest feelings.

If you have taken the wrong path up to this point in your life together, maybe you need to go back to the zero point and have a new course from the beginning to the end of the connection. Connected, will not occur in contact surfaces. Rubbing limbs and entwining and orgasming, which are often reserved for men, are never considered hookups.

Thousands of marriages take place where the people around them congratulate this auspicious connection and go home thinking that everything is in its exact position, without knowing that the connection never actually happened. A man and a woman have been led to a common room as two strangers, while they have not received any training to reach the connection stage. The orderly environment has made them two accepting and submissive robots who are supposed to sleep together according to the dictated rules and be deprived of reaching the connected ring throughout their lives. They will raise children who in turn will follow the same path and the same rule.

A deep feeling of arousal is the ultimate love. Loveless contacts will never lead to deep arousal and genuine orgasm. What guarantees the sensuality of the relationship is a process that takes place from the first meeting to the mutual understanding of another human being (who is our equal and our rank, and whom we respect), during a slow process.

In a sensual relationship with the other party, we understand his values and reach a common meaning of existence and ideas of life, and our biological experience, which is basically in line with this, becomes more compatible.

The further we go in the path of analyzing things that are considered lustful, the clearer it becomes for us that lust is the feeling of excitement that we experience when we find another human being; especially a human who has common values and understanding of the meaning of existence with us. We enter the world of unity with him from the valley of alienation. We understand and accept all his ugliness and beauty, goodness and ugliness, weaknesses and strengths. Without comparing him with other human beings, we accept and love him as he is. We go to bed with him and actualize this union in action, and finally, orgasm, like the result of previous interactions, is the culmination of this meeting.

Such a person fills the gaps in our existence. It takes us out of the great loneliness built into our creation. We see a manifestation of ourselves in him. Therefore, after the orgasm event, we hug him and think about the whole path that has brought us to this moment.

If such a perfect process has not been followed, we will run away from the bed or turn our backs on it and will be faced with some kind of torment of conscience and sense of emptiness. Such is the feeling of orgasm with temporary sexual partners. Such is the painful sense of emptiness and identity-less-ness that comes to a person after masturbation. Because in such a situation, a person reaches orgasm without a suitable person filling the empty part of his soul, and the feeling of guilt is due to the emptiness of his soul in the absence of a true lover.

The reason why sexual acts are so painful in cases like homosexuality, intimacy with animals, intimacy with children and street women is because of this painful vacuum. In fact, orgasm has a psycho-physical nature. Orgasm is a spiritual and spiritual category that if it occurs regardless of its exalting aspect, the whole existence of a person cries out and complains about the frenzy that has happened to him.

When a woman does not reach orgasm or the ideal conditions are not available for her to have an authentic flirtation. A man experiences this feeling of emptiness to different degrees. He plays with his phone. He leaves the place or tries to forget this unpleasant event by any other means as soon as possible.

The horror of rape, which is condemned in all cultures, is because of this. In traditional semi-straight sex, the man reaches orgasm and the woman, although physically, inevitably agrees to this work; but he is suffering in his life. This is a degree of aggression. However, in common rape, both the personal and physical privacy of a person has been violated, as well as his spiritual and emotional side.

Reject Requests for Sex and Relationship

Let us use the above hypothetical example as a basis for another discussion. Now, it is assumed that in the continuation of the formation of this several-day relationship and after finishing the familiarization dinner, the man makes his proposal implicitly or explicitly to have a sexual relationship. In the first premise of this scenario, we saw that the woman is inclined to have a temporary romantic relationship with the man. After experiencing this short-term sex, she decides to follow her destiny and wait to meet an ideal man who fully matches her personality for the rest of her life.

But in the second assumption, after the end of the evening dinner, the woman feels that she does not have enough inner desires and romantic feelings to enter into a sexual relationship with the man. Here the question of rejecting the offer of sex is raised.

The woman turns to the man with the same dignity and sobriety that she has had during these few days and says: "I prefer to be good friends and our relationship remains in this state." This is a logical and civilized answer. Obviously, it is not easy for a man to hear a negative answer. He has invested a lot of his feelings and emotions. He has revealed his inner tendencies that he usually keeps hidden under normal circumstances. He put himself in a weaker position and told the woman that he wants to have a sexual relationship with her. But for any reason, there is no attraction leading to sex for women.

The man is in a bad position. Contradictory feelings come to him. The lack of self-confidence, the feeling of being broken, the illusion of not having male attractions and the kind of judgment that women may have about him, do not stop him. He interprets hearing the rejection as a negative judgment of the woman. She questions her male charms and feels that she is going through a bitter experience in life. But are all these things true?

If we reduce the rules related to finding a partner for marriage to this issue, we will see that not only for a stable relationship in the form of marriage, attractiveness and psychological criteria are important, but also for a short-term relationship. So, if a person gives a negative answer to our relationship request, it doesn't necessarily mean that all self-confidence collapses and questioning male attractions and generalizations. For any reason, one person may not be attractive to the second person; but for the third party, it should be highly attractive.

In other words, we just picked the wrong person who isn't compatible with us anyway. Sexual attraction is dependent on several factors, and when these factors are in agreement with each other, sexual attraction takes place. Failure to achieve this does not mean questioning all our capabilities in winning the hearts of others. As in our evaluations of different people, different criteria come into play automatically, or pre-consciously, this is also true for others. If we don't find him attractive in the face of another person and push him aside, does it really mean that he is unattractive to all people? If we look at it this way, the frustration caused by hearing the rejection answer will be moderated and will disappear very soon.

If someone rejects our chest, it is because the self-conscious discovery and intuition mechanisms based on the hidden data of the subconscious have worked naturally and he did not find us attractive. This is what we have regularly done to others. This is the hidden mechanism that helps us find the right match. Now, when it comes to others, should we generalize it to the whole and get frustrated?

Sexual attraction, like our other desires and desires, is internal and automatic. Let's assume that we don't like the taste of strawberry ice cream. This issue is institutionalized within us for any reason. Does this mean that strawberry ice cream is bad for everyone? Of course, as the famous saying goes, "There is no conflict in an example." Comparing sensuality and attractiveness with ice cream does not mean equal valuation between these two phenomena. Rather, it is only a means to explain the problem.

This example can be mentioned in other fields as well. Areas such as artistic taste, liking surrounding phenomena and people's natural tendencies toward affairs and phenomena are among these. The internal mechanism of man by which he performs the act of pairing is similar to polarization in that the central magnetism of different people does not affect him in the same way.

All compasses work based on the Earth's internal magnetism. But when we talk about a human unit, it means that his center of attraction may be different from other people. Something that does not apply to the center of gravity of the Earth. If we don't cause a person's sexual compass to rotate, neither his compass is broken nor our center of gravity is wrong; rather, these two, for some reasons, are not subject to convergence.

That's the only problem.

In other words, when "sexual attraction" is done by someone, this issue cannot be a basis for moral judgment or judgment regarding physical and personality attractions. This is just a simple, random heterogeneity that occurs naturally millions of times between different humans. Our offer of sex to someone we are not qualified to attract is just plain bad luck that doesn't matter much.

There is a standard and specific scientific answer to explain a sexual dysfunction, which has been answered by psychology long before. Just as there are exact answers to most physical and scientific phenomena. In other words, when someone rejects our request to sleep together, he has done this unconsciously and without making a judgment about us.

Psychological science has determined that the mind plays a major role in sexual attraction. Because this hidden force operates based on a reserve of hidden data and other internal factors, in fact, no judgment has been made at the external level. So as much as we believe in the mechanism of action within ourselves and trust and respect our choices, we should accept this issue about others as well.

If we consider the set of these arguments and factors in a realistic atmosphere, we will see that our reaction to the negative sexual response will be completely logical and in accordance with moral standards and without unrealistic conclusions. This is the case (both when we give a negative answer and when we hear a negative answer).

Chapter Three
The Glory of the Sacrifice of Bodies

Late Sex, Its Causes and Consequences

To get into the "late sex" discussion, let's develop the above scenario in a different way. In this scenario, our target couple gets married. They have all the conditions to enter into a lasting relationship. Their temporary sex in the hotel has led to the formation of a stable relationship. They have moved into a single house and now they have been living together as an official husband and wife for a long time.

All stable lives that follow the necessary standards and are built on the right grounds will be subject to the passing of time after a while. The reduction of sexual attractions, daily troubles, repetition of repetitions and many factors, cause a drop in attractiveness indicators and physical tendencies of husband and wife.

Our couple has been living together for ten years now. But now there is a slight problem in their relationship. A problem for which a solution can be found based on marital education and scientific achievements such as psychology.

The presence of children is one of the factors that may cause the relationship between husband and wife to suffer. Our couple now has two children. A seven-year-old boy and a two-year-old girl. It is obvious that a major part of the energy, feelings, emotions, hobbies and needs of life are directed to the children by the parents, especially by the mother.

At the beginning of the relationship and in the early years, they had routine and successive plans to experience sensual moments. A man used to fantasize about every part of a woman's body. Thinking about his wife's white and round breasts, which have a round halo around the button, has always taken his mind and made him impatient for another sex-capture.

But now the situation has changed for some time. The woman has come out of the bathroom and is lying half naked on the bed, and while one of her breasts is sticking out of the bathroom towel and showing itself free and free, the man is still looking for something on his mobile phone, and the woman is wandering around with it as one of his nails. This is despite the fact that from the very first dinner in the hotel restaurant for many years, the man could have warm fantasies about these breasts in his imagination without having the woman naked in front of him. Imaginations that caused a wave of warm sensual feeling to start from his waist and move upwards by passing through the internal corridors of the body. He always felt that this deep feeling had little to do with the nudity factor. Rather, it is his unquestionable love that has made him so impatiently dependent on this balanced organ.

But now the naked woman is sleeping next to him in the best possible position and in the quietest time, but his feeling is so thin that he is not even able to change his position and turn toward her. He remembers that when they were in the hotel for the first time, every woman walking in the hotel room had sent a wave of warm blood to his brain. He was a thousand times more impatient than now to give up this prominence, even off the shirt.

But what happened now is that even holding his hand, in this ideal situation, evokes much less emotion than when losing hands with him in the formal environment of a lecture hall.

This crisis becomes much more when we know that women are in a more complicated situation compared to men. The decrease in feelings between husband and wife has caused their sex schedule to take place later and later each time. Lately, sex has become an obvious and routine rule in the life of our scenario couple. Problems like this are normal in the process of long relationships. But depending on its severity, it can be considered as a dangerous factor.

When the parties enter into a stable relationship, many factors enter the relationship at the same time, which leads to mutual coldness. In a stable relationship, the possibility of flirting becomes an easily accessible or always available option. Therefore, it is quite obvious that expecting a fiery relationship in the tenth year of marriage in the bedroom at home is just as unreasonable as the relationship that took place in the first days of dating in a hotel room.

Sometimes reluctance will occur outside of soft. In the sense that one of the parties is sufficiently enthusiastic about flirting; but the other party does not have such a desire. Such a situation will make the problem worse. Because if the situation repeats, we will see demand on the one hand and neglect on the other hand. As mentioned in the second assumption of this scenario, here we are also facing the problem of rejecting sex, with the difference that the general criteria governing the relationship have completely changed.

In the previous scenario, we heard the answer in a situation where no relationship was established at all. But in the present case, after a long period of successful marriage, we have entered a state of unwillingness and rejection. It is natural that the arguments we presented to rationalize the rejection in the above scenario are no longer effective. On the other hand, hearing a rejection from a spouse is far more painful than hearing a rejection from someone who is asking for a relationship for the first time.

Sexual deprivation and hearing repeated rejections from someone with whom we have made a pact for a life full of happiness and empathy can lead to humiliating and uncomfortable feelings.

Based on the previous assumption, it is no longer possible to invite the "blown" person to self-restraint with the previous reasons. The type of encounter with this problem and its consequences can be different depending on the cultural and geographical situation and depending on the beliefs and personality of people.

Before dealing with the whole issue and what methods are there to improve the quality of life and increase sexual attraction between men and women, we will first try to put forward different hypotheses and examine the approaches.

The first assumption is that the man has considerable sexual desire and the woman has become cold for some reason and does not want to have sex.

It seems that in societies that follow more modern laws, legal and social systems do not interfere much in such a situation. Because the rules of democracy do not want to interfere in the private affairs of citizens. But in underdeveloped societies, the matter is completely different. In the Middle East and among strata religions, there are completely one-sided and biased positions. A woman's obedience to a man's wishes is absolutely mandatory. The insulting word "submission" is a one-sided concept that refers to maximum acceptance by a woman. Obeying a man has no meaning. Only the woman must obey and the man can punish the woman if she does not obey.

In the geography we are discussing, the woman is under the ownership and guardianship of the man. Words like "Nakaha" and "Nikah" mean to have a one-sided sexual relationship. In marriage, the man explains the conditions to the woman, and the woman, willingly or unwillingly, accepts the understood conditions in the form of binding legal and religious contracts. The workflow in the marriage process is not similar to the explanation of charges in court cases. A man explains a situation to a woman. The woman agrees, and then throughout her life, she is forced to obey it based on the same initial contract.

"Compliance" means the woman's adherence to the contract she signed in the beginning. Therefore, in half of the world, the issue we are discussing; it means that the man's response to rejection is irrelevant. Because a woman does not have the ability to refuse an answer. On the other hand, the woman's response to rejection is culturally irrelevant. Because usually a woman does not demand. If he is a demander and he hears a rejection, the rules of marriage have clearly specified that this issue is one of the rights and authority of the man. In customary and unofficial sources, it is stated that a man can use this authority even as a means of punishing a woman.

Because marriage is the main basis for determining the limits of the rights of men and women, and the issue of rejecting the answer is also raised under this discussion, we will take a closer look at the foundation of marriage.

It does not seem that many documents are needed to prove that the marriage contract is one-sided. It is obvious that in the rule of marriage, there is no role for women as an independent unit.

The rights reserved for women are so unequal and inhuman that they cannot do anything for themselves by relying on them. To understand the one-sidedness of the marriage rule, it is enough to look at the oral culture and linguistic data in Persian, Arabic, Urdu and other languages that are written with the Arabic alphabet.

The word "manakah" which is the infinitive of "mufa'ala" in Arabic language, has almost no use in Arabic and other Eastern languages. Bab al-Mafaalah indicates a work in which two parties or involved parties have the same partnership status. For example, when we say "struggle" it means that two sides or two sides of a fight under equal conditions in terms of independence of action and possibility of activity. Like the equal conditions that the rules set for the fight of two wrestlers.

The same is the case with the word "discussion" which shows that two sides engage in verbal discussion and debate under equal conditions. These words are widely used in the cultural geography of the mentioned languages. But when we come to the word "manakah," even though this phrase is present in the grammatical structure of the Arabic language, in terms of frequency of use, it has almost no public presence. Because "marriage" means equal and equal participation of both parties in the category of "marriage."

But marriage is a completely one-way affair in which the man is the agent and the woman is the object. To understand the problem, it is enough to search the words "marriage" and "monakah" in the Google search engine. The results obtained for the word "nekah" are about 7 million and 500 thousand and for the word "monakah" or "monakhet" only 5 thousand. The reason is that conflict, which refers to a two-way action with equal conditions, has no relevance at all in this cultural geography.

Therefore, in Eastern culture and under traditional and religious marriages, a woman does not have the right to respond negatively to the demand for sex. He must be submissive and accountable under any circumstances. The obligation and necessity of this humiliating situation and sexual slavery for the women of the East is so deep and continuous that it is as if this fixed situation is deeply engraved in the rock of knowledge of the behavioral culture of the East.

To the extent that scientific theorists such as psychology and sociology, who are aware of the results of this complicated situation, do not even have the courage to criticize and attack it.

But the situation is different in the West and developed countries, especially in the new century, which is the century of knowledge and expansion of awareness.

Therefore, leaving aside the assumption that the man wants a relationship and the woman does not want to, we will examine two other situations. These two assumptions are as follows:

Second assumption: men and women have lost their sexual desire under the same conditions, and this risky factor threatens their lives.

The second hypothesis: the woman has kept her desires and the man has lost them, or vice versa. We will examine this issue in the next section.

Coldness of Temper, Impasse of Sensual Affections

The normalization of flirting and the decline of sexuality have been on the agenda of Western researchers for a long time. The result of this research is the instructions that can be used to give a more beautiful mood to the marital space and extra warmth to sexual relations.

Of course, all this is assuming that there is a romantic feeling between the husband and wife. Otherwise, no guidelines can prevent the gradual disintegration of a relationship.

It has been a month since the last time our target couple had sex. The man is lying on the bed and is reviewing the last experience. Compared to the fiery and blissful experiences they had before, their last experience was nothing to ponder. But if we compare it to the general standards of a sexy experience, it was not bad. Reviewing these images, he turns once more and takes her hand. The woman does not show a teething reaction. He gives a short smile and gets back to his work. Does the man wonder if the woman is also reviewing their last sex experience? He really likes to ask him this question; but it is not clear why he is not reckless and rude like in the first days.

In those days, they shared all their feelings with each other in every detail. They talked about their sexual interests. For quality sex, they would plan and after it was over, they would talk about Cam and his bag. But now many things have changed. It is as if a hidden curtain has been drawn between the two; So that the possibility of talking about sexual feelings and the details of a desired, planned and exciting sex has become impossible.

The man gets up. Open the window. Suddenly, a strange burner enters the room along with the outside air. He, whose upper body is naked, is surprised by the cold air, immediately closes the window and returns to the bed. He remembers that when their last sex was over a month ago, he got up and opened the window like now. At that time, despite his nakedness, the temperature outside was almost the same as the room temperature. With this comparison, an aura of sadness takes over him. How much time has passed! Is the coldness of feelings that prevailed between him and his wife similar to the coldness of autumn days? Fresh blood rushes to his brain. He goes to his wife. He takes her hand more seriously and says:

"Are you sleepy? Or that you might be awake for a while?"

The woman says: "I don't sleep much. But I had a lot of work today. Almost twice as much as other days. That's why I'm so tired." Next, he takes out his phone and starts checking the incoming messages.

Completely disappointed, the man stops talking and tries to amuse himself by looking at pictures of their last trip on his cell phone. But his thoughts turn to the coldness of their husband-and-wife relationship, and he quickly begins to analyze the data and compare the woman's current behavior with the past. Suddenly a thought comes to his mind like lightning. Don't get another man's feet in the middle…? But before this thought is completely settled in his mind, he pushes it away. He looks at the woman.

The profile of his face is innocently visible in the semi-dark space of the room. He remembers that night, when for the first time on the couch of the hotel room, he had seen the same profile in the halo of light published on the TV, the childish hairs on his skin were completely visible, which gave his face a certain innocence. A kind of girly, schoolboy personality that was sometimes complemented by a palpable awkwardness. But now the same face under the light emitted by the mobile phone, without those soft fluffs, inspires solidity and at the same time "mystery."

He feels that he loves this creature deeply, but what happened to him? Without making any other effort, the man quietly crawls under the blanket and the woman, who is ready to sleep, turns her back to him and becomes quiet and motionless as if she has found the ideal position.

Poetic Feast of Sex

The importance of sex makes us emphasize that this process should not be considered as an emotionless routine action along with other daily actions. Sex is actually the most special emotional event between a man and a woman. If we pay attention to the details and creativity that can be achieved with practice and precision, sex can become an attractive poetic feast.

Creativity can prevent sex from becoming a repetitive and boring routine. If it is clear that in the current situation and due to the lack of concentration, the sex feast will become superficial and without quality, it is better to leave it to another time.

In order to indulge in the sex feast, we should pay more attention to spiritual needs than physical desires. Female nature is such that sex for her means a deep and serious event. He never sees sex as fulfilling physical needs. Of course, depending on the circumstances and for the sake of getting rid of the physical condition of the man, she may give in to superficial and low-quality sex; but this work has no value and credibility for him.

Men with character and dignity never ask for intimacy without their partner being fully in the emotional flow of sex. Because such behavior is completely selfish. Social taboos and religious teachings encourage women to conform to men's wishes, under any circumstances; but when we talk about dignified and characterful behaviors, external patterns and rules lose color.

A man and a woman who have drawn ideal conditions and equal relations in their romantic relationships, leave almost all external rules and taboos behind the bedroom door and enter into a relationship based on their behavior patterns.

The process of sex in its ideal form should include the introduction, the text and the ending. Activities such as dance, music, singing, double play and a convergence at all levels can be complementary and quality factors. In addition, spontaneity and spontaneous flow are among the most important factors that can determine a quality sex.

Brain signals sent to certain sex organs are only a small part of the sex process. Completely following these signals and not paying attention to other influencing factors can ultimately lead to a short, emotionless sex without pleasure.

In the process of ideal sex, the bedroom or flirting place becomes a sacred and valuable place. In such a situation, sex can approach states such as meditation, revelation and discovery and intuition. The infinite world of each party is so vast that with each spiritual revelation of sex, they discover unknown parts of each other's being.

One lifetime is not enough to discover all the hidden corners of a woman's existence. Only superficial and capricious men who are unable to discover the spiritual worlds and verify the element of behavioral culture, after a few superficial relationships, think that they will not find a new component in their sexual partner, the initial seeds of most divorces that are emotional and sexual in nature are formed here. Complications such as polygamy, prostitution and the like also lie here.

Sacrifice of Bodies in Ideal Sex

In this book, wherever ideal sex is mentioned, it is meant to be sex that takes place with all one's heart, without any suspicion of exploitation, and in an equal position based on complete and mutual feeling. We all know how elusive such a relationship is, especially for women. The general education of men in the patriarchal society has been such that it has reduced the status of women to the level of a tool for pleasure. Almost all legal, ideological, moral, political, social, etc. systems have endorsed this situation.

This is a great mistake that history has made in dealing with women. It is natural that compensation is very difficult in such a situation. Even in the most emotional dealings with the category of women, which is in phrases like "heaven is under the feet of mothers" or "a woman is like a flower that should be loved and protected from harm" and similar, a fatal error has been made.

Many times these errors are made with all the good intentions of the announcers and promoters.

When we come to sex, as the main center of gravity of the relationship between a man and a woman, the issue becomes more complicated. In the field of literature and artists' view of women, there are cases of human view. In some of these works, you can see the precise cases of the correct physical relationship. In this view, generally, the issue of sex extends from the surface to the depth. The level is a starting point and a tool to achieve "unification of the soul." So, sex starts from the level and the sacrifice of the levels, reaches the discovery and intuition of the souls and finally returns to the level and physical caress and finally ends. Sohrab Sepehri has described this relationship well in a poem

> Ah, what a glory in the sacrifice of bodies!
> Oh noble cancer of solitude!
> May my body be a gift to you!
> Someone came
> to the muscles of heaven
> He extended my hand
> A person came to light the morning religions
> It was in the middle of the buttons of his shirt.
> From the dry grass of old verses
> window weaves
> He was young like the days of thought.
> His throat was filled with the blue characteristics of the ponds
> Someone came and took my books.
> He drew a roof of flowers on my head.
> The evening widened me with repeated shutters.
> My table was showered with spirituality.
> Then we sat down.
> We talked about the painful minutes.

From the words whose life was spent in the middle of water.
Our opportunity under the right clouds
Like the confused body of a sudden dove
It had a good volume.
It was the middle of the night, from the turbulence of the fruit
The design of the trees became strange.
The wet string of our sleep was wasted.
next
The hand at the beginning of the water body.
Then in the wet guts of Narun Bagh
it was morning

In fact, when we talk about ideal sex as spiritual discovery and intuition, such a quality can open the biggest windows of consciousness for two people, it is a kind of religion and mystical light. It means meeting the soul and feeling of someone whose "morning light of religions" is hidden in the middle of his shirt buttons. It means creating a spiritual opportunity under the right clouds. An opportunity that, if love is involved and the relationship does not mean the negative and commercial things of today, can always have a happy volume like the confused tone of a sudden pigeon and never be repeated.

In ideal and romantic sex, the lover's fingers can always stretch to the muscles of heaven. In unifications and "closenesses" of love, you can always weave a window from the dry grass of old verses. A window that leads two bodies and two souls to the wet life of words that live in the middle of the waters. Here, in the sacrifice of surfaces and the skin contact of two friends, an eternal glory is achieved that will never be boring.

Only then can we have a better world with the help of the eternal force of love that is mixed in our companion femininity. In this case, half of the people on earth will not be deprived of their share of honest pleasure. In this way, the huge capacity that women have to participate in improving the conditions of the world will be released, and as mentioned in the poem above, our opportunity will be happy under the right clouds, and the earth, which is our place of residence, will become a paradise. Perhaps this is the paradise promised to believers in most religious texts.

In this case, it is not necessary for the man to give her sexual equality and full share of carnal pleasures. It is enough to allow a woman to explore and work hard enough to discover her inner and physical abilities, and to cultivate the capacities of her rebellious spirit. In order to create the space described above, neither a man has complete and unilateral power nor a woman has the full ability to realize it. These two, in turn, are unique and it is in the meeting of these two that the miracle of nature occurs and existence is discovered with all its beauty and grandeur.

In order to reach this ideal world where men and women are present in their most natural form, it is necessary to break the dominant attitude toward women in the first place. This attitude is so deep and rooted that even the most free-thinking men can find traces of it.

We refer to a sentence by Osho, an Indian philosopher and theoretician in the book "Woman," which says: "A woman should be loved and not understood."

When such a view of women prevails, it is never possible to cross the realm of male dominance and view women as tools and "commodity-like." When we say "a woman should be loved," in fact, there is a prevailing view that everyone has accepted as a principle. In the sense that the listener and the speaker of this sentence has implicitly accepted that a woman is, at her best, "like a beautiful flower" created as a gift for a man to entertain or love and benefit from. This woman has certain characteristics that should not be ignored at all; rather, he should be loved as a beautiful being.

Refreshing Sex Requires Creativity

Along with the routine activities of life, it is necessary to look at sex as an activity that requires practice and creativity. Otherwise, even with love, the dust of time will settle on the fabric of sexual relations. Humans try to refresh different aspects of life at different times to avoid boredom caused by the "dust of habits."

Changing the decoration of rooms and the reception hall, changing the shape of life tools, changing the necessary necessities, making a difference in the routine mechanisms are among the activities that are done to remove the dust of habit from the living surfaces. Sex is also an example of this issue and if you don't pay attention to the little things, even with the initial love, it will be affected by the passage of time and its quality will decrease.

Creating creativity in the sexual relationship and trying to keep the materials and behaviors sensual will make the romantic intimacy of sexual partners not decrease gradually.

Can Sexual Playfulness Be Permanent?

Humans are naturally prone to change. Therefore, with the prolongation of relationships, the possibility of slow and qualitative changes in sexual relationships is inevitable. On the other hand, when couples are deeply involved in the issues of life and managing family affairs, and everyone is trying to play their role and manage things during the day, they inevitably leave the bedroom space and the tangible emotion that exists inside it. Under the influence of the emotionless environment outside, the emotional and sensual signals subside.

Usually when a man and a woman return home at the end of the day, even if we exclude or ignore the existence of children, it becomes difficult to immediately return to the sensual state necessary for a passionate night. In other words, the behavioral culture that is necessary for our presence in the society is in conflict with the behavioral culture and emotional auras that are needed in the atmosphere of socializing with the spouse.

Leaving each of these spaces and entering another space is usually not an easy task. Therefore, people prefer to keep the same feeling of the previous space when entering another space. In this case, priority is always given to the outside space. That is, when a man or a woman enters the house, he prefers to stay in the same mood that he was in the whole day. Because in this case, it will be much easier to enter the office environment the next day.

This is a subtle point and even many people may not have felt it; but deep psychological facts are usually manifested in the stomach and we may be oblivious to them.

An example of this phenomenon is that usually the atmosphere of the weekend or public holidays is more emotional and sensual than during the week. Even the atmosphere that prevails between men and women during trips and work breaks is usually far more emotional and sensual than other times. By understanding and knowing the functions of changing the space, psychologists recommend a night stay in a hotel or attending a couple's campaign in nature to increase sexual attraction.

While the husband and wife are forced to resort to the style of small business management to run the family and apply various management and discipline skills and regulations, on the other hand, the tender and emotional nature of love makes them marginal during the application of management. Especially the application of any type of law and regulations is associated with a significant amount of exercising authority and imposing rules. Especially, for the disobedience of children and the optimal flow of affairs, sometimes, authority and imposition become inevitable.

These make the husband and wife, as in the past, not have enough time to focus on charm tricks. The more the number of children and family population increases, the more the husband and wife will enter the emotionless and emotionless atmosphere.

Flirting requires a great deal of concentration, energy, creativity, openness, imagination, playfulness, and sometimes a loss of control. This space is clearly in conflict with categories such as time management, discipline and strictness. A husband and wife cannot enter the emotional space needed for flirting and joking at night, like theater actors, and immediately after that change their feelings and enter the daily management style.

For this reason, they prefer to remain completely in the form of a strict and emotionless manager, and this will mean the beginning of the process of the subsidence of their desires and the collapse of their emotional world.

Many times, the reason for avoiding flirting for husband and wife (the same old lover) is not that they no longer enjoy flirting, but because flirting weakens the ability of the parties to bear the heavy burden of managing life. The opposite of this problem is also true. In other words, the heavy burden of managing the house can reduce the energy of the parties to focus on an all-round courtship.

Sex is like a work of art. Like a poem, in order to write or read it and deeply understand the meaning of the word, a calm and worry-free environment must be provided. If we compare family management to the behavior of a marathon runner, we will see that it is not possible for a marathon runner to simultaneously enjoy a poem and be immersed in the love of words.

When a husband and wife enter the heavy atmosphere caused by the number of children, management of the family and worry about the future and livelihood, they practically leave the initial romantic atmosphere that they had in their loneliness and freshness of love. Conservatism, creating distance and considering non-emotional relationships due to economic considerations and difficult life conditions, brings the space in between into the phase of exchange and give and take. In this situation, when one of the parties wants to express his sexual need, it is as if he is revealing his weakness, a weakness that can seem humiliating.

Therefore, each of the parties may prefer to hide their sexual need and postpone their next erotic event to another time and an incident in the future, and in this way, the distance between intercourse increases each time. It is precisely because the couple in our scenario, when they look back, they see that more than a month has passed since their last union, and there are currently no suitable conditions for a romantic event to occur.

Rejuvenation of Sexual Attraction

As we said, the studies conducted on the cooling of sexual relations have included achievements and results. Now the first question that arises is how to prevent the decline of sexual sparks between a husband and wife (or a man and a woman in general) in a stable relationship? And if this decline has occurred, how can it be restored?

Sometimes the decline of sexual activities is due to the occurrence of some hormonal changes and physical changes for which medical science has solutions. But most of the cold relationship cases are not related to medical issues.

Porn movies and sexual fantasies remind us of an undesirable idea that, although it is not moral and practical and has bad consequences, it reminds us of one issue, and that is to avoid the obsolescence of elements. When the dust of boredom and obsolescence settles on the surrounding behaviors and objects, very quickly, the sexual act loses its attractiveness and importance.

In fantasy and porn movies, it can be seen that sexual partners, by involving a third party in their sexual act, breathe freshness and novelty into their surroundings. The presence of the third person is exciting for them because he has introduced a new factor and element into the space. Therefore, without requiring the presence of a third person, this formula can refresh the atmosphere governing the relationship. The presence of objects, changing the environment, changing behaviors and actions, etc. can be a factor to create freshness and remove oldness.

The normal flow of life is like a boring mist that gradually buries the desires of husband and wife under it. Refreshing factors must arrive to revive these desires. What was said about the third person, which is not acceptable to most people, indicates the importance of the external factor, which can show the couple by looking at it from another perspective that the situation is not much different; rather, they must remove the dust of darkness and boredom that has settled on their glasses of reality over time.

There are other things that are not exaggerated and extreme like the one above; but it is an attempt to remove this dust of habit. For example, some couples publish their nude photos anonymously on the Internet. Reviewing these photos from another angle and as an outsider becomes a factor to stimulate the sexual tentacles of couples who have never looked at each other from this angle.

There is also a milder form. That is, some couples are interested in making videos or photos of their relationship and viewing it on digital receivers. In such a situation, it is as if the couple sees each other naked and provocative for the first time. This action can move the sexual tentacles of the couple and give movement and freshness to their sexual relationship.

The mentioned examples mean that one of the solutions to get out of sexual stagnation is to change the perspective of the lover or sexual partner as a whole. In the sense that it is necessary to look at the lover this time as if we have never seen him before. When the lover and the beloved watch their sexual activity in the home player, as a third observer, they can achieve beauties and charms that they are unaware of in conventional practice. These methods, which are less welcomed and socially ugly, generally have a theatrical aspect, and basically sex is a theatrical act in which both parties participate. Now, if they can watch the same show that they have performed, the possibility of mockery will multiply. Because in the state of being a spectator, visual pleasure is added to the process in a wide way, while visual pleasure is very limited in the act of sex.

So far, we have talked about a general principle to show that the dust of habit and conditioning that falls on the sexual act of couples is an inhibiting factor and can be removed. But there are other different methods to get out of the conditioning crisis in sexual action, which will still guarantee the confidentiality and privacy of the relationship and will bring freshness and excitement like the above methods. It is natural that couples can invent and use similar examples depending on their creativity and imagination.

A Night in a Hotel or Anywhere Other Than Home

Part of the problem with boring sex is the repetitive elements of the routine. The same bedroom, the same walls, the same bed, the same objects and the same constant event. Obviously, repetition can be boring. This boredom ultimately has a negative effect on the effectiveness and attractiveness of the relationship. Now, if couples can remove the repetitive elements and replace them with new elements, they will experience more excitement.

Spending a night in a hotel is one of the useful ways to increase the excitement of sexual attraction. As we said, some men turn to unknown women and even prostitutes to escape sexual boredom. Although the quality of sex with such women is very low due to the lack of romantic element and usually it is not repeated more than once, it is clear that the excitement of such a relationship is due to the non-repetition of the elements. In the first place, this excitement is caused by the special adventure that lies in the essence of this action. Components and elements of the environment are non-repetitive. Even the sexual partner itself is non-repetitive. Although the sexual partner and lover are not supposed to change in our scenario, all elements of the scene can be changed.

Spending a night in a hotel means that all elements of the scene will be fresh and unique. The room, the bed, the doors, the walls, the windows, the towels, the soap, etc. are all new in the hotel room. Therefore, the occasional experience of sex in a hotel room can be an attractive erotic adventure. Many faithful couples who try to keep their sensual freshness for each other use this trick.

"When we never change the carpet in our bedroom, we shouldn't expect our sex to be mundane and unmotivated," writes Alain de Botton. In his opinion, hotel rooms are attractive and sexy for couples and stimulate their sexual adventures, because all objects and phenomena around have a color of novelty and difference.

Defamiliarization in Sex

In the field of literary criticism, there is a theory called "defamiliarization," which in Persian is also referred to as "alienation." This theory was proposed more than 100 years ago by Viktor Shklovsky, a Russian formalist critic. Here, while making a short reference to the above theory, we show that if people use this theory as a basis for changes, they can renew their relationships according to the principles of aesthetics, psychology, biology, and the like. Especially since we have mentioned elsewhere that sex can be considered an artistic act. Because it has a lot of compatibility with the field of arts.

Viktor Shklovsky is looking for an answer to the question of what can continue the poetry of the poem. Poetry is made of routine tools and specific concepts. It is obvious that after a while most of the poems become similar and lack charm and beauty.

This is what happens in the art of sex. The artist or the lover gradually falls into the abyss of repetition of deeds and actions, and sex becomes ordinary and sometimes boring. Viktor Shklovsky's answer is reflected in the theory of "art as a technique."

From the point of view of the "defamiliarization" theory, the poet must separate it from ordinary and everyday language and discover new areas for words in order to create distinctive aspects and give poetic language to words. Poetic speech is a structured speech with a form. So, you should be a formalist and look at it in a different way. It is necessary to give it a different and attractive nature by creating distinction and "breaking the habit." This is the same idea reflected in Hafez's famous poem:

Search for your desires in unusual things
Because I got focus from those messy hairs

The key point in "extraordinary affairs"; it means to differentiate the mechanisms and components involved in a phenomenon. This is the same "being different" that is mentioned in Saadi's words with the phrase "abnormal things." In this way, we can gain focus from the popular "messy hair." The secret of gaining focus is in different elements and data, otherwise this is the same woman who made the most important sexy memory of our life on the first night of flirting.

In the field of literary criticism, there are other theories that often complement the theory of defamiliarization. For example, according to the "foregrounding" theory for norm avoidance and highlighting, some elements can be highlighted to be remembered well. For example, enlarging some fonts and words in a text leaves a different effect on the mind. This rule is based on the principle of "disturbing the balance" and getting out of conditioning. Because conditioning and the spontaneous and involuntary flow of processes lead to habituation.

This issue is also abundantly mentioned in daily behavior. For example, it has often happened that we leave the room and go to the kitchen, pour a cup of tea and drink it and start doing something else. We have done this so spontaneously and with conditioning that after a while, we doubt whether we have done the "act of drinking tea" recently or not.

Due to not taking relationship techniques seriously, many erotic and romantic events between couples flow like the same conditioned drinking tea. These relationships will definitely not have value and credibility in the calendar of emotional relationships between men and women. Messing up the rules can cause failure in this neutral and linear process of "conditioning." If we show each of the erotic events between the couple with the word sex and highlight a few of them based on the rule of defamiliarization or foregrounding, we will come across such a picture:

Sex-**sex**-sex-**sex**-sex-sex-sex-**Sex**-sex-sex

As can be seen, several events have been transformed into a different event based on the rule of foregrounding (highlighting) or defamiliarization. According to the theory of defamiliarization, the secret of having a passionate and regular sex life is to differentiate and avoid the same and automatic formulas and methods.

For this, there is no need to change the playing field. Football fields are almost no different. I love the same football player. The green field of a lover's feelings is the same ground that is prone to play. If he doesn't have enough talent and ability to play a good game, he won't make a difference in any other field he goes to. Changing the playing field does nothing. The rules of the game and, as the formalists say, "the technique of the game" must change. They say: "Art as a technique" and in our discussion we should say: "Sex as a technique." That is, just as Viktor Shklovsky's idea can be generalized from the presentation of poetry to many fields, this idea will also be well answered in the field of sex. Sex is not only related to art, but the highest arts are inspired by it. If we take a look at Persian literature (regardless of the part that is related to the sexual deviation of a certain period and the flow of Shahid Bazi), it is always about the romantic relationship between a man and a woman.

The remarkable point in the theory of defamiliarization is that it is said that the ultimate goal of art is to reveal the feeling that is obtained through the perception and intuition of the surrounding phenomena, not from science and awareness of it. This version may work better in the field of sex and flirting than in the field of art. We know about sex, the angles of the lover's body and all the factors that surround two people; but most of the cases of this science does not lead to discovery, intuition and understanding, but it is an obstacle and deterrent. In the example of watching sex on a home screen, this change of viewing angle has been desired.

Alienation helps us to distance ourselves a little from our knowledge and knowledge and to look at the surrounding elements from a new perspective and to discover and approach them more intuitively. When Alain de Botton talks about the increase of sexual attraction and enthusiasm in a hotel room, he actually wants to refer to the issue of renewal or defamiliarization.

When we enter the room and see the beautiful body of our spouse or lover on the hotel bed, it is an intuitive moment. All elements are foreign. Even though this is not the same person as before and the moment we are in is like the lasting moments of the first flirtation. In other words, alienating the object can change our perception toward it.

We come out of a shell of scholarly routine and approach the scene from a perspective of discovery and intuition. This is where sex becomes far more attractive and beautiful than thousands of times before, which has flowed spontaneously and without discovery and intuition.

What made the first flirting event on the first night so attractive and exciting? Obviously, all these factors exist now; but under the fog of habit and repetition, they have been forgotten. It is enough to push this dust aside so that they will appear again soon.

In the words of Sohrab Sepehri: "Life is not something that leaves me and you on the edge of habit." Life is the formality that once was pleasant for us, why is it not pleasant now? This is because we have forgotten it due to negligence. In the continuation of this poem by Sohrab Sepehri, definitions of the scene of life are presented, all of which indicate novelty and difference.

> Life is the attraction of the hand that picks.
> The new life of black figs is in the mouth of summer.
> Life after the tree is in the eyes of an insect.

Life is the experience of a moth in the dark.
Life is a strange feeling that a migratory chicken has.
Life is a train whistle that turns a bridge in sleep.
Life is like seeing a garden through the blocked window of an airplane.
The news of the rocket going into space.
The lonely touch of the moon.
The thought of smelling flowers in another country.
Life is washing a plate.
Life is finding a village coin in the atmosphere of the street.
Life is a mirror square.
The life of the flower is eternal.
Life beats the earth in our heartbeat.
Life is a simple and identical geometry of breaths.

A creative couple looking to keep their sex appeal going can have a fun road map for a lifetime based on each of the sentences and phrases above. It is natural that in order to reach what is reflected in these sentences and take it to flirting moments, again, according to Sohrab Sepehri, "eyes must be washed." It should be seen differently. The thought of smelling flowers in another world is available to us as a couple. Spending a night in a hotel or pitching a tent in the yard or on the roof and flirting in a different way is actually the same as smelling a flower in another world. Otherwise, the flower is the same flower and still has the same freshness.

Do not forget the mirror square. Watching the bodies in the square of mirrors and in the midst of the infinite environment, can be attractive and blissful. It is possible to create a situation where habits fall by the wayside and every experience is just as fascinating and wonderful as the first.

If you have a garden, building a tree house and having sex among the branches can be an eternal and lasting memory. Have sex on the highest peak of a mountain. In the bathroom, in the toilet, in the car, when you have stopped by a promenade at night. In the dense forest covered with elms and countless wild plants, while you worry about being bitten by insects and vermin, the unknown bliss of a mythical experience awaits you.

These can be experiences that even your sex life is not enough to do them all. You can't have such amazing experiences with a street woman, a prostitute, and a woman in a hurry. These are possible if we change our perception of the beloved.

Artistic Sex, an Opening out of the Dead End

The way artists use to describe and reinterpret the surrounding phenomena makes some of the most ordinary objects and subjects completely new and give it an attractive nature. They can even make some painful and uncomfortable phenomena acceptable and normal. The essence of art is in the presentation of different phenomena. When we spoke from the point of view of formalists like Shklovsky, we were talking about this rule. With the difference that formalists make, routine phenomena appear attractive and fresh by means of "defamiliarization."

We mentioned elsewhere that sex is an artistic act. That's why when we talk about artistic sex, it means differentiating conditioned and sometimes painful phenomena.

Perhaps in order to better explain the function of art, it is necessary to mention an example that Alain de Botton discussed in the book, *Art as Therapy*. Alain de Botton's argumentative structure is formed around the effect of art on the renewal of events and phenomena. He makes a similar argument in his other book, *How to Think More About Sex*. This argument revolves around the painting "Bundle of Asparagus" by Edouard Manet.

He says that in 19th century France, usually only people who cared about asparagus were either cooks or had a special interest in different types of food. But when in 1880, Edouard Manet chose a bunch of asparagus as the subject of his painting and created an extraordinary work, asparagus was no longer the same phenomenon as before. He gave a different nature to a bunch of asparagus with the help of painting technique.

Now the question was whether there had been a change in the ordinary nature of asparagus? The answer is negative. The change in the audience's attitude toward asparagus was caused by the effects of this painting. Now that ordinary boring plant had become a phenomenon whose charm was endless and could be a source of inspiration for many years.

The same is true about sex. With the difference regarding the coldness of the romantic relationship between husband and wife, we are not dealing with the boring asparagus plant from the very beginning. This relationship was once fiery and artistic. But over time, the dust of habit has settled on it and now it has become an ordinary asparagus without excitement and charm.

An artistic look and, as a result, artistic sex, can once again remove this boring dust and revive the attractive and beautiful nature of the relationship. During this artistic look, that ordinary asparagus plant can once again become a work of art and a constant source of inspiration for the parties.

What should we do if we apply all the proposed solutions and it still does not work? Does a person have the right to be offended and bitter if flirting with an old lover remains cold and devoid of fiery passion?

The modern culture and relations of the present age give this right to man. Because this divine gift is one of the absolute and fundamental human rights. Man should experience a sensual life full of pleasure and happiness. There is almost no one who encourages a person to be austere and give up his desires and urge him to continue the relationship despite the unbearable coldness of the marital relationship.

In terms of psychology and social studies, there are signs of depression and mental illness in a cold and unhealthy relationship. The scientists who researched and studied the subject of sex in the current century believe that sensual vitality has standards that deviation from these standards means lowering the indicators of life.

The main focus of theorists such as Masters and Johnson is that sex is the main engine of marriage and relationship continuity; Of course, with the quality criteria mentioned in psychology and sexology.

According to researchers, sexual health and the quality of sex is a social health indicator. The pioneers of sexology, who for the first time brought the discussions about sexual health and its standard patterns into the public domain, took a bold step in explaining these theories, creating a revolution in the field of correcting the distortions caused by dysfunctional sex. They publicized these issues, and as mentioned, they took it to television and public media. The society's reception of these discussions was also an important issue. The extraordinary sales of these two researchers' books and the popularity of their television show showed what a sensitive point they touched and how much hidden dissatisfaction there was in the society. A hidden dissatisfaction that could not even be expressed due to social taboos and the ugliness of such issues.

According to sex researchers, in the modern age, a married man or woman not only has the right to enjoy sexual vitality throughout their married life, from the beginning to the decline of their sexual power, but having such a gift is a sign of a person's physical and mental health and finally it is a sign of community health.

With the beginning of this series of discussions, other medical and psychological topics were included in the discussion, which were considered as side effects or causes involved in sexual failure. Issues such as painful contraction of the vagina, orgasm disorder in men and lack of recognition of orgasm in women, inability to ejaculate and premature ejaculation, complications caused by old age and methods to strengthen the power of ejaculation were among these topics.

Therapeutic suggestions and methods of strengthening the relationship, along with various formulas and tables including useful suggestions and exercises, were the result of a series of researches that became popular in this decade, especially in American society.

The achievements of these discussions and their results were not only in practical guidelines and health and psychological recommendations. Rather, the most important achievement of this course was creating awareness about the nature of the problem. Mankind, before this, was not even aware of the form of the problem or if he had a decision, he did not have the courage to raise it. Now, in the shadow of these debates and destigmatization of it, women and men knew that they were dealing with a real problem and they should look for a solution.

Now, how effective could this solution be? It was a separate issue. The main problem was that the couples were socially mature enough to talk about it while their children were asleep in other rooms.

The Philosophy of the Originality of the Body and the Issues Surrounding It

The female body is the most important controversial tool in all areas related to sex, morality and freedom. The body in general, and the female body in particular, is a wonderful and beautiful phenomenon. The female body, as one of the masterpieces of creation, has always been associated with misunderstanding. In the sense that the first interpretation of it is the factor of being lustful.

Although the female body has been a great source of inspiration for creativity and the driving force of life in all the aesthetic themes of the human race; but at the same time, it is subject to oppression and tyranny.

Poets have exaggerated and exaggerated in describing the beauty of women's body and face as if no other phenomenon in life can compete with it. At the same time, in real life, the female body has been insulted and insulted and often used as a tool. In the field of wars and big battles, women were always considered as spoils of war by the conquerors and were looted and raped.

Women have always been under tension and insecurity because of their beauty, because they are defenseless in front of men's muscles, and still men have not learned to respect women and their bodies as equal beings.

According to the religious text of Tantra, the main foundation of life starts from the body. The joy and happiness of a person is possible when there is no opposition and stubbornness with the body. This doctrine is completely against the moral systems of religions. The philosophy of authenticity of the body believes that all the pillars of existence, including religion and ethics, can be imagined as a background for the authenticity of the body.

live in peace because they follow the philosophy of originality of the body. The tensions that man constantly faces in his life are due to forgetting the originality of the body. When the originality of the body is at the center of philosophical thinking, all the natural and innate needs that are based on the body become a priority. Under this belief, sex can become a relaxing factor of discovery and intuition; because it is not dangerous or controversial. When sexual energy is released in the body, it can discharge harmful emotions and lead to physical health.

The conceptual philosophy of sexuality has been able to set precise frameworks for this field while explaining the place of sex with respect to the originality of the body. Philosophers like Alan Sobel, an American philosopher, and Judith Butler, a post-structuralist philosopher and an American feminist, have been able to define the limits of human physical action in the field of body and ethics, and confirm the human ability to increase sexual skills.

Therefore, there is no problem for humans to recognize the originality of the body, philosophically and morally and even in the field of social rules.

The philosophy of sexuality has determined where the position of sex is in human nature and what is the nature of intercourse in terms of ontology and epistemology. This philosophical system determines how sexual power can have an effective function in improving mental health in daily behaviors and traditions such as marriage, family, and complications such as homosexuality, prostitution, and the like, while following legal criteria.

On the other hand, by acknowledging the complexity of sex, which is true to nature, biological science shows how it can be effective in improving mental and physical health and increasing the quality of life. In other words, the relationship with sexual quality and not restricting the body and paying attention to its authenticity can create a basis for self-knowledge and reducing stress, increasing self-confidence and strengthening the physical foundation.

A list of the benefits of sex and lack of control of the body has been presented by various sciences, which shows how miraculously creation has worked in regulating the physical quality and state of the body with the emotional state and sex hormones. Strengthening the body's immune system, reducing the risk of prostate cancer, improving sleep, increasing body metabolism, mental stability, reducing stress, improving heart function, creating a sense of satisfaction, increasing self-confidence, improving brain function, and...just some of the positive effects of healthy sex, according to the originality of the body.

Sex in which the body, as a unifying factor, should be in a normal state and away from restrictions.

When the body regains its true originality, it releases sexual energy during courtship. This energy flows throughout the human body and the body reaches a mysterious state, the trance caused by orgasm is an example of it. Any attempt to eliminate the body and its natural reactions will lead to a reduction and incompleteness of the process.

Sex increases the speed of blood circulation and breathing of the body. This human action, the body as a masterpiece of creation, if it can regulate and execute spontaneous processes, will bring a combination of the best performance.

During sex, by increasing the depth of breathing, carbon dioxide hidden in the cavities and alveoli of the respiratory system is pushed out, which results in complete oxygenation of the brain and other organs. The feeling of lightness after sex depends on the body's spontaneous processes.

The body should be unconditionally free. Religious texts often prohibit people from this issue. But texts like Tantra write that there are no boundaries for human physical freedom. Because people who are sexually repressed are less intelligent. In other words, there is a direct relationship between people's sexuality and their intelligence. The best state of man is that his sexual power does not conflict with his physical body. Otherwise, this conflict can be traumatic.

According to the teachings of Tantra, a person should always be friendly with his body and have the most sincere attitude. The close relationship between man and the body allows the body to flow positive energies throughout the organs and play a constructive role in life. According to the writings of Tantra, man needs to touch his body sometimes and be in close contact with it. Otherwise, the body can be an expensive burden on the shoulder of the feeling and life in it will be reduced to the minimum possible.

Loving the body, whether from a man or a woman, means praising and loving the most important masterpiece of creation. If a person does not love his body, how can he expect someone else to love his body? A body deprived of its owner's attention emits vibrations that repel others.

The approach of religions to the body is completely against the direction of nature and the teachings of Tantra. Religions advise people to cover their bodies as much as possible in the presence of others and even in private. Religion looks at the body in such a way that the body is the source and center of all sins and transgressions.

One of the signs of not liking the body is that some people try to change its external shape with exaggerated arrays and clinging to artificial devices. When a person accepts and loves his body, it means that he acknowledges his beauty. In this case, there is no need to use excessive cosmetics.

This is because the Tantra text constantly emphasizes that a person should treat his body romantically and love it. Man should respect his body and accept it with all its requirements. Loving the body will lead to maximum care of it. Because of this, devotees and those who mistreat their bodies do not like their bodies and have not been able to cope with it. Addicts and those who continuously destroy their bodies are also most likely to have fundamental problems in the matter of self-love and the issue of the authenticity of the body.

The five senses are an important part of the body. According to Tantra, the senses are the gates that connect the human body to the outside world. Man, with the help of his senses, opens his eyes to the realities and beauties of the world. When experiencing the pleasures of sex, an authentic person tries to use all his senses.

Those who have sex in a dark room without light still lack the confidence to show their body. Absolute darkness means that man has one of his most important senses; That is, it completely deprives the sight of understanding the beauty of the lover's body.

Religions are unbelievably opposed to the senses. This opposition is caused by not recognizing the originality of the body. Limiting the body and trying to limit the senses is for this reason. The hijab that some religions are trying to promote is in line with this way of thinking. It means depriving the sense of sight from understanding the beauty of women and keeping the body, which is a source of inspiration, hidden. A source that has been praised in all aesthetic aspects.

One of the important senses of the body, which can be a suitable communication channel for understanding external phenomena, is the sense of hearing. Religious taboos are strongly against a woman making sounds that are signs of pleasure. Here too, ignoring the originality of the body and the originality of pleasure is working. Performing the task of sex in the darkest possible space without sound is a sign that the process is not alive and dynamic.

A person who has limited or blocked his senses is actually the same dumb dreamer who perceives external and internal processes incompletely. When a number of senses are disabled or remain inactive, the understanding of the process of physical pleasure will be very incomplete. Because for religion, in principle, physical pleasure is not important and only the transfer of sperm and the production of children is important, the more the act of sex is free of borders and without passion and excitement, the better.

Religious systems teach man to suppress his physical senses. In the first years of life, the child uses the senses with all their capacities. Touching, smelling, tasting, seeing and hearing are the child's communication ways to understand and analyze the surrounding phenomena.

Freud believes that a human child establishes some kind of sexual connection with the mother's breast through the sense of touch and contact. If the intelligence of the senses is transferred to adulthood, the quality of physical contact between men and women will definitely be better.

But when this same child grows up, due to wrong upbringing, because of the imposed teachings of religions, which are also promoted by parents, a mist of indifference and habit is drawn over his senses. After puberty, he loses his discovery and intuitive process in relation to the surrounding environment. In such a way that the body loses its originality and the mind replaces it.

As we know, the field of mind is the field of abstract affairs. When the act of sex takes place in a semi-abstract situation, the deep emotional connection that comes from a deep understanding of body states does not occur. We gave an example about this before. It happens many times that we go to the refrigerator. We pour a glass of water and after drinking it we go back to our work. After a while, we basically have doubts about whether we have done the act of drinking water a few minutes ago or not. Even if we are convinced that we drank water, we have no memory of its details. In fact, drinking water is an instinctive action due to the repetition of routine processes that took place due to the needs of the body and our senses were not involved in it. Our language has never understood the coldness of water. Our hands have never felt the coldness of a glass of water. Our eyes have not experienced the beautiful clarity of water. Our ears have not heard the beautiful sound of water falling inside the glass, and this spontaneous action took place in the worst possible way.

This can be the case for many issues that humans are involved with, for example, smokers may have smoked a pack of cigarettes throughout the day and not even understood the pleasure of one of them.

It means our abstract presence within a process. Our body was not present. Our senses have no external existence. Our action was actually an abstract action, not a physical one. The reason why many sexual relationships between couples are dull is because they are done spontaneously and without the presence of deep senses. A routine, abstract and subjective action that is actually no different from our perception of a porn scene on the monitor screen.

Tantra, unlike religious texts, teaches man to be intelligent and present when facing external phenomena and to understand them with all his senses. When we gaze at a tree, its deep understanding as a beautiful external phenomenon requires the deep activity of all human senses, along with abstract perception.

The reason why sex life is boring is no different from the reason why other things are boring. There are many people who do not understand the pleasure of "eating" while eating. Bites go into the mouth one by one and are chewed and swallowed. While a person is either chatting with someone else, or is immersed in his imaginary and mental worlds, it seems that someone else is eating food and not him. This is the situation described by the phrase "being present and absent."

During sex, we are touched, but we have no real understanding of the process of being touched. We touch; but receiving a sense of touch is not created in us. The whole process, from start to finish, flows in a state of mindless, boring gunk. Then comes the orgasmic phase and...the ending, which leads to sleep, playing with the cell phone, or soaking in the bathtub, sex with this profile seems to be no different from the act of defecation. While if we use the deep teachings of Tantra and similar texts as a criterion for action, even rejection can be an attractive process with better understanding and acceptance. Loving the body and the originality of the body means the same. Every phenomenon related to the body is important and significant in its place.

In this way, it is not out of place to say that humanity has reached a point where it has to be taught the alphabet of life from the beginning, in the captivity of mindless routine processes. Walking, breathing, seeing, eating, tasting, drinking, watching, having sex, flirting, flirting and all the usual and routine behaviors of life must be taught to man so that his life regains its true freshness and quality. achieved, in this way, his sex life will find a new meaning according to these transformations.

The result of all these things can be shown in the key phrase "observability." "Observation" is the opposite of dullness of behavior caused by boredom of habits.

Leave the Habit and Discover Another

The teachings that man needs to add freshness to his behavior should ultimately lead to freeing him from his sensuous habits. Boring sensory habits have caused a kind of dullness and boredom, and this boredom has caused a crisis in all human relationships, including the relationship with the spouse.

Humans can find new ways to explore the surroundings. Maybe going back to childhood and looking at the world like a child is a good solution. A new way to love must be discovered. Inventing new ways to love will bring variety and novelty. Deviating from established habits can change the shape of flirting. This is what religion is completely against. Religion recommends stillness. Repetition both in the field of thoughts and opinions and in the field of action and behavior. In such conditions, sensitivities gradually disappear. Man turns into a mechanical and robotic being, with predictable and boring behaviors.

When a person turns the game of love into a magnificent feast, each courtship as a new and unique event finds an authentic and unique place in the archives of his memories. New tasks can be added to the flirting process every time. Dancing, running in the garden or forest, or walking outside the house, before making love and any experience that is different from the previous experiences, causes you to get out of the cycle of boredom and is a suitable exercise in accordance with the teachings of "Tantra."

Repetitive and boring cycles are against the spirit of life. In fact, it is death that is receptive and compatible with boredom and depression. Life with all its elements is in deep contrast with boredom and conditioning. It is interesting to note that during the centuries, man has never experienced a break or decline. Otherwise, all these developments and transformations in life would not have been created.

However, many people are not inspired by the fate and history of mankind and soon enter a cycle of interruption and repetition. While there is a lot of potential for diversification and creativity. You can always create a different experience. Life has enough talent for this diversification. Because no day is the same as the previous day.

It is enough to put aside the dominating intellectual mechanisms. Thirty years old does not include exactly the same feeling and situation as thirty-one years old. Night is a different thing compared to day. Saturday is completely different from Friday.

In order to understand all this, it is necessary for a person to use his physical senses with all his might and not to allow his sensitive tentacles to slow down. A human's emotional system toward the surrounding phenomena can be weakened in case of inattention and lack of concentration. The human mind is designed in such a way that when faced with routine processes, it ignores many of them. When the human mind realizes that it is going to experience the same dry and normal process once again, it instructs the body to be indifferent to this process and save its energy.

If the quality of "energy storage" in the mind is not managed intelligently and under constant practice, it will be harmful. Alzheimer's disease is actually a mechanism of spontaneous destruction of the brain. Conditioning and captivity in routine processes can be the main cause of Alzheimer's disease.

It is enough to start removing habits. Eating naked once can give a different meaning to this meal. A change of route from work to home can give a different meaning to a city trip. Maybe we need to experience eating with Japanese chopsticks instead of spoons and forks this time. If we hold the spoon in the left hand during a meal, we put the brain into a "situational challenge" crisis. The posture challenge is one of the proper and serious exercises to prevent brain conditioning and laziness.

Thousands of different experiences are available to humans. These experiences can also be extended to the field of private relationships. In the words of Sohrab Sepehri: "Eyes must be washed, one must see differently." Sometimes it is necessary to "let the feeling eat."

The exercises and recommendations that exist to remove the dust of habit will also have another benefit. This benefit comes from avoiding imitation. Most of the time, because of this, people suffer from repetition and boredom of everyday life, which is on the track of imitation. In order to get off the rails of imitation and get out of the safe shore that man has prepared for himself and does not have the courage to leave, starting simple experiences can be effective.

Imitation means extinguishing the flames of creativity and existential originality in humans. Imitation is a type of psychopathy that forces a person to accept the intellectual and ideological views of others in a deadly passivity and use them as a model for their practical and intellectual life. For this reason, imitation is a deadly poison for creativity and originality of soul and originality of body.

Religions are in favor of imitation and try to take away the creative power of thinking and criticism by interfering in the most private personal relationships of people. Humans who, in the dictionary of an "obedient and submissive herd," without any sense of responsibility regarding their human identity, follow the path and follow religious leaders. These are the most desirable followers of cults.

The basis of human identity originates from his individuality. Modern and contemporary man has given great priority to individualism in defining his biological relationships. For this reason, it can be seen that religions, while remaining in the past centuries, are hostile to all the enlightened and enlightening approaches of the new era.

When the originality of the body is ignored, man becomes a common noun. From the point of view of the opponents of the originality of the body and the originality of individual identity, man is defined as a mass in the dictionary.

A common noun means a phenomenon or entity that does not have an individual identity. In the Persian language, "horse" is a common noun that refers to a species of creature. But if we want to talk about the individual and personal identity of a particular horse, we must mention his special name. For example, let's say "Rakhsh" or "Shabdiz."

In the definition of man, without individual originality and physical originality, we are only faced with a generic name that has no identity. It is therefore easy to issue a series of general instructions to the individual identity-less "mass," which the religious leaders define as "imitators." If we want to solve the problems of every human being with all the details and his individual feelings and emotions, according to his unique physical and emotional structure, the imitation mechanism will be ineffective.

In the imitation mechanism, a person should not have personal questions. For example, he cannot say: "When I was in the bathroom, I encountered this phenomenon…" He should say: "When a person is in the bathroom and faces this phenomenon…"

In this way, when a question about the origin of personal identity and the originality of the body arises for an impersonator, since there is no answer for him, he must remain silent.

Man is an observer and seeker. A healthy person, who has grown and lived in a suitable environment, seeks to discover material and mental phenomena around him since childhood.

The direct result of this searching spirit is scientific achievements in the field of natural and theoretical sciences. If a human child has not assumed a static identity in a conditioned path, he can achieve a self-made and personalized consciousness in search of distant horizons that can transform the quality of life.

Resilient and cortical forces try to suppress the dynamic and reactive human identity. They are worried that the human seeker may question their fixed and inflexible teachings. Therefore, they try to minimize human creative power.

This difficult situation is double for women. Regarding women, in addition to religion, social and moral taboos and the population of men are also factors suppressing the dynamics of questioning women.

Removing the Imposed Masks

In the free relationship, which occurs based on the natural discourse of nature, usually many of the above factors are absent. Therefore, the free romantic relationship is always full of physical passion and full of sensuality and pure pleasure. But as soon as the husband and wife enter the cycle of life and are engaged in the affairs for a while, they quickly distance themselves from this space.

Sciences such as psychology have worked on this issue. Many books have been written and humanities scientists have suggested solutions to prevent the feeling between men and women from getting cold.

Looking at these findings, some highlights stand out. Including the fact that over time the parties put masks on their faces and do not behave with honesty and breaking emotional boundaries like in the early days of love. They no longer talk about their interests and inner desires. The sex incident is not only delayed, but its quality and details are reduced and it is often dependent on an incident and regardless of any planning.

The masks that the husband and wife put on their faces are the inevitable result of entering an atmosphere without feelings and fears caused by economic administration and raising children. A couple who are sleeping alone in their room and the children are not waiting for daily services in other rooms, have a much better space for romantic behavior. This does not mean recommending the complete elimination of children from life. Although the management of this issue is very important, having children is not everything.

Daily rules, considerations, excuses and bio-social requirements, if not consciously managed, will cause the husband and wife to gradually put masks on their faces and look at each other from behind these masks in daily encounters, even during night meetings.

If thinkers like Osho believe that marriage is the deadly poison of a love relationship, they make such an assumption considering all the effects that this dry social institution can leave behind. Love and sex are sacred and spiritual matters, and the more they are involved and challenged with worldly affairs, they gradually lose color.

Escape from the Archetype of the Holy Woman

Another reason why a free romantic relationship is far more attractive and sensual than a relationship between a husband and wife is the dominance of a halo of maternal archetypes in the view of women. When a man enters into a permanent and contractual relationship with his wife and begins to live under the moral rules governing the family, a part of the mentality and images deposited in his mind is unintentionally realized in the personalization of the holy face of the mother to transfer it to the wife.

According to Freud's psychological views, the male child is dependent on the mother in the stages of his sexual development. This dependence is such that men remain in its control until the end of their lives. This dependence, which is referred to as the Oedipus complex, includes various stages of the child's sexual and emotional development. According to Freud, the male child is dependent on the mother and considers the father as his enemy, and the female child is under the influence of the father and in competition with the mother in the stages of her emotional development. This trend is called "Electra complex," according to this theory, the girl has a complete dependence on the father and considers the mother to be her enemy. However, it has been said that sometimes the opposite may happen. These theories were later developed by Carl Gustav Jung.

Men's attachment and return to the mother's bosom, which is associated with the wife's bosom during the marriage period, is caused by another complex inside the man, which Jung names as "the mother's complex."

Coping with the mother complex is one of the most difficult psychological changes for a man. This complex, which has a referential and regressive state, is a strong element inside every man, which, if not controlled, can make his life face serious challenges.

After puberty and separation from the mother's lap, the man tries to close his emotional umbilical cord with the mother, he often succeeds in this field and acquires a fighting and "masculine" spirit, which is caused by this desire for independence. But there is always a risk that he will succumb to the "mother complex" again and start the regressive period of returning to the world of childhood. A time associated with mother's care, crawling under the blanket and benefiting from maternal caresses and before that benefiting from the mother's body as a source of sexual inspiration.

The man, in his hidden biological memory, has good images of the safety of the mother's presence. The security that starts from the womb and continues to the time when he was sheltered in his mother's arms. At that time, the duty of fighting with the outside world and its dangers and assuming all the responsibilities and cares was on the mother. In this way, many times men look for this safe and happy time in their wife's dictionary and the wife's motherly aspect is overcome.

No man is interested in having sex with his mother. The Oedipus complex is a constant state of alarm in the mind of men. Such analogies that a man makes between his wife and mother cause him to avoid sexuality and create an aura of non-sexual sanctity around his wife.

By developing the mother archetype theory, Freud shows that the mother has complete control over all aspects of the boy's life. The archetype or archetype of mother includes different dimensions such as good mother or bad mother. In human beliefs, both Western and Eastern, mother is the origin of many human virtues. The archetype of the "burning candle" that gives light to others, and the person who has heaven under his feet, and images of this kind, which have many examples in the cultural geography of Geth, help to create an aura of holiness in the mind of the man.

Many men under the influence of this holy aura, prefer to have a sensual and brash sex relationship full of breaking boundaries and red lines, apply the maximum (apparently moral) standards and have their sexual adventures with women other than their wives. to experience.

It is the case that usually men do not talk about their sexual experiences with their wives in the company of friends. What happens between a man and his wife is one of his secrets. But it is enough that a male gathering is formed so that the participants talk with all intensity and heat about their sexual experiences with other women and describe it in full detail.

In terms of social taboos that have accumulated in the minds of such men. A good woman is a woman who suppresses her bodily needs as much as possible and renounces her sexual pleasures. Archetypes, laws, superstitious views, collective unconscious, religion, etc. are among the factors that confirm the isolation of women and emphasize the need to suppress the sexual instincts of women as mothers.

When a woman enters the family and transforms step by step within this customary system, the possibility of sexual and sensual signals in her becomes more limited. The process goes like this:

unknown woman a woman we know a woman who is our friend a woman we like a woman we love a woman we have a sexual relationship with a woman we have sex with a woman we are married to a woman who is the mother of our children a woman who is our mother.

We see that as we move forward in this hypothetical line, the woman's situation worsens in terms of her erotic moods. He has to move toward self-censorship in his sexual interactions with his wife. Because the change in the man's condition that we described above obliges him to apply more censorship. This is how, in two equal events, a man expects from a temporary sexual partner to be as rude and reckless as possible and not observe any red line in terms of rudeness and insolence; but under equal conditions, he expects his wife to not even make a sound, to be calm and quiet and to finish the task without any sudden and emotional reaction.

To apply these patterns and frameworks, the man categorizes the woman in a degrading way. Within the framework of conjugal and family norms, he and his wife look for Florence Nightingale, the Greek Athena and the Virgin Mary. But in his imaginations and mental and sensual adventures, he is looking for Alexis Texas, Mehsti Ganjavi and Maryam Magdalieh. It is natural that these contradictions will lead to the separation of two souls and the decline of the physical aspects of love.

In order to find his ideal woman, a man must be a combination of all mythical women and all female archetypes and not just a part of them. He should find his ideal woman by referring to his inner intellect and philosophy without being influenced by taboos and outdated social views. For this, it is necessary for him to put aside his usual mental equations and accept that his ideal woman is the woman who sleeps next to him every night. It is enough to discover her hidden dimensions and in a relationship of discovery and intuition without the presence of the shadow of his mother, consider his wife only as a wife.

A repressed woman who was once a lover and is now suppressed under the influence of archetypes of decency and sanctity, her instincts and natural femininity, if she is discovered, in the words of Sohrab Sepehri, she can be a "flower capable of eternity" or a "mirror square." Then he will be surprised to find that she is the beautiful and defiant woman with all the sparks of charm and sensuality that he has been looking for in his dreams. When Saadi says: "friends are at home and we have gone around the world," perhaps he is referring to this aspect of men's attitude toward women.

In order to understand such an experience, a man must first of all abandon the categorical view of women. It is enough for him to consider the bed and time of sex as the most sacred time and place of his life. A man can never have a successful sex life when he puts his money, daily calculations, office secretary, cell phone, social networks, and in a word, his unrefined mind to bed and is censoring his woman with a ridiculous prejudice.

One must be sure that, in the end, women are no different from each other, as Plato says about Diotima. The bodies are all the same with little difference; but when we go beyond the beauty of the body and reach the beauty of the soul, the worlds will be completely different. The only difference is in actions and reactions.

Even Sophia Loren is in the end an ordinary woman who slept with ordinary people. To discover the differences, the Sophia Loren hidden inside her partner must be discovered. Creation has been designed in such a way that there has been no significant difference between women even since the beginning of human life, from cave dwelling until today. Differences are made by belongings, edges, objects and actions.

We can have the same properties and actions. From this point of view, issues such as fetishism, which social psychologists refer to as a behavioral problem, can actually be tools to strengthen the relationship.

You can benefit from all these things and create a beautiful sexual world. A man should know that the most respectable woman for him is not his mother. His wife is equally honorable and holy. It is true that the social rules have strongly condemned sex with incest. Perhaps this is the reason that the disorders and genetic abnormalities caused by sex seriously threaten human life and social health. After all, it is still not clear whether Adam Abul Bashar's children had sex with their siblings or not.

Regardless, sex can be considered sacred and spiritual; because it is the deepest form of relationship between two people. Of course, based on the structural rules of creation, these two people should preferably be of the opposite sex. If we see our ideal woman in the dictionary of mother, we will never be able to spend an hour blissfully in a hot tub with our spouse or permanent sexual partner.

These solitudes require crossing oneself. Convergence among the "square of mirrors" requires reaching the highest degree of self-confidence and mutual acceptance. When we fully accept the body and soul of the other party, suddenly an aura of "becoming" surrounds us. In this case, all the private creations and visualizations that a person can have in their most private moment will take on a two-person nature.

Obviously, we are talking about the beauty of these solitudes. When beauty dominates, many boundaries are removed. The field of sex is not the field of censorship and rules. The assimilation is complete. It is abandonment and selflessness. The body reaches orgasm after passing through the most wonderful moment of its existence and coming into contact with the person who is currently the most intimate person on earth.

Regardless of the extreme and immoral aspects of the world of pornography, deconstructive sexual creativity is neither obscenity nor lack of decency. The wife is the most accurate sexual partner of the man. The attempt to censor him and the dual behavior at home and on the street indicates a moral imbalance.

The problem is not promoting blasphemy. Even animals do not engage in extreme and ugly acts in sexual behavior. For example, shared sex in animals is almost never seen. Most animals do not have sex in secret. Most animals have exclusive sexual partners. Most animals respect their sexual partners. Most animals consider their sexual partners perfect and superior. There is an intermediate but desirable way to have ideal sex; but when we see the wife in the mother's dictionary, it is no longer possible to achieve that ideal level.

It seems that humans can use animals as their best teachers to draw their policies in sexual matters and to optimize the culture of sex and to correct stereotypes. Animals never display sexual behaviors with their partners. Although others can watch their sexual interactions; but as far as they are concerned, they don't care in the slightest what other people think about their sexual act.

Men are more interested in dividing people into friends. First: "people to have sex with," second: "people to love." There is nothing wrong with this category in itself. The problem starts when some men try to put their wives in the second category. This view is more or less present among women. For women, there is also the "good boy or bastard" complex. The same dichotomy that exists for men regarding the "holy/harlot" pattern. But the boundaries of this division are fainter in women.

Women, while accepting that loving, supportive, and well-drinking men are theoretically attractive, but at the same time, they cannot deny that they are heartless bastards who walk away as soon as the love game is over and walk away from them as far as a continent, are more sexually attractive. What binds the whore and the bastard in these two scenarios together is that both are practically and emotionally unavailable, and as a result, they are not constant witnesses and reminders of our sexual idiosyncrasies and weaknesses.

The act of flirting is sometimes more private than we want to do with someone we know well and see all the time. Perhaps it is based on this feeling that Sigmund Freud went a little further and said that many of us find it difficult to flirt with a long-term lover.

Freud first identified, more clearly than anyone else, a much more complex and profound reason for this difficulty. If we note that the logical continuation of this feeling is sex with intimate partners, it is well understood why men do not like sex outside the norm and the peak of sexual pleasure (neither for themselves nor for their wives) in the face of their wives.

Writing an article in 1912, Freud uncovered a fundamental challenge that all of his patients seemed to be dealing with. The problem was that when they fall in love with their lover, they are not interested in having sex with him, and when they have a desire to have sex with someone, they cannot fall in love with him.

In this study, Freud estimates that there are two unavoidable facts. First, this complication is related to our educational system during childhood. Another thing is that this issue can destroy our sex life in the long run.

The reason for the first fact is that the first people who teach us love in childhood are those with whom we cannot flirt in any way due to the strict prohibition of taboos.

The reason for the second fact is the detailed discussion that we are raising. This means that in adulthood, we usually choose those who are similar to those whom we loved in childhood. In this way, in their choices, men, without knowing it, guided by hidden forces, choose someone who is more like their mother or favorite people of their childhood. These similarities are related to some important and bold aspects of personality that even we are not aware of.

Logically, the result of this discussion and this enigmatic situation is this: the closer we get to our beloved and the more love we feel for him, this hidden intimacy will remind us of the deep intimacy of family bonds. According to instincts and sensual desires, we will be far away from him. Because the more she becomes like our mother, the more she becomes holy. With the explanation that most men mistakenly and under the control of taboos think that sex and sexuality are unholy. The main problem and not of this puzzle is here and it can be opened here as well.

If the combination of a high level of love with an aura of our childhood memories plus a high intensity of sensuality and pleasure is gathered in one place, the most ideal situation for a lover and lover or husband and wife and any other couple is realized. Unraveling the main spiritual knot of men is to recognize this knot and this hatred.

The main source of this distaste is that a man thinks that if he wants to respect his wife to a real extent and classify her among the people he respects, in this case, he will face a "conflict of respect and lust" in the sexual act. will be the reason that many sexual relations between a man and a woman in a stable relationship often takes place on the surface and does not have enough creativity and dynamism, also comes back to this issue.

If a woman completely disarms herself and tries to reach the depth of sexual satisfaction, she will be attacked from two sides. The purity of the sexual act, which is possible to get out of the outer layer of the body and reveal all the deep sexual desires, makes it possible that his wife does not respect him enough. On the other hand, social taboos attack him as if he does not have enough decency. This conflict has remained unresolved until now, and since a man is not supposed to ignore the original and real desires and the peak of sexual pleasure as his inalienable right, he is looking for this experience elsewhere. A woman should also censor herself and suppress her desires and needs that nature has institutionalized in her as an inalienable right, and in this situation, she should burn and make trouble.

This situation, through the first, is clearly seen in the oriental woman and the institution of marriage and traditional family. In fact, many poisoned marriages, which remain until the end of life, continue in such a context. Society does not like women who get divorced and protest against such a situation; but women who remain in the aforementioned situation are defined as good and noble women.

The above-mentioned crisis may not occur in the first months or years of marriage and in the period before and after the honeymoon; but as soon as the child's voice was heard in the hallway of the house, the woman has become a mother, and because an incorrect definition of sanctity and decency and "mute mother" has been defined for her, it seems that the natural life of a woman as a "woman" is in this space is running out.

This is where the house becomes a prison for the oriental woman, where she must forget her carnal desires and devote herself to the sacred duty of motherhood. This status provides a definite, but unwritten, license for a man to seek out other women to pursue his sexual adventures.

There is a hidden philosophy behind religion's support of male sexual adventures that lies in this cycle. Religion obligates women to suppress sexual desire and encourages men to have sexual adventures, and since religion must solve this contradiction, the solution is in matters such as "polygamy" and concubinage and "sexual exploitation" and the like.

The conflict between the status of motherhood—femininity—gender is perhaps the most important complication that has endangered the life of women and the vitality of their lives in some parts of the world.

The authoritative position of the father has also increased the severity of this crisis. The archetypes depicted by Jung are a good representation of such a situation in human society. According to Jungian archetypes, the position of parents in the collective mind is drawn as follows: the father, heroic, powerful, idealistic and the mother, selfless, selfless, noble, the candle that burns.

Perhaps in the oral culture and marginal subcultures of the society, we have clearly seen that the young and professionally ignorant man has tattooed on his arm or painted on his truck with some hearts and flowers that Mother is the king of sadness Where does this pattern come from? Why is the mother eternally the king of grief? What is the meaning of this sadness?

This sadness is actually the same sadness that Eastern women feel under the influence of the same reactionary archetypes; but the dominant are condemned to live with it.

Mother He is the king of sadness because he has to ignore his life and bodily needs and physical desires that are deposited in all his cells and expose his family to burning and destruction as fuel for the fireplace so that those around him can enjoy its warmth and enjoy life and happiness. Pay yourself.

The physical life and physical joys of the oriental woman are ultimately limited to the first few months of marriage, and since another oriental model considers the mother as a "means of reproduction" as soon as the woman's menstruation stops and there are signs of the presence of life. A third was revealed in her womb, her mission as a living being is over and all her rights are lost.

At the same time, nature has provided more capacities and capabilities to enjoy physical life for women than for men. The issue of women's frequent ejaculations, the issue of the capacity for sex in realms beyond the sexual organism, are just two of the potentials of women to enjoy bodily pleasures.

These two female capabilities have been destroyed by men throughout history. The capacity for repeated ejaculations in women, especially in closed and religious societies, has been suppressed in such a way that many women in their entire lives not only experience frequent ejaculations, but do not experience even one ejaculation. The issue of a woman's vast physical power for sexual experience, which is spread in all her physical cells from the tips of her feet to the top of her head, is also destroyed by men's carelessness and selfishness, and finally it is extinguished.

There comes a time when this suffering body, following its suffering soul, accepts that the only way to achieve catastrophic peace is to suppress all these capacities. The taboo of talking about this issue also fuels the issue that a woman can never share her inner self with someone else.

In addition to religion, mythology also has a similar attitude toward women. Human mythology seems to have a masculine nature. In Greek mythology, the view of women is almost consistent with these relations.

Athena, in practice, fully accepts the patriarchal order of the world around her. According to her father's orders, she never married and remains a virgin. Therefore, virginity, which is the symbolic form of "prohibition of sexual activity" for women, is a sacred thing in his character. Even though he is in love with Prometheus, he never has a physical relationship with his beloved, and this makes the Greek culture refer to Athena's love for Prometheus as the highest and most noble love. Love for a woman is sacred if it does not rely on carnal desires and does not lead to physical flirtation. This is especially true for women. Of course, in other cultures, love that does not lead to flirting is great and will remain in history. Part of the attraction we see in love without flirting is related to the tragic aspects of the issue.

The love of Lily and Majnoon is tragic and sad. Because it is associated with failure and permanent regret and has a bitter end. This love is not beautiful; but it is lasting and effective. Despite the fact that Weiss and Ramin's love is beautiful, sensual and attractive; but the public perception of it is not a holy and tragic love.

Tragedy is an important factor for the durability and authenticity of a phenomenon. For example, it is said that if Christ was not crucified, most people in the world would not be Christians now. In fact, the religious leaders who died in their bed and while talking with their relatives did not have an important element to influence the society and history from the tragic side of their lives.

Therefore, regardless of the role that tragedy plays in drawing the main lines of a romantic relationship, the sanctity of non-physical love is something that will eventually spread to the real and true layers of women's lives in the world and through the first way of the women of the East. Hayat has drawn them.

Mankind and Its Masks

If we examine the issue of man's failure in relation to the opposite sex from another angle more precisely, we can consider the issue of man and his masks as a major flaw. How many couples marry each other and live happily ever after! They live together and even death separates them from each other; but in all this long life they never meet each other. They can never reach the root of each other's existence. The protective guards, created to protect the inside, are never opened. They never touch each other's souls. They never speak to each other's hearts. They never manage to discover each other's existence. They live together like two strangers, or in better words, like two acquaintances, eat together, sleep together, have expedient or sensual sex. They talk to each other, have children, lay their heads on the same bed and are together in all moments of life; but if we don't say "stranger," just like two acquaintances who are supposed to be friends one day, their lives will end.

This is the reality of millions of marriages that are called "successful marriages" in the customs and laws of societies. These are people who have not understood the necessity of discovery and intuition of each other. Their needs are similar to the food on the table. If needed, mating takes place (not in a romantic way, but in a routine and automatic way). The basic necessities of life, housing, clean clothes, one or two good and healthy children and finally a constant care for finances and the like are all they have in mind.

Those whose lives lead to divorce realize the existence of these shortcomings and problems. They feel that their needs are not what we mentioned. They understand the necessity of surrendering to the soul of their partner, and if this surrender is not possible, there is no other option than separation. These are the people who cannot live with their partner despite the presence of an invisible fence between them. They object to the presence of this hijab. This protest comes from what they see and understand. Otherwise, if someone does not realize the existence of a veil and a barrier between his life partner, he naturally does not feel the need to solve this problem.

In this way, the lives of the first type lead to divorce and are recorded in the daily and normal relations of the society as unsuccessful lives and marriages, and the lives of the second type are recorded as a success in statistics and sociological social relations. According to Hafez, in the meantime, man is oblivious to his own work and cannot put aside the "veil of the face of life":

> The veil of my face becomes the dust of my body
> I am blessed to remove the curtain from that face
> Such a cage is not a melodious punishment
> I must go to the garden of paradise, where I am a bird of grass
> It was not clear why I came, where I went
> Reluctance and pain that I am oblivious to my own work
> How do I circumambulate in the holy world?
> that in the composition, the board of my body

Love is composed of soul and soul and one cannot remain loyal to the cage of the body. One should leave the cage of the body in the freshness of the body and be free in this amazing metamorphosis

If there is a smell of joy in my blood
It's amazing how painful it is to be circumcised
See the style of my golden dress like a candle
which is the secret burning inside me
Come and take the existence of Hafez before him
that despite you, no one will hear from me that I am

Man is defined in the core of his existence and not in his surroundings. In fact, the surroundings of man is the place to start to enter the core of his soul. Around man is the place where his material life is present and his central core is the realm of the main substance of his existence. To get closer to a human being, one must reach the main center of his core being.

Husbands and wives who have lived together for years may be just acquaintances. Maybe they have never known each other. With this quality, the more you live with someone, the more you forget that the centers remain unknown. So the first point to understand is what Osho states more clearly: "Do not mistake familiarity for love. Maybe you flirt, maybe you have sex, but sex is also around. Until the centers meet, sex is just the meeting of two bodies. Sex is also dating—physical dating, but still dating. You can only allow someone to enter the center of your being when you are not afraid, when you are not afraid. So I tell you that there are two ways of living: one is rooted in fear and the other is rooted in love."

"A fearful life can never lead you to a deep relationship. You remain afraid and don't allow anyone else to enter. He is not allowed to penetrate into your being. You only let him so far and then that wall comes and everything stops."

This uncooperative behavior is the result of a fearful mind. The fearful mind is constantly thinking about what might happen in the future during this relationship. But the self-confident mind, which is watered by the juice of its inner abilities, thinks in the moment and now and is not bound by calculations. As we said, love is in conflict with calculation. But people who do not have successful relationships always live in an aura of determination and caution. They draw a plan. They plan.

Security guards are built to prevent their partner from accessing the corners of their soul.

If you can live in the moment and have the success of being in love, all these worries and misunderstandings will disappear. Get out of the daily routine and you will achieve the blossoming of love. Of course, love is love in its true meaning. Millions of people have this misunderstanding that they interpret lust as love. While their behavior shows that love is completely absent in this scene. Conventional arguments, exploitation, control, jealousy, boundaries, dominance, sense of ownership, sense of superiority and dozens of other concepts that are abundant in people's lives are all signs of the absence of love.

Conservatism in opening the boundaries of the relationship is like giving a book to someone else and only giving the audience the right to read the introduction or parts of it. The importance of being open about all the content of the book, when facing the life partner, is because almost no two books can be found that have the same content. But "conditionalities" and superficial and false connections mean that all humans on earth have the same content and there is a general idea about the content of all books on earth.

If a human being is a book and hides his soul inside a hard cover and an external shell and does not allow others to see his content, how can we expect him to have a wide interaction with the audience? Perhaps the resistance against revealing the content of the book of life. Everyone should be aware that there is no valuable content in this book. Otherwise, the most important feature of any book is to be read by the audience.

If we leave conditionings aside and each person has a specific plan for their relationship, then this conservatism and fighting for privacy will not have any meaning. If love becomes a real behavior and purpose of life, then we will no longer allow an external layer to hide the privacy of the relationship. The relationship will no longer mean satisfying biological desires, sensual pleasures or fulfilling physical needs. In this case, a meditative state will prevail for the relationship and both parties will continuously move toward each other and climb to the peaks of love.

Such a relationship will be a maximal and ultimate relationship. If you are in love with someone, you will be immersed in his outer realms at first. Then you will move into the inner and spiritual realms. After delving into the horizons and souls of his being, you will begin to converge and become one with him.

But why do people, instead of optimizing deep connections and internalizing relationships, repeat the wrong path they have gone before with religious ceremonies and making the rules of marriage more difficult. The reason for this approach is that paying attention to the internal institution is a completely personal matter, and social networks and religious institutions are not able to extend their scope of supervision and authority to human beings. They can't get to the inside of humans and influence human attitudes there.

This issue is true not only in the area under discussion, but also in areas where the authority of religions is more. This is because there is no standard for evaluating human faith. Social complications appear in the shadow of this weak function of religion. Pretense and hypocrisy spread, and religions deliberately prefer a kind of symbolic hypocrisy over honest and sincere action. Because they only care about the apparent plurality of their followers and those who follow their rules.

For religions, the inner quality of a follower is not very important. This is because the rules of customary and religious marriages give way to the real needs of communication between men and women. Although this method leads to divorce and breakup of relationships in a large way. For the custodians of ideological systems and customary structures, it is important to say how many people of a society have married in the form of their approved system. The second half of the glass does not matter to them. They do not pay attention to the issue of how many of these marriages have led to divorce and brought unfortunate social consequences. Even if all traditional and religious marriages lead to divorce, they see no need to revise their traditional mechanisms.

It is for this reason that religions do not show happiness in ways such as mysticism, Sufism, and various methods of discovery and intuition that are prevalent in different parts of the world, including the Eastern regions. These systems of discovery and intuition pay attention to the inside of man, while religions are completely concerned with the external action and demonstrative behavior of their followers.

For them, it is important that a marriage takes place and a child is born, which is classified only geographically among the followers of a religion. What fate this person will have or what bitterness may come to him in this world is not important for the guardians of religious rituals. They are indifferent to the personal destiny and individual identity of humans and only care about the category of counting and quantity.

Chapter Four
Sexually Defective Activism

Kamasutra, Understanding Sexually Defective Activism

In the treatise of Kamasutra, we see that the author provides guidelines that include the same points regarding the optimization of flirting activity. He suggests that instead of being a passive body below, the woman should be on top and take the initiative. This issue seems correct in terms of the nature and physical creation of women. A woman is a fragile and delicate creature. The heavy weight of the man when he is on top gives the woman the feeling of being "trapped." This is the starting point of relationship failure. In such a situation, a woman's physical potential and creative power in sexual activism are turned off.

Vatsayana, around 400 BC, had the aristocracy to understand the flaws of such a relationship. In this treatise, which was written to explain the principles and criteria of sexual and sensual relationship, he explains in detail that love and sex is not a one-way and physical relationship and that many other components such as love, philosophy, attitude and pleasure play a role in it. He believes that strengthening and optimizing sexual power includes techniques and principles that, like any other field, humans (especially men) should not be ignorant of.

Based on the ancient philosophy of ancient India, Kama Sutra focuses on the reality of sex as one of the four pillars of existence on the planet. For this reason, the state of sexual intercourse and the principles of lovemaking are very important in achieving the fundamental goals of life. These principles are based on the correct methods of hugging, kissing, caressing and even biting and pinching, slapping and the like, some of these principles spread to areas such as fetishism.

In this regard, women's reactions, whose limitations we considered as a deadly poison in creating a deep sexual relationship, are taken into consideration. According to the author, moaning and noises like this are part of the reality of sex, which should not be censored by relying on taboos or other limiting factors.

At the beginning of this work, it is emphasized that men should read this book and apply its principles in their personal life and romantic relationship. It seems that at the same time, it was well felt that most of the current defects in the relationship between men and women depend on the ignorance of men.

He also emphasizes that achieving maximum success and creating a successful sexual relationship and realizing the ideal sex is related to the form of sexual relationship and meeting the basic emotional and romantic conditions and requirements.

Of course, in all cases (as we have mentioned many times) the role of men is very important in creating an ideal sexual understanding. It is for this reason that in Kamasutra, while paying attention to this issue, it talks about "good and bad man's inclinations." But in general, the main approach of this text is the involvement of psychology and paying attention to the complexities of human behavior (both men and women) to achieve the peak of sexual pleasure.

An interesting point that the Kamasutra makes is about adultery. He forbids adultery because he believes that in the act of adultery, pleasure belongs only to one of the two parties. Based on this argument, it can be said that adultery has occurred in all sexual relationships where only one of the parties is subject to sexual consent, even if this relationship is in the form of a traditional marriage.

Although there is no detailed and documented information about Vatsayana, it seems that he was quite serious in terms of pragmatism and criticism of social customs and taboos that are rooted in religions and social relationships. In this sense, he can be compared with Osho, the Indian philosopher who has similar views, and even from the social aspect, he can be compared with Hafez Shirazi.

His educational views are completely in conflict with social taboos, especially in the Middle East. According to the social taboos of the East, a woman should not only stay under and not make a sound, but she should also keep her eyes closed. These taboos falsely state that any kind of action and reaction of a woman in the act of sex means that she has moved away from the state of decency and "being a lady."

One of the most important teachings is that a man's view of sex should change in general, he should be aware of women's sexual capacities and potentials and apply appropriate behavioral requirements. He must learn that lovemaking is not an immediate event to satisfy his quick and short-term needs, but a deep and revolutionary event that takes place with the full participation of both parties.

A man should learn to avoid looking at a woman as his tool and property and a means to fulfill his desires and gradually internalize this different view. He must learn that love and sex are two sacred institutions and the experiences gained from this passage are among the most important achievements of a human being in his lifetime.

Men should learn that sex is the moment of liberation from any mask and impurity. The moment when the fear of being intimate and showing the real face should be put aside and the woman can show her authentic and true self and both sides stay away from any kind of deception and self-restraint.

A woman should have the possibility and assistance from men to be in a state of pure assimilation, as she likes, based on her nature at the moment of sexual climax. This is the moment in which pure experiences such as mindlessness, "spacelessness" and "timelessness" can be obtained. At the moment of ejaculation, all processes stop for a while. There is no time, no place, no rules, no morals. There are no boundaries. Any attempt by a man to draw red lines in the experience of sex is at odds with its existential nature.

This situation makes sex similar to other experiences such as meditation and revelation; The experience of a pleasant playfulness for the woman, an experience that she cannot get in other conditions and situations. Therefore, it is his absolute right to understand this discovery and favorable intuition.

Eastern panic men have a hard time with such an approach. They do not allow their women to experience the peak of sexual pleasure. These obstacles and restrictions have caused 98% of women in this region to not experience orgasm. Of course, this issue is clearly different in Western countries. It seems that as long as public patterns such as decency, loyalty and acceptability are based on imposing red lines on women's sexual behavior, solving the problem of women in the East will be far from reach.

When talking about the East, it does not mean that the West has always been an exception to this rule. Before the 20th century, the condition of women in the West was also miserable. Sometimes this situation has been more complicated. But with the beginning of the 20th century, with the help of serious research and scientific information from scientists, especially psychologists, Western women became aware of their situation.

In the first place, the research led to enlightenment about the physical nature of women. In these research processes, it was shown that the sexual motivation of women is not limited and depends on the sexual organ, but the peak of sexual pleasure in women is more than men, depends on psychological components and is aimed at the range of all organs. In other words, the Western society was surprised to find out that the female genital organ is not sensitive and does not feel anything, contrary to the previous idea. Even the genital organ known as the clitoral plays a minor role in arousal. In addition, this organ is a completely separate muscle from the female sexual organism.

The problem that caused women throughout history to give in to sex as a routine and emotionless thing without recognizing their sexual capabilities and to manage their married life was that a woman can act close depending on the conditions that are imposed on her. To do and reproduce mechanically. In such a situation, she is just a mother, whose actions appear in a machine state before giving birth, mostly, far from emotion. After giving birth, she enters a different emotional state when facing the child. Of course, this is if she has a desire to be a mother. Otherwise, sex has brought nothing but trouble to women. In fact, the woman acted as a child-producing machine, which required constant suffering and bitterness caused by repeated pregnancies and subsequent bitterness. In such a situation, in the best case, giving into sex and consequently pregnancy is considered a woman's duty.

But this duty does not take the place of feeling and love. In many cases, despite the fact that she hates her husband, a woman gives her body to him so that the process of family development and reproduction can flow naturally. In such a situation, the man is not respected by the woman. Because the view of men and society toward women is not in the form of respect. This issue has caused the man not only to not feel the need to satisfy the physical needs of the woman; but in many cases to suppress these needs.

The situation of women in the West was also in this way until Masters and Johnson's research discovered strange facts about the power of successive ejaculation of women for the first time, and a new window was opened for women in this part of the world to assert their rights.

Relationship Management; See a Therapist

If the importance of a perfect relationship was well understood, most couples would go to psychotherapy centers during their life together, just like they go to a hairdresser or a clinic, to avoid possible voids in their souls with periodic check-ups.

The psyche of humans is exposed to challenges and increased burdens throughout their lives, which over time reduces the capacity to tolerate and accept others. Periodic and regular psychotherapy can prevent tensions and communication crises by removing these heavy burdens.

It is not known why there is an idea in society that people who visit mental therapists periodically are crazy or have some aspects of madness in them? While no one has such a problem due to routine visits to medical centers and medical check-ups. It doesn't create an image of epilepsy, cancer, MS or terminal illnesses.

Humans prefer to hide small and big mental problems and disorders from the eyes of others and do not experience being in a psychiatrist's office or a psychotherapist's office, or if they do, do not make it public.

The lack of attention to the state of mental health makes people think of solutions in times of crisis, which often make it difficult and sometimes impossible to return to a normal state. Because mental health, like physical health, starts from a small point and gradually grows. Prevention is always better than treatment and treatment in the early stages is easier than treating the acute stages.

Changes in the relationship of couples are slow and hidden. These changes happen inside people without them being aware of it and gradually spread. They never realize that every word, gesture and behavior is meaningful and can be signs of disorder and intolerance of others. Every small movement and behavior that leads to resentment, even brief, will mean a decrease in the desire for a relationship and the depth of flirting and the quality of love, which means the secret growth of cancer of "incompatibility" and even hatred.

An experienced therapist can notice changes in behavioral relationships by receiving detailed information in the process of periodic care and categorization and analysis of frequent data. He can suggest a list of possible considerations and a set of appropriate precautions that can be applied to prevent dangerous holes in the relationship levels.

He will ask the couple in question to bring a list of behavioral data with them at monthly or weekly intervals so that he can predict possible pitfalls in the future path based on the meaning and meaning of this data and to avoid falling into these pitfalls. Show a rule.

The longer the visit is delayed, the more likely the healer will encounter souls that have suffered serious damage. Deep resentments can create scratches on the soul level that are highly repairable and likely to become permanent (due to delay in action). No matter how skillfully the psychotherapist tries to remove and repair the annoyances, there will still be traces and signs left. In the words of the poet:

If the thread is broken, it can be closed
But there is a knot in the middle

If such conditions prevail over the relationship, the couple in question will enter into a vicious cycle of suffering relationship where each part of this circle completes the other. The collapse of tensions in the soul will cause a gap in flirtations and sex. While flirting and closeness are one of the drugs and factors to remove challenges.

Most likely, the psychotherapist will tell our couple that in order to reduce the unpleasantness and coldness of the relationship and remove the dullness, they have to modify their behavior, not send negative signals, strengthen commonalities, increase the levels of empathy and honesty, and even change the mechanism of periodic flirting. manage.

Delayed sex or any kind of flirting can cause the body's cells to be charged with sexual energy. Since the body with all its cells is completely dependent on the soul and emotion, this vicious cycle can continuously produce negative energies and more adversity.

The help that a psychotherapist can give to a damaged couple is to make it clear to them that the other party is not an undesirable, spiteful and malicious being; rather, he is the same old lover who is now a sad and damaged creature who feels a deep sadness inside himself because of the misfortunes that have happened. Sadness, most of which is due to being away from the beloved. In fact, if this clarification takes place, instead of blaming each other for problems and disturbances, both parties will realize that they are both sitting in a common boat that goes up and down on the turbulent waves of life. None of the occupants of this boat is the other's enemy or his ill-wisher, but both of them are in the same situation that they can only succeed with the help of empathy and love and becoming one.

If there are no centers related to psychological and relationship management in the streets and alleys of the city, parallel to every store, grocery store, hairdressing salon, and sports club, it means that mankind has not yet come to understand the importance of psychological issues in their lives. A problem that we see clear signs in is the frequency of divorce statistics in big cities and numerous social complications.

Children of divorce are products of broken relationships. Psychological pressures on the society due to the spread of loneliness in the new generation, the loss of the spirit of interaction and friendship and thousands of other complications are the direct results of the absence of these centers and offices.

People mistakenly think that it is impossible not to go to the local store, car wash, restaurant, and bar every week, but life will go on without problems without going to specialized psychotherapy and psychotherapy offices. The fact is that this case is completely the opposite; but no one pays attention to it.

Mankind with all its scientific power and tremendous achievements in the field of discovering the dark spots of galaxies and penetration into particles, is still in knowing itself and finding a solution to regulate individual relationships between people and to achieve a discovery and intuitive knowledge about the subtleties of the human psyche and how to face the other is at the beginning of the road.

Mankind has been able to make achievements in regulating social relations and creating order in collective relations; but at the same time, compared to the optimization of romantic relationships and the intuitive discovery system of emotional connection between two people, it is faced with the poverty of knowledge and collective experiences.

Man has tried to push all that is related to romantic spirits and individual feelings into personal and hidden areas. If such experiences were shared collectively and in collective action, based on extensive scientific research, there would be a greater ability to understand the characteristics of a personal relationship.

Sexual Impotence and Premature Ejaculation

Impotence is one of the most common causes of cold relationships and leading to divorce. However, it was impossible to talk about it, at least until Masters and Johnson's research took place. Even now, talking about impotence is a dangerous taboo for men. They prefer to accept the collapse of the family and do not even admit their impotence to their doctor and psychiatrist.

It is not unlikely that this reluctance is caused by the same false male pride that he has prepared for himself over time, through the same vast propaganda, and because he deeply believes in it, he is spiritually dependent on it. Impotence is difficult to admit because men base much of their pride on this imperfect ability. In another part of this book, we showed that biologically, women's sexual power is many times more than men's. We also showed that men have denied and suppressed female potentials to implement their dominance scenario.

The feeling of shame is caused by sexual impotence, even though men generally do not have a significant ability in terms of sexual performance compared to women. Male impotence is a major biological defect and when it is supplemented with a secondary medical defect, it results in a huge identity crisis for the man.

The damage that impotence causes on the relationship between men and women can be examined from several aspects. First, failure in bed is a dignified phenomenon for a man. Generally, he has allowed this failure to women routinely and systematically. The automatic and self-centered performance of the man has trained the woman in such a way that she basically does not look at sex as an action based on mutual success. However, when impotence becomes the cause, the man becomes so agitated that he prefers not to maintain such a relationship. Because more than sexual pleasure, the issue of his self-esteem is involved.

If extensive research was done on the causes of impotence, it would probably show that mankind did not face the issue of impotence at the beginning of life. Impotence can be a complication of modern life.

Some of the conducted research raises hypotheses. Including the fact that impotence can be related to the issue of masturbation. Or the human use of some products of the modern age and various detergents and various medicines have had a destructive effect on his natural reproductive system and the natural process of sperm production.

Man's special attention to the genital category and sexual system has increased the sensitivities of this system and left it out of its natural state. Watching porn movies, which reproduce sex in one's imagination without the flow of a physical process, causes abnormal impulses in the erotic mechanism and causes it to have a situation recognition error.

Modern man has irrationally learned to exercise sensual fantasies about another person without the presence of another and in an aggressive manner. Maybe no one imagines that this brazen act is also a form of rape. Violating another person's privacy without their consent and knowledge, especially if that person is a woman.

In the natural process of sex, the dreaming mechanism of the body stops. The body in the physical realm is carrying out a meditative process from the first stage to the last stage. But when sex is without the presence of another, it is only dreamy. The human mind encounters unwanted jumps in the state of dreaming, and the last stage of sex; That is, it restores orgasm. In this way, the human mind, by removing the usual and physical prerequisites of the process; From talking to caressing, nudity, flirting, cuddling, cuddling and sexual climax, it imagines the orgasm stage at once. This brain shortcut, if repeated continuously, causes a routine habit in the brain.

The next time, when sex takes place in the act and with the physical presence of a second person, the mind repeats the dreamer's previous process, which includes a shortcut to orgasm, and this means premature ejaculation.

Premature ejaculation is as important as impotence and erectile dysfunction in the destruction of sexual relations. Men are naturally unable to satisfy the sexual needs of women due to the fundamental weakness in their physiology. A sexual intercourse usually lasts no more than a few minutes based on the normal sexual ability of men. Meanwhile, women's sexual ability can continue a sexual relationship for hours. The ability of women to ejaculate frequently is something that naturally less men are able to respond to. Regardless of whether men have tried to suppress women's sexual excitement, premature ejaculation can be the end of a minimally conventional relationship between a man and a woman.

Female Abilities and Male Disabilities

A woman's physical and romantic potentials are not limited to these matters. Considering the quality of her creation, a woman can act much deeper and more creatively. Because sex for a woman is not a limited process and relies on the sexual organs, but starts from the first caress or the first romantic and caressing look and continues long after the last ejaculation. This performance range, in men, starts only around ejaculation and ends completely at the moment of ejaculation. This structural contradiction, which is rooted in physical qualities and the difference in the creation of men and women, is perhaps the most important serious challenge between the two sexes in two-way communication.

The results of scientific investigations, regarding the comparison of the sexual abilities of women and men, indicate that women have at least two great advantages over men due to their capacities. These potentials make a woman have the ability to have a much deeper and better sexual experience. The potentials that show his competence to play the field in the sex process. Until today, the historical relationship between man and woman has flowed completely opposite to this rule. We mention the natural advantages of women compared to men below:

Multiple Ejaculations Versus Single Ejaculation

The most important obvious advantage that the woman's creation has given her is the ability to have multiple and consecutive orgasms in one sexual act. If there are perfect emotional, environmental and romantic conditions, a woman can reach the peak stage of sexual pleasure and experience orgasm several times. In addition to the mentioned conditions, the sexual partner's abilities are also important in realizing this. Assuming that the man does not suffer from sexual defects such as premature ejaculation, erectile dysfunction, lack of physical energy and weak constitution, he can last a process in about three or four minutes. This period is not enough to actualize women's capabilities. In fact, this time is not even enough to turn on the powerful sexual engine of a woman. Although there are various medical and pharmaceutical ways to create a kind of physical equality between men and women, in natural conditions, this structural conflict in the creation of men and women cannot be denied. The truth is that to create this equality and balance in the field, men have always needed the help of medical products.

Regardless of the duration of the operation, sudden male ejaculation is another problem that increases this conflict. A woman, unlike a man, is neither emotionally nor physically exhausted when she reaches orgasm. Because of this, it is always the man who leaves the scene half-done, and the woman's fielding has never been a problem.

Male orgasm means the end point of the whole process. Because after orgasm, he doesn't have the power and emotion to complete the process. But if the woman orgasms earlier, she can continue the process and make the man orgasm in the same situation.

All this proves the undoubted superiority of women in the sex process. The fact that, along with his other abilities, shows a great superiority that indicates the great weakness of men in creation. It is not known why the intelligence of creation deposited this male weakness and female strength in the creation of these two sexes. If we do not accept that this is a mistake in the dictionary of creation, we must look for the philosophy of this conflicting structure.

Sense Organs – Sexual Organs

A woman's extraordinary ability in sex is not limited to the sensitivities of the sexual organs. Even multiple ejaculations, which only women benefit from, are not the only reason for the difference between men and women. A woman's vast abilities in sexual act lie because of the extent of sexual act in all her organs and in all the hidden corners of her feelings. In fact, a woman's sexual organ during flirting is wide from the tip of the foot to the part of the head. Caressing and touching each of these organs can be a completely sexual and emotional act in order to complete the process.

This is despite the fact that such a mechanism is not embedded in the creation of man. The small area of a man's sexual territory in his body is directed to or around his genitals. This small territory ends in a quick and one-time ejaculation in a short process. But that's not all. Ejaculation is the end of the short-term sexual process in men. It can even be said that for a while, a man's sexual desire after ejaculation gives way to disgust and sometimes hatred of any kind of caressing or cuddling and being touched.

This, of course, depends on the type of two-way relationship between sexual partners. If love is not involved, the end of sex means the end of sexual enjoyment. This formula works much stronger on men. But if a deep love is rooted in all the sexual and spiritual parts of both parties, then the occurrence of ejaculation will not mean disgust, depression, regret or indifference.

Irrespective of all these, the capacity of sexual action in a woman is such that after ejaculation, it is the turn of caressing and flirting. Just as the female sexual organs are wide from the tip of the foot to the top of the head, the process of courtship-sex-ejaculation and its delay is much wider for women. This issue makes the timing and length of the process one of the most challenging issues for men. Regardless of premature ejaculation, which should be mentioned as a common complication, premature ejaculation in general is a feature that makes sex a fast and controversial process. The speed of ejaculation in men is rooted in their philosophy or existential structure. both physically and intellectually and other physiological and material requirements.

All these things make sex in a woman a deep, rich, profound and therefore stable experience. Understanding an experience with this breadth and depth makes a woman's need to repeat the action, overtime, far less than a man's similar need.

But the description we made of the deep and special potential of women in the sex process is unfortunately not an obvious and common thing. That is, for various reasons, some of which we will mention below, throughout history, women have been deliberately and forcibly deprived of the capacity granted to them by creation and deprived of their inherent rights.

Inequality of Women in Sex

Due to being deprived of these two characteristics, the man tries to compensate for the aforementioned deficiency by having multiple sexual partners and multiple sexual acts. If studies are conducted in the field of complications such as sex addiction, premature ejaculation and the like, it will be clear that these complications are considered male complications, which are all rooted in the aforementioned weakness. But in general, several major factors cause women not to enjoy the gift of equal sex, which briefly includes the following:

The First Factor: Male Impotence

A man's inherent inability to arouse a woman's body with all its inner strength has made very few women achieve their natural and self-evident utopia. In fact, even if a man makes an honest effort to motivate a woman to the maximum, he will not be successful in this matter due to his inherent inability. If such a success is achieved once in a while, it will be considered as an extraordinary and adventurous experience, which is not easy to repeat.

Usually, the sense of responsibility in men is not enough to consider this issue as a form of self-sacrifice for the maximum satisfaction of their partner and take it into consideration.

Any phenomenon that has the nature of self-sacrifice in routine life, can soon be removed from the cycle of stable affairs and placed in the corner of oblivion. In this way, by nature, a woman cannot expect her partner, as a wife, partner, or boyfriend, to pay attention to her physical requirements and capacities.

Now, if a man suffers from multiple disabilities such as premature ejaculation, lack of skills, ignorance, irresponsibility, false belief, etc., the situation of a woman will be much more complicated. One of these beliefs is that a man thinks that a woman is a sex machine and a man can use her as he needs.

The Second Factor: Cultural Crises

When it comes to cultural crises and problems, the class and social system of the world can be separated with bolder demarcations. This issue regarding religion and religious beliefs is not so bold. Things like free thinking, intellectualism, belief in the equality of men and women and recognition of the needs of female physiology, etc. have a direct relationship with cultural development.

Societies that are more culturally developed accept these things to a significant extent and perform better. For example, writing and reading many books in the field of couple crises and solutions to face them is more common in developed countries. Social forces and customary laws have more power to counter restrictive religious beliefs and social taboos. Democracies also try to have more support for progressive forces as one of the foundations of pluralism (which is a requirement of libertarianism). Forces that try to recognize women's basic rights (including their biological capacities) operate more freely.

Therefore, in societies that are culturally backward, women cannot enjoy their rights.

It has been said that about 98% of Eastern women have not known the peak of sexual pleasure. Many of these women are born and grow up within the framework of the same rules and taboos and old patterns, get married, endure men's sex (sex machine) and pregnancy (reproductive machine), perform obligatory service to the family and husband. They provide (housekeeping machines), grow old and die.

Maybe the situation of these women is not too unfortunate; because they sometimes have never experienced ejaculation in their life. They do not know anything about their ability to ejaculate repeatedly. Most of them do not imagine that they can be at the top and take control and initiative. Therefore, if someone does not know that he has a property, he will not have any anxiety and sorrow about it, and he will not seek to take possession of his right.

The Third Factor: Religious Restrictions

Religious teachings, especially in the Middle East, clearly state that a woman is not only under the possession and guardianship of a man, but as a sex machine, she must always be on standby to be serviced when needed.

It has not been seen that any of the religious teachings mention the sexual rights of women. By referring to some of the fundamental texts of Eastern religions, we will see that it is clearly mentioned that men can use sexual deprivation as a tool to punish women. In addition, the legitimacy and even the legality of polygamy, in itself, is considered a factor for imposing sexual deprivation on women.

According to what was mentioned above, a man is basically unable to meet the sexual needs of a sexual partner in terms of his creation and physical factors, in accordance with the emotional and physical needs of a woman. However, in many religions, a way has simply been opened for men to benefit as much as possible from multiple women.

What was said about the clear difference between the Orient and the Western societies, after the industrial revolution and the sex revolution, has a lot to do with the issue of religion.

Religious restrictions do not even allow women to discover themselves. In Eastern societies, a woman is considered a part of the house and not a part of the society. The philosophical interpretation of the woman belonging to the house is that she is at the base of the pyramid and the man is at the top of that pyramid. At the base of this pyramid, which is called family, there are things that are all aimed at serving the top of the pyramid and ultimately serving the quantitative expansion of society.

In this structure, the woman is also part of the base of this pyramid. Religious people are strongly fighting with the complications and results of modernity because the same rule of the former and the latter continues to exist, and pushing women to the corner is one of their important and main strategies in advancing this struggle.

All these things make the Eastern woman have a difficult way to reach the position where the Western woman is now.

The Fourth Factor: Social Taboos

Another reason that has made women unable to benefit from their potentials and capacities is social taboos and the wrong perception of the patriarchal society for many centuries. In the sense that from the point of view of the conservative society, either because of the dominance of religion or because of the dominance of reactionary views, a woman is not defined with her potential as a congressman and agent.

As it was said before, from the point of view of taboos, a woman is like a sex machine, which must perform the task of "giving" sex in the same way as her other tasks. Duties such as laundry, ironing, cooking, cleaning, shopping and the like.

Obviously, a woman with this attitude cannot be active and take the initiative. He must be passive, receptive, silent, silent and restrained and has no right to comment on the time, quality, length of the process, place, number, quantity and requirements of the process. All this depends on the will or in better words, depends on the diversity of the man. It goes without saying that in such a situation, talking about women's initiative and "sex in all physical and mental parts" will seem pointless. Suppressing the completeness of women and turning them into the second sex, without any power of discernment and decision-making, is the essence of this reality.

Perhaps nature has made a fatal mistake against women. The appearance of the matter is that by putting several extraordinary powers in the woman's body, he has created her more powerful; but as we have seen, this power is not considered an advantage in a major part of women's society; rather, it has caused harm and failure.

The problem here is that to fulfill the ultimate goal of creation, i.e. reproduction, based on the logic of evolutionary biology, only male ejaculation is sufficient. Even sperm injection seems to be enough. That is, the role of a woman in the reproductive cycle starts from the ovary and with the help of other reproductive organs; Like the uterus and placenta and other parts, it is completed in the best possible way.

This is the cruelty of nature about women. In fact, nature has used the element of pleasure only as a reward for the man, and no part has been considered for the woman in this equation. If this possession was supposed to be complete, the means of realizing it should be deposited in the man's body. If the nature of guaranteeing the health of the child and ensuring the quality of reproduction and the realization of factors such as the intelligence and beauty of the children were postponed to the woman's indulgence, what a beautiful paradise would be realized for women on earth! If it was so, the society of men would do everything to make women benefit from sex. Medical and biological sciences and the human knowledge system worked with all their might to improve the quality of women's sex as much as possible.

Man's Physiological Weakness, the Reasons for an Enmity

Man's inabilities compared to women's abilities have made him use aggressive strategies to solve his constant crisis, instead of looking for a peaceful solution. It has always been said that the best defense is offense. In order to hide his disability, the man has tried to keep his sexual partner in a state of permanent suppression by using various tools, some of which have been mentioned above.

For a man, it is only important to suppress his sexual tensions. Sometimes he only needs a few seconds to do this. One-sided scientific considerations that have published results without considering the woman show that a man needs three minutes in the best conditions to complete the process of arousal to ejaculation. If we consider sex as a detailed book that includes the introduction, text and conclusion, this three-minute time, in which the man's sex book closes, is actually not enough time for the woman to finish the introduction.

A man is deprived of "quality sex" and "deep sex" due to physical disability. This deprivation and deficiency, for which apparently there is no solution, makes him feel jealous and spiteful in many cases. Enmity between men and women can be observed in the oral culture of the Tudeh, both in a humorous and serious form. This humorous short story is an example of millions of stories about the constant hostility between men and women in Tudeh culture:

A couple is moving with their young son inside the car.

The son says: Father! Last night I dreamed that a monster was standing behind the window of my room and was trying to enter my room.

The father says: My son, don't worry! it is nothing! Because when you get married, you have to sleep with the same monster every night in the same bed!

The woman listens to this conversation in astonishment without saying anything.

Analyzing the dimensions of this hostility requires scientific and research work. But apparently, the main motivation of this hostility is different from men and women. Because of his own weakness, the man has harbored jealousy and resentment against the woman during the millennia they have been together. The woman also looked at her life partner with caution and historical misunderstanding because of the oppression she always endured from the man. This repression, in turn, stems from the same historical lack of self-confidence of men vis-a-vis women. The lack of self-confidence is caused by the biological weakness of the man…As we can see, this cause-and-effect sequence has created a dynamic and active circle of action and reactions, within which men and women, in a state of suspension and obligation, Life goes on.

Suppressing and restraining women's power, relying on such means as taboos, religion, ethics, and the like, is just a cover to hide men's weakness.

A woman's body is aroused later, but when this arousal occurs, it is deep and extensive. The continuation of this stimulation (if it is given the field) leads to a kind of desirable rebellion in the body and non-conventional behavior. Screams of pleasure and arousal, unusual dialogues, fetishistic tendencies, repeated ejaculations, different peaks of arousal, are the things that the traditional man tends to suppress.

On the other hand, a routine, calm and predictable rule is going on. When the man is done and his "three minutes" are up, the woman is still just starting to get excited. At this time, in a humiliating act, the man turns his back to his sexual partner and goes to sleep.

Now, depending on the woman's awareness of the painful tragedy in which she is caught, she may have different reactions. It is possible that this woman will be suppressed to such an extent that the process of stimulation will be turned off in her. Most Eastern women have this situation. In their opinion, the peak of sexual pleasure in the form of ejaculation is only for men and women are only silent spectators of this short-term pleasure.

There are other women who are aware of their body capabilities. Some of them have even experienced orgasm in one or two happy memories. These may be longing for repeating the same event over and over again in a permanent longing. They may shed tears every time a man finishes his work and turns his back on him and starts snoring.

There are other women who not only have this knowledge; rather, they consider it their indisputable right to achieve the peak of sexual pleasure according to their abilities, and thus it is the duty of their sexual partner to make the woman participate in such a peak at the same time as the peak of sexual pleasure. This group of women is definitely not religious and they do not accept social taboos either. They definitely react to male sexual behavior and do not tolerate being ignored.

This reaction can be an attempt to improve the man and get training and techniques to optimize the quality of sex. Maybe the desired solution is to end the relationship and break up. The lack of fundamental studies makes us not know how many marriages occur as a result of sexual tensions and neglect of women to men; but this issue is definitely one of the determining variables.

From the point of view of a knowledgeable woman, disrespecting a sexual partner is a possessive treatment and instrumental exploitation. For him, the ideal of good sex can be associated with the simultaneous ejaculation of a man and a woman. But it is more ideal that before the man ejaculates, the woman has the experience of a small ejaculation once or twice and then it is decided with her final orgasm.

In a few men, it may be such a power, but in the rest, it is not possible without recourse to medicinal aids. Therefore, it may not be bad for a man to benefit from medical achievements to overcome his weakness.

but this is not the whole story. Because the process of sex is not defined only in orgasm. For a woman, making love is a spiritual and long process that begins with courtship, kissing, caressing, and flirting and does not end with orgasm. For a woman, the behavior of the sexual partner after orgasm has a special meaning. Reluctance and indifference after orgasm is not a problem that a conscious woman can accept.

From the woman's point of view, the ideal process of flirting starts long before bed with a euphoria and a good mood, and continues with the approach, and by sharing this good mood, during a long process, it approaches its end as mentioned.

Sex is not a reward for another job, not an end to a long war and conflict, not a bribe to comply with a request, not an act of hypocrisy, or something to make the petition not empty. Sex is not an addiction to repetition, nor is it an emptying of body toxins, nor is it a way to relax muscles and a way to sleep. Flirting is none of these things, but in a stagnant and toxic relationship, a couple who are only together to avoid divorce, it can be all of these things.

Sex is like writing poetry. First of all, an inspired mood should be created before styling. When this feeling and motivation starts and penetrates through the heart and feeling to the cells of the whole body, the woman is ready to accept flirting. At such a time, a woman's body is like an instrument ready to accept romantic wounds so that all her emotional strings vibrate and that deep emotional music enters the process of playing.

Forced sex and instrumental use of a woman's body is not in accordance with creation. Sex in an optimal state starts from the boundaries of consciousness, then it is completed in a meta-conscious process. For this reason, in an ideal situation, sex is one of the most perfect two-way communication in the universe. It is natural that these two people must be a woman and a man. Physical condition, age, development, intelligence and mutual understanding are among the components that are effective in flirting. In other words, sex is subject to its own criteria. The structural conflict between consciousness and awareness of creation in the creation of women and the behavior of human beings through laws and religions shows the depth of this heterogeneity.

In the essence of a relationship, there should be no suspicion of effort. In the example of poetry and poetic inspiration that was mentioned, inspiration, as the main factor, is always necessary before the creation of a literary work. Sex is like a poem that is written spontaneously and does not take place from prior planning and based on needs, tricks and utilitarianism. A couple in love naturally dances, dines, plays and walks in nature or even does household chores together. In the meantime, sparks of flirting may appear spontaneously, in the form of a kiss, a flirtation or a whole process. There is no imposition. There is no suspicion of hypocrisy and pretense. Deception (even the smallest tricks of husband and wife) does not play a role in this. The flow and spark leading to the fire may be strong enough to feed the couple's feelings for days on end and keep them in a state of ecstasy and pleasure.

In a spontaneous two-way relationship, the rules lose color. Accepted rules say that it is acceptable for a man to be on top. Especially in backward societies, such a phenomenon is taken for granted; but perhaps some never thought that this rule might be wrong in general.

According to the rules of physics, the man who is heavier, taller and more muscular should be placed below and the woman should be above because of her elegance and light weight so that she does not feel suffocated and imprisoned under the heavy burden of the man. Also, because of her strength and creativity, women can take the initiative and manage the process much better than men.

Apparently, due to the same physiological shortcoming, the man wants to take the initiative by being on top and announce the end of the process whenever he wants so that his defects are not revealed and he turns to suppression to avoid the feeling of responsibility. Naturally, it is important to be on top to apply repression.

The Fifth Chapter
A Bridge to Transcend Oneself

Love Is the Astrolabe of God's Secrets

The utopia of sex will be out of reach without love. What brings the identity of femininity to the fore is practical love. This is why we say that platonic love cannot be imagined independently. Based on the belief that "physical love is a bridge to reach God," which is mentioned in its place, any type of love relies on the experience of physical and sensual love. This is the bio-social driving force, the struggle for survival and the flourishing of female identity. Therefore, in defining the nature of love, Dr. Ali Akbar Siasi mentions it as "one of the various signs of social tendencies" which "is often considered among lusts."

According to Plato's point of view, the foundation of love and belonging is based on the recognition of beauty and the re-understanding of goodness and beauty. He says about this: "The human soul has seen the truth of absolute beauty and goodness (that is, good without veils and hijabs) in the world of singles before entering the world. So, in this world, when he sees the external, relative and virtual beauty, he remembers the absolute beauty he has seen before, and he is overcome by the sadness of separation and takes away his air of love, he is seduced by the world and like a chicken that he is in a cage and wants to fly to him."

"The emotions and worlds of love are the same as the desire to meet the truth, but physical love is virtual, just like physical beauty, and true love is a dream that hits the wise head, and just as virtual love causes the body to come out of sterility and produce children, and is the reason for the survival of the species, so is true love. It frees the soul and intellect from sterility, it causes the understanding of the truth and the realization of eternal life, that is, the attainment of the knowledge of the beauty of truth, absolute goodness, and spiritual life, and man reaches the perfection of knowledge when he attains the truth and essence, and the observation of his beauty, and the unity of the universe. And it should be clear, wise and reasonable."

The foundation of Sufi beliefs is also based on the authenticity of love. According to them, the universe is based on love, and the vibrancy that makes the whole universe move is because of love. Therefore, true perfection should be sought in love.

If we put the theory of Plato and mystics next to the central theory of mystics and philosophers like Mulla Sadra who consider human love as a prerequisite for transcendental love, the result will be that love cannot be divided into types. Rather, it is a process that includes elements. If love is the main source of life and the driving engine of creation, then the helplessness of mankind in the face of sex, husband and wife relationships, sexual failures and social vitality should be resolved with the help of love.

In our place, we will say that in some mystical and philosophical views, love is not only the driving force of life, but also the main goal of creation. Different branches of mysticism and different philosophical categories introduce love as the main base of human evolution on earth.

In his poems, Hafez often introduces love as the most important approach to creation, without which the mechanism of existence would be incomplete and the human mission on earth would remain incomplete:

Fall in love, one day, the world will come to an end
Without the fact that you have reached your main goal in this world
He even goes as far as to believe that love can replace all phenomena and themes of life:
As soon as I performed ablution from the fountain of love
I ignored the whole world and the things in it

Alain Badiou, a French philosopher, in defense of love, advises people not to be afraid of love. He refers to the views of theorists such as Kierkegaard, Marcel Proust and others who consider love to be a glorious adventure in life. Quoting Plato, he says that whoever does not start with love will never understand the essence of philosophy.

Bridges to Cross Oneself

With all these abilities and considering that a woman has countless other capacities for an ideal and romantic life, one of the most important images we have of her is the ultimate self-sacrifice for the well-being and happiness of others. The people around the woman who have the highest benefits from her sacrifice include her husband, sexual partner, life partner or children. In the next circle, there are other relatives who benefit from the woman's sacrifice to varying degrees. He ignores his life so that others are in complete peace and favorable condition physically, psychologically and socially. Love and sex are two valuable possessions of a woman, which she often sacrifices.

A woman's self-sacrifice can be compared to a bridge that a woman crosses and sacrifices her life for the people around her. In the meantime, sex, as one of the major pleasures and carriers of pleasure and happiness, includes this sacrifice. Perhaps you can see a small replica of this situation in the movie *The Bridges of Madison County* by Clint Eastwood.

The story that takes place in the movie is one of the most prominent creations of cinema regarding the uncertainty of a woman between the two paths of tradition and love. The female character, who has lived with her husband and children in a traditional family for fifteen years, now, in the absence of her family and husband for four days, in a completely random situation, meets another person and a deep love is formed between them. The two live together for four days, which is a clear example of a perfect romantic relationship. The woman is revived in these four days. He gets out of his traditional and passive form and feels that new windows of life and love have been opened for him. A woman tears the ancient skin of passivity and fossilization, and horizons open beyond her eyes that show the depth of the heart and feelings.

He has experienced love. He has understood unity and "closeness" and closeness. But this short period is coming to an end. The family returns from the trip and the lover is on the verge of separation forever, and the woman experiences a critical moment in the situation of making a big decision between staying with the family or going with her ideal man.

In the last meeting, they have under the same roof, a series of conversations takes place that tragically shows the position of the woman who is stuck between the traditional family and the family tradition and crossing the dependencies and opening a new door in life. In the end, she decides to sacrifice herself to the traditional morality and the moral tradition of the society and so that her husband, who is a "good man," is not harmed, and so that her children do not suffer losses, she continues her old life and her lover leaves forever.

Now the woman is dead and she has left the memories and extended narratives of these four days for her children, who review the mother's memories. The girl and the boy, who both have families and both families are on the verge of collapse, at first are reluctant to accept this fact, but in the end they sympathize with this issue and even their thoughts and feelings are affected by the story of the mother. They both reach a stage of contentment and forgiveness where they return to their family life and forgive their partner for what he was before.

The Two-Way Nature of Love

Love is a two-way event. Love does not happen in a vacuum. Therefore, one-sided platonic love is not really love. Some psychologists classify passionate one-sided love in the category of sadism or masochism. Love only happens by being in the presence of another. Being together brings a wave of joy and happiness.

Happiness, if it is channeled in the path of forming a family or creating a stable relationship, can create a huge potential for the survival of the relationship. In love, there is a great harmony between feeling, soul, heart and organs. They feed from the juice of each other's existence, and the essence of life flows in the veins of each other. Love is a type of comprehensive integration in which the parties transcend their individuality and gradually transform into a single whole. In this case, love is no longer lust. No more sex. It is no longer a woman's body and a man's body. It is the presence of another that creates a feeling of happiness. With the help of love, the parties achieve a kind of undisturbed immortality and their existence in the realm of love continues in an evolved form.

Love Is Plurality but Unity

There is no single version of love that can be extended to others. Herein lies the difficulty of love. Love is like a relationship with God. Just as there are as many exclusive versions of God as there are people on earth, the same rule applies in love. That is, there are as many versions of love as there are people on earth. The story of Moses and the shepherd in Malawi's Masnavi and Moses' criticism of the shepherd's prayers and the shepherd's innocent and naive love toward his beloved and God is a beautiful example of diversity and plurality in love and relationship with God and the beloved.

The version of love that made our neighbor happy may not work for us. Love is the phoenix of the peak of Qaf, and there are different truths and different phoenix according to the number of travelers for it. Each path, in its own context and depending on its personal and inner behavior, can reach the truth and become a Simorgh of love. All these steps and rituals are related to the existence of a person. It is related to his personality and thoughts. It depends on his inner education. It is directed to his worldview.

Some people (especially men) may never achieve the alchemy of love due to the reactionary upbringing and decadent mentality that is the result of childhood upbringing. Because of this, women in regressive societies, where the educational principles of regressiveness are applied during the childhood of men, are often deprived of finding a suitable partner who is able to understand each other, at the same level, and love.

A man enjoys being superior because of his mental content, and to cover up this feeling, he calls it love. He is tormented by this feeling and tries to compensate for it by providing women's welfare. What a strange familiar sentence that we constantly hear in movies and series and in the daily life of the people around us: "Did I miss something for you?"

The speaker of this sentence does not understand enough to know that what a woman needs in the first place is love and then welfare and comfort. Love may take the place of prosperity; but the opposite is never possible.

Men, due to the same educational system and the faulty cycle and cause and effect chain that we mentioned above, have a habit of exploitation. Most of the time this is not even intentional. It is by instinct. The collective unconscious, born of centuries of wrong education, has formed an unconscious mechanism. This unconscious feeling is so strong that even when there are sincere glimmers of love, it begins to possess love itself. After the sense of possessiveness, the feeling of jealousy comes, and after that, violence, which is the child of jealousy, appears. In such a situation, love (if any) instead of producing joy and happiness, brings suffering and bitterness.

This love is poison covered with a layer of honey. Hemlock is a sweet show that will never sweeten the palate of the lover and the beloved. When in the darkness of life's facts, the naked soul of a jealous man falls out of the curtain, life gradually sinks into the ominous shadow of deep-rooted misunderstanding and the decline of the relationship begins.

The boring repetition of this experience has led to the emergence of a deep misunderstanding between men and women. Sayings like "men are all the same" are prejudices caused by repeating this experience and this lack of mutual understanding. This is how many people decide to never fall in love. Love fades and phenomena like pets take the place of male-female relationship. Loneliness and isolation, like a progressive cancer, destroys the human soul.

The World Health Organization has warned against the accelerating growth of isolation in global societies. According to the opinion of this organization, in 2023, this global problem will threaten the health of the world community much more than any psycho-physical disease. A simple relationship with a puppy, love for a cat, falling in love with a car, etc. as unnatural behaviors take the place of a rational relationship between a man and a woman. Because humans (especially men) have not been able to cope with the complexities of relationships with the opposite sex and the practice and tolerance of love. For this reason, they have chosen simple relationships without the need for tolerance and practice.

Man has ruined his soul under the domination of possessiveness. It is enough to look at the theme of romantic songs. Even the best of them are constantly expressing a morbid sense of possessiveness. Perhaps the most recurring concept in love songs of the last decade has been this phrase: "You should be mine." Why? because I love you so I deserve you to be mine.

In these songs, no artist talks about the soul of a woman. It is always about long hair, black or honey eyes, and balanced bodies. While the essence of a woman's existence is not summed up in the combination of organs, eye color and hair style. The soul is the missing element in the regressive view of men and women. Phrases regarding the expression of possessive ownership are the cornerstones of expressing morbid interests in the musical vocabulary of today's modern societies. This, in turn, is a form of violence. Sometimes the face of violence is internalized and cannot be seen with the naked eye. Covert violence fuels open violence at other levels of society.

Today's modern man, who has suffered from self-centeredness and vicious business, tries to manage his love relationships based on the same business vision. For this reason, human life undergoes the degeneration that we are currently witnessing. The collapse of the foundations of families and relationships and the frustration of humans from creating a healthy relationship with the opposite sex is the result of these attitudes and the desire to close love from the heart of life. Otherwise, love can be the most important event of any person's life on earth.

Love is an inspiring connection with the transcendent elements of creation, which brings man back to his original roots and softens his soul. It is not for nothing that Christ said: "Love is God" and mystics believe that "Love is God." Mystics believe that any type of behavior to reach the origin or in other words "Transformation in God" is love. Love is the life-giving element that brings man to the alchemy of knowledge.

This is because love is not for cowards. Love requires great courage and great sacrifice. In order to transcend the ego, man must rise from the ashes of another human like a phoenix, whose existence is from the ashes of another phoenix, in order to understand love and continue the generation of phoenixes.

The background of this great transformation is the departure from individuality. Because love is the dissolution of a person in another. When your individuality remains strong, you are in love with one person and the lover of another person. In this case, we will not achieve the quality of unity. Love in which there are two parties who stand on both sides of the scale and constantly weigh their spoils from life and everyone takes their share, no matter what, it is not love. Conventional marriages widely try to legitimize and magnify this participation of the parties.

The phrase "Al-Majaz Qantara al-Haqiqah" means that a person can begin the process of understanding divinity with the love of a person. We will show examples of this belief in the words of mystics and philosophers such as Suhrawardi and Ibn Sina.

If we look carefully, the lover is the window and perspective that reveals the infinity of the sky in front of our eyes. The reason for the inconclusiveness of today's love is that people fall in love but at the same time cling to their individuality with all their might, while love is not a place of conflict between people; rather, it is the place of transformation of tones and the point of connection and unity.

The starting point of love is like the point created by a stone falling into a pond. If the space and conditions are right, the radius of movement of the circles of love can expand and include all aspects of your being. But as soon as a secondary obstacle is created in the path of its movement, the regular movement of the rays immediately breaks down and love suffers a decrease and decay. The factors that we have mentioned under the title of mercenary view, self-centeredness, depriving the lover's freedoms, possessiveness, jealousy and the like are among the obstacles that can cause this destruction.

Love and Spiritual Refinement of Society

Spirituality happens inside a person. In the sense that although religious teachings are likely to be effective in improving a person; but if there are no internal prerequisites in a person, pretending and acting like a parrot to religious teachings cannot alone be the cause of human happiness.

The index of spirituality in man is determined by his encounter with nature. A person who has all the manifestations of being religious or spiritual in his face, but when passing through his yard, can kick a stray cat in need, there is no doubt that he is thousands of miles away from the standards of spirituality.

You cannot be a transcendent and spiritual person and slaughter a sheep in a religious ceremony. You cannot be an exalted human being and crush a butterfly that is stuck at your window and throw it in the trash. The pillars and natures of existence are surprisingly in deep correspondence with "lack of love." A person cannot be in conflict with these natures and at the same time be a perfect and loving person.

No lover can ignore the army of ants passing under his feet while walking. The sublime soul of man, who has the talent of love, cannot ignore these things. Since love springs from the inspiring source of nature, it is constantly refining and refining the human spirit.

The teachings that mystical and intuitive systems give to their followers are more in line with the nature of creation than the teachings of religions. This difference is clearly evident in the non-violence of mystics, and the promotion of violence among sectarian religions. The conflict between religious leaders and mystical leaders is also related to this issue. Oftentimes, this equation can be used to evaluate love and humanity: wherever there is violence and brutality, there is definitely no love, spirituality and humanity. It is possible that the long and wide reasoning systems of religions try to question this hypothesis. Because religion itself is full of violence and violence. Wars between religions are proof of this claim. But to understand the truth of this idea, each person can very easily refer to his own experience and personal perception and find the answer.

Somewhere in the story of Laila and Majnoon, the relatives of Qays Bani Amer (Majnoon), with the intention of proposing to Laila, go to Noflian's residence and are faced with a rejection. On the way back, Majnoon, who is disappointed with his lover, wanders aimlessly in the desert and runs on fours. After some time, he reaches a hunting ground and sees that some deer are trapped, and soon the hunter comes out of the ambush and intends to kill the deer. He goes ahead and gives his horse to the hunter to vouch for the deer and releases them. Majnoon says to the hunter:

> He who is not a man is a wolf
> Killing a deer is a great unseen for a human being
> This eye, although it is not a good eye
> But it is a sign of the black eye of the lover

This is the spiritual characteristic of a lover. The system of nature is compatible with love. Therefore, the lover has the greatest compatibility and identification with the creatures of existence. Love, as the intellectual manifesto of Rumi, is the main focus of his mystical thinking, he prioritizes love so much that the audience imagines that without love, there would be no world at all. He considers the return of man to love as the return to the essence of existence. A person without love is the same "singing reed" whose burning is due to being cut off from nothingness:

> Anyone who is far from his original
> He is looking for his roots

All human disorders are due to the same fire of love. The same love that has been deposited in man and he has a mission to find this fire throughout his life. For this purpose, he tests different methods and methods. The simplest form of this search is trying to mate in marriage. But the main issue is love:

> The fire of love is a reed
> It is the excitement of love that is in the cup of wine

In order to reform society, it is necessary that love is the road map of man. Otherwise, human society will be full of defects such as greed. To understand the truth of happiness, one should take help from love:

Every person who is disturbed by love
Existence is cleansed of evils and ugliness.

Man's solution is to find a companion so that he can accompany him to the home of love. If this is not the case, even with all the riches in the world, a person cannot eliminate his inner poverty:

Whoever is separated from his loving companion
Despite all the facilities, life will be troubled.
If someone does not care about love
He is like a bird without feathers, so woe to him

Now the question is why the mirror inside man is not polished and polished? Why has man suffered from all kinds of darkness and destruction? The reason for this is the absence of love. Because in the absence of love, the rust of corruption tarnishes and pollutes the inner mirror of man.

Do you know why the mirror of your life is not clear and polished?
Because the dust is sitting on it.

But we continue to deceive ourselves. We think we are in love. And this is the ultimate ignorance. If you imagine that you are in love and you are not, you will be in the center of ignorance, trouble and not at all looking for freedom from the existing situation. Your problem is in the absence of love; but you are not aware of this problem at all; because you think you benefit from the gift of love. Because of this, there is no place or opportunity for the manifestation of love in your life.

In order to get out of the state of lovelessness, man must start a new effort. He should not take it for granted that he has understood love. One of the signs of the existence of love is: Every human being is so full of undiscovered secrets that a lifetime is not enough to find them all. If after some time of acquaintance and relationship, you suddenly feel that you are tired of him and there is nothing new in him, it is certain that you have reached a dead end in the vacuum of love. Love means opening new ways inside. Marriage, sex and lust, means remaining in the periphery. If you are tired of someone, it means that you have always been around him and you have never found an opening to penetrate inside with the help of love.

Love Can Be Learned

Humans have a potential capacity to love. His ability to optimize relationships with life partners is high. But this is not always true. Because love is a basic skill that needs to be developed through training like all other skills. Humans seem to believe in a kind of unplanned and spontaneous action in the category of love. The skills of making love have been discussed in various books, and in the following chapters, we will talk about one of them titled "The Art of Making Love."

No one is born without the ability to love; Even the most hard-hearted people could be loving, professional and kind people, if their upbringing and life progressed in such a way that their emotional capacities came to the fore at the beginning of their lives. It has been said that when Hitler was a teenager, he planned to become a professional painter; but apparently due to the non-acceptance of his works, he returned from this path and became the source of the death of millions of people and the destruction of a continent.

So, if making love as an educational category and as a biological art was given more attention, the quality of human life would probably be better and there would be no news of the current wars and violence. Every person needs a favorable environment to exploit their emotional capabilities. If the personal space of each person expands according to his inherent potential, we will have better people on earth. People's personal and family life is significantly postponed to this issue.

One of the skills that a person can learn is to respect the other party and not disturb their privacy. He should not violate the individuality of another, and love is not an excuse to impose monopolistic demands and demands.

A standard life based on romantic relationships requires attention to the absolute freedom of the other party. There are moments when he needs solitude and solitude. If he is sad, he should be given a proper opportunity to deal with his emotional waves and fluctuations. These are just some of the skills that a person must acquire to start a relationship.

Relationship Between Marriage and Love

Social patterns such as marriage, which have arranged instructions and descriptions of ugly duties for women, make the crisis between men and women more complicated. All the old concepts and taboos that act as the engine of this ugliness are anti-woman elements that should be completely revised. Committed and intellectual men who have reached such an understanding never base their behavior patterns on traditional theories and approaches. But the problem is that the number of such men in human society is undeniably low.

Social science researchers believe that marriage is not a correct approach for communication between men and women. While marriage can be an evolved form of a relationship between a man and a woman, the wrong models that have been promoted in the form of marriage have brought this legal social relationship to a dead end.

The reason why many romantic and emotional relationships end in divorce may lie in the nature of the marriage rather than the nature of the relationship. Marriage puts men in a superior and unequal position by drawing a wrong policy and justifying the domineering behavior of men toward women. For this reason, even if in the early days and years, there is a strong romantic relationship between the two parties, the poisons caused by these unequal obligations will gradually poison the love.

Rarely, a man will have enough intellectual independence and courage to ignore the benefits that the rule of marriage has traditionally brought to him. He gradually begins to exploit this power of his action and gradually pushes the equal feeling between himself and his lover to the unequal state of "dominion."

Of course, this category can have strengths and weaknesses. From an abusive male attitude and tyranny and sexual slavery to more balanced situations that fluctuate depending on the type of upbringing and socialization of men in different societies. But any amount of this arrogance and superiority and creating a feeling of duality is harmful for the durability of a stable relationship.

In its essence, love is free from restraint. Love in its purest form can continue in a completely human context and away from any kind of male domination. Love is averse to any kind of possessive attitude.

Ownership in its essence carries the philosophy of "being an object of mamluk." When the relationship between owner and mamluk becomes dominant between man and woman, there is no doubt that soon the roots of love will dry up. The mouth of love is a great feeling of oneness and identification. In the state of being one, neither side is superior to the other. But as soon as this variable changes, "oneness" turns into "duality." One person is superior and the other is inferior to him. One is the owner and the other is owned. One person is dominant and the other is subordinate. One person has countless advantages and the other is deprived of his rights. And…

For a marriage (traditional or white) to last, two people must love each other. In fact, even the concept of "lover and beloved" is meaningless in the equation of love. The lover is in the active position and the beloved is in the passive position. So if we traditionally think that a man is always in love and a woman is always the beloved, there will still be a problem due to love's escape from dichotomous labels. A lover is also a lover while being a lover, and a lover is also a lover while being a lover. This television in the romantic identity implies the durability and survival of the love equation.

What is manifested in the principle of "Ana al-Haq" of the mystics, and Mansoor Hallaj is the symbol of it in the literature and mysticism of the East, is mixed with this category. The marriage and unification of the lover and the beloved in the way that Hallaj is a symbol of it, or in the expression of Rumi "the union of light," can depict the state of love in different degrees.

> He said lover to lover in exam
> One morning, my lover
> Tell the truth, do you love me more or yourself?
> He said that I have transformed in you
> As if I am full of you
> All that is left of me is my name.
> And all that is in me is only you.

If we are going to consider a different and different foundation for marriage, it will be in this way that man and woman should love each other and at the same time have the freedom and independence of their actions in the best possible way. Marriage should not create any religion for women against man in its dictionary and also the independence of man should be preserved in it. Men and women, while having complete social relations, are free to stay or not stay with each other at their own will and only with the help of love.

In the form of such a marriage, sex can be an evolving factor of this relationship, not as a duty for the woman and a privilege for the man. In such a relationship, sex will not only be considered reprehensible and absurd; rather, it will be a factor to increase satisfaction and serve to strengthen the foundations of mutual love. Peripheral matters such as reproduction and economic benefits should be considered as optional options and dependent on specific circumstances, in the context of marriage, and not its main purpose. Marriage should not consider pregnancy as a woman's duty. This idea completely contradicts a popular belief. A belief that advises young couples to "have children" to strengthen the foundations of their marriage. If the foundation of marriage is not strengthened by itself and with the support of love and deep understanding, it cannot be strengthened with the help of children.

Fortunately, the advancement of medical knowledge and drug therapy has made pregnancy change from an unconscious, obligatory and a kind of duty to a conscious choice. This issue has created a kind of safe margin for women who at some point in time, or in general, are not interested in pregnancy and childbirth and raising children. Because if reproduction is inevitable and one of the definite consequences of sex, it can be mentioned as a threatening factor of love.

The existence of children in a weak and unreliable family actually leads to the equation becoming more complicated and adding a burden on the shoulders of the marriage organization. If we liken marriage to a building, the presence of children should be considered as mortar and pestle that transforms the external image of the structure. Maybe it is another fault that imposes more weight on the thin foundations of the structure. The above popular idea has caused the issue of children of divorce in societies where divorce is common due to the aforementioned reasons, or in the less advantaged classes in the form of working children and children with defective social identities and independent of any standard education and destiny, to a deep dilemma.

Non-democratic governments that seek to expand their domination and authority through population growth have turned women's wombs into a political factor. In such a structure, even in a situation where the family's minimum livelihood is not provided and the family does not have a proper foundation, people are encouraged to reproduce by accepting obvious and hidden risks.

Plato believes that one of the most important wisdoms that a person should have is the wisdom related to the regulation of society and family. According to him: "The greatest wisdom is wisdom and knowledge that is related to the regulation of family and community affairs, and it is called self-mastery, righteousness, and moderation, and it establishes the state of governments and families in a proper and orderly manner."

But it seems that in vast areas of the world, governments and families are far from this collective and human wisdom. That is, governments try to change this wise system in favor of their own interests by influencing families and setting up mechanisms in which the requirements of happiness and biological indicators are absent.

It is like this that in some of these societies, forced marriages and as a result forced and frequent pregnancies have reduced the female identity to the extent of other mammals. In such an environment where there is no practical authority and women's feelings and personality are constantly targeted by threatening factors, it is obvious that the healthy buds of a love will not grow.

Complications such as child marriage, child marriage, increasing social unrest due to uneven population development are part of the social achievements of politicians who try to increase marriage in any way possible and keep the social problems caused by marriage hidden.

Solving social problems through the presence of love (as we have explained in the above pages) is completely achievable. However, a look at the history of male-female relations shows how idealistic the situation outlined above is. But as the famous saying goes: "The mountain begins with the first stone, and man begins with the first pain." Every road always starts with the first step.

The road to the advancement of women in human society starts with simple awareness movements. This movement in the global women's community has been started for a long time. What should be done is to join other women of human society in this dynamic wave. Otherwise, who does not know that throughout history, women have been sold as slaves, traded, buried alive, stoned, burned, and what bitter experiences they have gone through within the framework of the rule of one-way marriage.

All these behaviors were aimed at keeping women in a "commodity" state. A situation in which a man does not have to spend his heart, feelings and even his body to create a balanced relationship. He has preferred to remain on his safe shore and refrain from any kind of responsible behavior. If love and feeling is the main criterion of action, then a man has to pay a lot for a marriage.

Under current circumstances, marriage is an easy and legal way to acquire a wife. But since the free and healthy relationship of its romantic type does not have the bonds of a traditional and paper marriage, it currently works much better in terms of the quality of the relationship.

When two people enter into an equal interaction, automatically, the standards and rules, said and unsaid, start to operate around them. Sometimes, the parties review these rules with each other and remind them once more. Sometimes they put these rules on paper and sign them, and sometimes without saying a word about them, they allow the rules to flow and apply themselves so that the parties can decide about it at each stage and in each instance.

In all these cases, the open and hidden rules that flow around two people, include a series of legal, moral, human and romantic bases, at the top of which is privacy and respect for the human identity of the other party. Today, all these forms are defined in the form of "white marriage."

But in the rule of traditional marriage, all these criteria are changed. The lawmaker and marriage mediator puts the laws on paper and signs them. But these rules are completely different from the ones we mentioned above. The laws specify that a woman is supposed to serve a man and her identity and human status are not important. If it is possible that the careless glaze of apparent love can also give the exterior of the structure a deceptive color and shine, how much better! But if it doesn't happen, there is no problem to realize the traditional marriage.

It goes without saying that among these, there are also couples who have a deep and genuine love between them. But as we have explained in other places, any love within the framework of traditional marriage gradually fades. Because the imposed rules that make the man the absolute master of the woman will destroy the grounds of a true love. Because love does not last in the environment of master and subject.

For this reason, it can be said that throughout history, the highest damage to women has been inflicted from the angle of authoritarian rules of marriage. Marriage in itself may be tolerable for the woman; but the margins and appendages have poisoned the environment of traditional marriage more than what it is in itself.

Polygamy, which is often practiced within the same marriage, has created a corrupt environment for the creation of a form of religious prostitution for the benefit of men. Marriage is in conflict with the freedom of the female soul, in such a situation, this double injury and product has made the situation unbearably difficult for women. It is from this point of view that we see that a set of anti-woman vocabulary has been created in human culture, especially in Eastern culture. Words such as: Huw, Sugli, first wife, second wife, polygamy, submission, alimony, concubine, Tamattu, and the like are a prominent symbol of the history of male separation, all of which appear in the dictionary of marriage.

In other words, prostitution should be considered as the offspring of marriage. In fact, without marriage, there will be no prostitution either legally or illegally. The truth is that if the correct definition of prostitution is given, no law can formally change its nature and serve men's interests.

The fact that religions are apparently against prostitution and in practice widely promote it, means that men's history has widely exploited religion in order to secure their interests, along with other exclusive possibilities. The relationship formed in marriage is the center of gravity of other patterns of social behavior, both practically and symbolically. If the woman enjoys enough of the gifts of democratic behavior, she herself will be the controlling catalyst for society's standard reproduction. Using the self-confidence resulting from his freedom, he will shape the education of the next generation of society based on human dignity. This is one of the potential advantages of marriage. But in a situation where a woman has given in to the disrespectful restrictions imposed in the marriage document and her human dignity has been questioned, how can she talk to her children about nature, equality, human identity, dignity, self-confidence, democracy and acceptance of others? These are all things that the rule of traditional marriage has officially and legally deprived him of.

Marriage and Love; Two Mismatches or Two Pieces of a Puzzle

One of the first reasons why marriage is not a suitable method for a principled relationship between a man and a woman comes back to the issue of love breaking away from the rules. The love of Ceylon is the directness of the soul, and like the free and aggressive waves of the ocean, without any rules or logic, it surrenders itself to the expanses of the sea and recklessly hits the rocks of the beach. The waves break apart, come back and restore themselves and repeat the process.

Now think if we want to say to these waves that they must be regular and move through the designated concrete channel and move with some behavioral logic from within this channel and reach the rock in a certain way and with the same specific method and rule, return to their place again. This artificial regularity will actually contradict the existential nature of the wave.

Marriage is full of rules. It is full of assignments and dos and don'ts, and it is full of promises and agreements that are written on paper and signed by the parties. Witnesses monitor this event, institutions determine executive guarantee for it. Money is exchanged. A path is determined that two people must move on exactly and channelize their love in these artificial frameworks. It seems that with the beginning of the first calculations and bindings, love flees the scene and often does not return.

If the weak points of marriage were limited to these, it would still be possible to overlook its shortcomings. But this is the beginning. The problem is that the institution of marriage not only does not have a plan for the functioning of love as a living and dynamic organism, but it is generally a one-way mechanism to oppress women. The institution of marriage is designed in such a way that it is the woman who should always be in love with the man.

This love (if we consider it love with tolerance) should always be applied by a woman to a man. A woman should worship a man as her guardian. He should be his servant and bear this issue as a duty and responsibility until the end of his life. For the woman in the institution of marriage, there is no possibility to review and change the course. The right to divorce is exclusive to men.

In many societies, the social identity and even the existential nature of women have been considered dependent on men. In some societies, a woman must remain single and mourn her husband's death forever. In some cultures, it is even better for a woman to be cremated or buried with her husband after his death.

All these are the drawing and general picture of what the institution of marriage has prepared for women in different degrees of severity. It is obvious that there is no place for love in this imposed mechanism. In fact, the institution of marriage does not place any importance on love as the driving force of a relationship. In the absence of love, as a sensitive and persistent element that is often not an easy task to achieve, the institution of marriage tries to subjugate the woman by tightening the shackles and increasing the restrictions and taking more guarantees.

It seems that the best solution to find the correct mechanism of the relationship between men and women is to pay more attention to nature and creation. Conventional relationship systems will not be successful without paying attention to the components that nature has deposited in the human body, especially in the female nature.

Many questions and challenges related to the relationship between men and women will disappear by listening to the call of nature and creation. The first issue is that men and women are naturally attracted to each other. But the point of contrast between this issue and the institution of marriage is that marriage, to define the relationship between a man and a woman, has a long-term and unchangeable plan, while the elements involved in the tendencies of both sexes are not the same and can be changed.

Humans may lose inner pulls toward each other. This process can be long or fast. Many of the things that social rules imposed on women in the form of marriage are factors that accelerate the speed of the disappearance of tensions. By optimizing these rules and by men's understanding of women's human nature, it is more likely that this trend will remain stable. Maybe it is because some thinkers like Osho believe that the institution of marriage is not compatible with human nature.

Marriage in most social structures does not attach much importance to the category of love. Although in some dialogues during marriage, there are references to love, feelings and empathy; but the experience of life in the form of marriage has shown that these statements often remain at the level of compliments and unreal conversations.

If love widely rules the relationship between men and women, many disorders will disappear. The lover and the beloved do not often enter into dry, non-emotional relationships, giving and receiving, and utilitarianism. The lover and the beloved never deceive each other, and because the lover sees all the sparks of existence manifested in the beloved, whatever he likes for himself, he also wants for the beloved in the first way.

The concepts hidden in the conversations during marriage, depending on how much it is mixed with love, can guarantee the stability of the relationship. Otherwise, men and women will soon come to the conclusion that by joining the framework of marriage, they have made themselves prisoners of restrictions that do not match their spirits.

When love is present, both sides find a unique nature. Neither will consider the other a burden or a nuisance. In such a relationship, the parties feel that they have discovered a missing part of their existence by discovering a new and fulfilling world. Otherwise, the relationship between the two parties will become unbearable during behaviors, speeches and mechanical activism.

In such a situation, the passage of time makes the burden that the parties feel on their shoulders from the presence of the other, and depending on the capacity and sensitivity of the soul and personality of each party, the relationship will go toward decay and in a certain time, which may last for years and decades. It will break apart. At the beginning of the work, factors such as novelty and the element of sensuality (even without love) and the fun of communicating with an unknown person may inject newness into the body of the relationship; but without the component of love, all this will eventually lose color and eventually even turn into hate. Because each party blames the other for ruining their life and destiny.

The relations between the parties and those around them and the financial and legal exchanges that are carried out in the form of an official document show that marriage is a business where each party seeks to obtain its maximum profit. At the same time, love not only hates business and business, but if there are any sparks of love, commercial spirit will destroy it soon.

There comes a time when a man and a woman have no feelings for each other. They hardly tolerate living under the same roof and sometimes they are estranged from each other.

Obviously, in the continuation of this toxic relationship, the parties enter the "emotional divorce" stage. In this case, the divorce is realized, even if it was not legally done.

Depending on the social and cultural class of the parties and depending on how much public awareness they benefit from, the management of such a relationship or its termination can be subject to multiple scenarios. Sometimes the two parties, realizing the difficult situation they are in, part very amicably and then they can be good friends.

Sometimes it has even happened that after breaking the bonds of marriage and reaching a state of freedom, which is compatible with their temperaments and intellectual logic, they go back to the previous relationship (which started with love and was broken by the lever of marriage). are), they return and this time in free and normal conditions, they make a fundamental revision of their love or old feeling and they are attracted to each other and in the absence of restrictions that pushed love back, they experience the blossoming of love again.

Sometimes, due to the behavioral culture of each party, separation occurs with deep hatred and enmity. The parties begin to eliminate all signs of the presence of the other in their lives. Destroying and removing images, cutting photos of two people, removing all signs of the other's presence from the living environment, and destroying common memorials, are among the things that take place in such separations. Such behaviors are usually done by couples whose love was absent at the beginning of their lives. Otherwise, the presence of love, even at the beginning of the work and its decline due to the imposition of rules, and the separation after that, does not allow the emergence of spiteful behaviors. Because love is always and everywhere soothing. Even if it has been long gone. The memory of love can be as effective and soothing as love itself.

An important point that is usually neglected is that love, relationship, sex and private relationships between men and women are completely personal. These matters are variable and informulable in each person. In this case, how can you define the principles and basics of this relationship with a general rule and expect it to be effective and suitable for all human beings.

Marriage rules are usually defined in such a way that it brings to mind the relationship of owner and mamluk and prisoner and jailer between a man and a woman. How can there be a romantic relationship between a prisoner and a jailer? If there was a romantic relationship before marriage, how can it continue in such a framework?

Of course, there are also romantic relationships that have continued successfully even in marriage. But the subtle point here is that in most of these relationships, marriage has only served as the outer layer and outer shell. Men in love mostly ignore all the oppressive privileges that the laws of marriage give them. Their relationship is the love relationship and all the negative and positive orders defined by the marriage system are simply converted into a historical memory of the lover and the beloved in the form of a document and are deposited in the archive.

In fact, it is not the institution of marriage that has defined or enabled the successful relationship of such couples. Rather, ignoring the rules of marriage has been the secret of their success. But the problem is that there are few men who are willing to give up the privileges provided by the institution of marriage in order to save their lives and continue the growth of love. It doesn't matter whether such a document is drawn up between two people or not, if the lover and the beloved return to the original and act according to the original nature of love and continue living, the marriage document cannot poison the sapling of their love.

One of the best interpretations expressed in this context is in the poem "Fath Bagh" by Forough Farrokhzad, which is one of the few masterpieces of modern Iranian poetry. In a part of the poem, the poet refers to the "loose connection of two names" and "an embrace in the old papers of a book" and states that unity is not dependent on the connection of two names in the form of an old and obsolete book of marriage and divorce, but on the nature and The flow of love is dependent.

The poet considers the existence of such a document unnecessary and unnecessary. The presence or absence of such a document is equally important. The lover and the beloved have managed to pick the "apple of love" from the "far away actor's tree." So getting the fruit of love is not an easy task. Love is out of reach. Without love, life is nothing more than a cold and sullen hole

…everyone knows
everyone knows
that you and I are sullen from that cold opening
We saw the garden
And we picked the apple from that branch far from the hand of the actor

This is something that others don't do because of restrictions and taboos. But the lover and the beloved do and do not avoid others knowing about their discovery:

Everyone is afraid
Everyone is afraid, but me and you
We joined the light and water of the mirror
And we were not afraid

Love requires courage. If you were able to pick the "Crunchy Apple of Love" from the "Actor's Out of Hand Branch," then you must adhere to its rules as well. The rule of love is irregular. Love flows in its own channel, and in order to realize it, it is necessary to pass the conventional criteria. The criteria that the society imposes on the lover and the beloved and are generally destructive to love, should either be avoided or, in the best case, ignored:

> …talking about the loose connection of two names
> And there is no hug in the old pages of a notebook
> It is about my happy hair
> With the burned anemones of your kiss
> And the intimacy of ourselves, during the dance
> And our naked shine
> Like fish scales in water…

So the lover and the beloved have managed to have a successful relationship without the necessity of registering themselves in the old papers of the Marriage and Divorce Office and without giving in to the outdated rule that the society suggests to regulate their romantic relationship. They have succeeded in discovering the true truth of love and relationship. Just like the truth that Simerghan unveils in Qaf Haqirat. They have approached the heart of nature and made this truth and success public by following the elements of nature and the originality of human existence, which is defined in love and purity:

> …everyone knows
> everyone knows
> We have reached the cold and silent sleep of Phoenixes
> We found the truth in the garden
> In the shameful look of an unknown flower
> and survival in an infinite moment
> that two suns stared at each other.

Now that two suns are staring at each other in a natural logic and flow and the true secret of love and relationship has been discovered, this issue cannot and should not be hidden. Because love cannot be hidden and it is more valuable than being afraid and trembling and talking about it in the darkness of human ignorance and in darkness and isolation. One should open the windows of awareness and put aside useless things and superstitious thoughts and taboos and give room to love:

> There is no talk of fearful chatter in the dark
> We are talking about the day and open windows
> and fresh air
> And the oven in which useless things burn
> And the land that is fertile on the other side
> And birth and evolution and pride
> Speaking of the hands of our lover
> which is a bridge of the message of fragrance, light and breeze
> They built over the nights

Therefore, it is necessary to continue to follow the pattern of nature. According to Rumi's words, "Anyone who stays away from his origin/interrogates his connected days." Human authenticity is also summed up in nature and love. So, life should be continued based on patterns derived from nature and on the bed of love:

> Come to the meadow
> to the great meadow
> And call me, behind the breaths of silk flowers
> Still the deer with its mate
> The curtains are full of hidden malice and innocent pigeons
> From the heights of your white tower
> They look at the ground

If we express the conflict between the institution of marriage and the authenticity of love in one sentence, perhaps that sentence is that if the human race used this poem as its main manifesto to regulate the relationship between men and women, many disturbances; Including divorce and breakup of relationships, they were destroyed. This manifesto can guarantee an organic and dynamic relationship between a man and a woman, both in the form of formal marriage and outside of it. The problem is the authenticity of the action between men and women, and especially men's attention to the importance of understanding this authenticity.

In this beautiful and humane manifesto, there is no mention of a man's right to possess ownership over a woman. There is no news about the types of restrictions imposed on women based on religious and customary laws. Religious laws are not involved in the regulation of romantic relationships between men and women, and there is no news of the influence of religious teachings on the most private aspects of the relationship between men and women.

In such a world, there is only friendship and pure love. The logic of the relationship flows based on the elements of nature. Lust and love are equally present between men and women. There is no ruler or judge. There is no dominant or weak in the scene. Sex is not a one-way exploitation by a man and a forced service by a woman. Everything is based on enthusiasm. No annoying or intrusive behavior is seen. Everything is based on the "custom of life" and who does not know that all the customs and rules of life directly or indirectly rely on the behavior of nature or are based on its influence.

It is interesting that mankind follows nature and the intelligence hidden in it in all its life affairs, including its scientific achievements and inventions; but when it comes to regulating the relationship between men and women, there is no sign of nature's presence.

In the world that the poet draws, the originality of nature has the first word. Referring to nature can be the savior of mankind in the field of feelings, emotions and love. Because the field of marriage is a completely emotional, emotional and romantic matter, therefore, modeling nature is completely superior to other approaches.

What was drawn above as the ideal state of men and women is very idealistic and represents the utopia of human communication. an ideal situation; but out of reach. Human society must work harder to reach such a world. The ruins that have been built on the relationship between men and women throughout history are so many that it is not easy to rebuild them.

One of the reasons why it is difficult to reconstruct the relationship between men and women is that societies have been built and organized by men throughout history. Men set the rules and founded civilizations, cultures and subcultures.

In drawing the rules related to the relationship between men and women, they have acted in any way that is appropriate and required by their own interests. They have established unnatural rules and followed them. All these infrastructures have caused that there is no ground for deep friendship between the female and male sex. All rules and relationships are based on a misunderstanding. They have learned that they must be "husband and wife" to be together. It was never said that they could be friends with each other. Instead of friendship, an "ugly" and uncomfortable relationship has formed between a man and a woman. A relationship that is "husband and wife" at its best; but there are other modes for it. Modes that look very ugly and disgusting in a deep human view.

Throughout history, men have demystified these ugly things. Men have often learned from their ancestors to think of possessing, owning, and even raping if needed as methods of possessing women. This is despite the fact that it seems very unlikely that concepts such as possession, rape, assault and the like exist in the female subconscious mind. So it is clear that the relationship between a man and a woman is a one-way relationship from top to bottom.

In such a situation, when we talk about the rules and principles of marriage, it is obvious that they all focus on male domination and subjugation. The reason for hateful social complications such as honor killings and the like is that men actually try to defend their territory.

A man feels that his property has been violated if the woman he wants is in contact with another man. The foundations of this argument are quite clear. We imagine that instead of a woman, there is a man in this relationship. The relationship between two men is firstly based on friendship, secondly it is not defined based on ownership. Therefore, if a man's friend breaks up with him and becomes friends with another man, the idea of violence and things like murder seems ridiculous. But this situation is quite common for women.

The relationship between man and man is not based on possession. It has been like this since the beginning of history. For this reason, we have not seen honor killings even in the case of sexual relations between two men due to the termination of sexual relations and the establishment of a relationship with a third party. Because the relationship between man and man is not based on ownership. Man-to-man relationship, even sexual, is based on equality. The two sides of the scale are completely equal and both enjoy equal status and equal rights.

So, we are faced with an unequal relationship in marriage. Marriage tries to regularize and systematize this unequal relationship and record them and even add to its dimensions.

If we look through the glasses of realism, in practice, the work of women who indulge in forced relationships (of course, if there is no love and friendship) is no different from prostitution. A man's relationship with a prostitute is also based on the rule of ownership. He takes possession of a woman for a certain amount of money for a certain time. In the absence of love, a man takes possession of a woman for an indefinite period of time in return for some money, property or reciprocal services and calls it marriage.

The main problem here is that men's minds are poisoned due to inappropriate historical upbringing and contain wide deviations. In their private circles, men use statements about women that are sometimes very embarrassing.

That rule and this perverted mind has caused the way women look at men, always with a certain amount of misunderstanding.

Maybe this is the reason for the old enmity and the sarcastic words of the man in our story in that car. This misunderstanding, in the absence of love, over time hides the relationship between a married man and a woman in a cloud of hatred and enmity.

Many divorces, which occur with a great deal of hatred, are the result of the marriage itself. Because marriage is firstly a property relationship and secondly a relationship based on need and economy. The way out of this difficult situation is for humans to accept that a certain amount of love and friendship is always necessary for any kind of relationship between a man and a woman.

The Achilles heel of women in marriage is lack of financial independence. If patriarchal social relations allowed women to have financial independence and appear alongside men in social arenas, men could not use their means of conquest to transform the rule of marriage into a rule of ownership. No one can have what he owns as a lover. You can love objects and necessities of life and goods; but you can't love them. In other words, the distance between a healthy and unhealthy relationship is the distance between loving and loving. Those who love their spouses, but are not in love with them, are in such a state of suspense.

For centuries, men have not allowed women to have education, business, employment and financial independence. For the simple reason that they are interested in loving women and not in love with them. Because love brings responsibility. Love means the unity and equalization of two people in all of your being. A person cannot love someone who has already reduced him to the level of objects. He has bargained for him and denied his values in order to pay less money. Determining the amount of dowry and shirbaha (bride price) and haggling over their material values are only limited symbols of a broad behavioral culture within which marriage takes place. The problems that are brought to the rule of marriage from a philosophical and emotional point of view include such cases.

Men's mistake has been that they have imagined that women need them only because of the problems of livelihood and economic dependence, and out of gratitude they may love their man to the extent of worship. But history does not remember that the price of a material good is something like love.

If the sense of ownership disappears, the relationship between man and woman will be defined by the concept of friendship and love. In such a situation, as depicted in Forough Farrokhzad's poem, relationships will revolve around different concepts and feelings.

When a man loves a woman, a woman will also love a man. In this case, both will try to make the lover happy and satisfied by resorting to all possible means. In such a situation, assuming it is impossible, if a woman finds her happiness with another man, the man will not only resort to force and violence, but will also accept the happiness of her lover and her feelings and interests.

It is true that separation is a complicated and painful phenomenon; but far from a possessive feeling, it will never lead to violence and disgusting phenomena like honor killings. It is acceptable that when a man and a woman separate, it is the man who is offended, his feelings are offended; but we should not forget that freedom is the greatest and highest human value. The possessive feeling that leads to pressure and violence against women is completely against the spirit of freedom.

The rules of marriage, in their most civilized form, unimaginably limit a woman's freedom and make her a prisoner without shackles. When a woman feels that pressure and the possibility of violence and cumbersome rules have potentially violated her freedom, she will always be in an aura of feeling imprisoned.

Citizenship rights and civil liberties follow this philosophy. A citizen may not face the dictatorial rules of dictatorial governments and governmental oppression and violence in his life. But it is certain that such a possibility exists for him and this possibility will always keep him in a state of fear and stress. If his neighbor faces violence and repression and is subject to organized oppression, and he benefits from a safe margin for any reason, this does not mean his freedom and benefit from the blessing of democracy. In fact, the possibility of facing oppression and deprivation of freedom is like the sword of Damocles over his head, even though it will not fall on his head throughout his life.

In the case of women who think that they are far from the possibility of violence and oppression in their personal lives, such a rule also applies. Women who live under the constraints of marriage in regressive societies, under the possibility of violence and a sense of majesty, there is always a feeling around them that they will suffer from complications caused by such an atmosphere. Now, whether this sword of Damocles falls on them or not, it does not negate the fact that such a sword is on their heads.

When there is no love and friendship in the relationship between a man and a woman, a woman's soul is offended from the inside. He endures for a while in the cramped cage that was made for him. Due to the tyranny and rigid rules of marriage, he continues for a while, but eventually, his patience runs out. At this time, even if he cannot express his displeasure, inside, he cultivates hatred that makes life unbearable. It is difficult and painful to imagine a woman who is forced to have sex with a man at the same time as he has internal hatred, caused by the tyrannical environment and subservient desires.

In such a situation, even the question of whether the man is good or bad does not solve the problem. A good man in an anti-woman social structure inadvertently becomes an intolerable dictatorship. It is even possible that a man is a good person, loving and tolerant; but he does not know how unequal and inhumane the rules imposed on women are.

In this situation, if two parties ignore the conventional frameworks with the help of love and friendship and define a specific individual framework for themselves, they can manage the romantic relationship between them and continue living based on their personal principles and standards.

This state requires understanding, knowledge and a kind of self-sacrifice from the man. This self-sacrifice does not mean that a man passes his desires; rather, it is the ability and self-esteem that makes her leave the imposed rights granted and draw her relationship in a different way so that under it, an ideal and normal life is possible for women.

Such mutual freedom is so effective in optimizing biological relations and humanizing the relationship that the parties will be surprised by this miraculous action. Such an ideal means the realization of the fantasy of heaven on this earth.

When the relationship between a man and a woman is regulated by a free flow of joy, the vicious cycle we talked about will be able to be repaired and restored. The lover and the beloved will have promises and appointments for their future and life, and they will definitely fulfill these promises and appointments; but when the jurists and preachers try to enforce these promises and appointments under the outdated laws of thousands of years, they are actually cutting the feathers of the dove of love, which is supposed to bring the green olive branch of happiness to the shore of this couple's life.

One of the most important behaviors that have been popularized by men in the form of subcultures, and unfortunately women have also fallen into the trap of this apparently civilized behavior, is that men must take the lead in getting married. The hidden philosophy in this social behavior is that the man, as the authority and decision-maker, takes the first step to marry a woman who is in a passive position. The false meaning behind this social act is that it seems that such an act is consistent with the dignity and modesty of a woman.

If we are to accept that men and women are equal in every aspect, women can also use their freedom of action and take steps to get married or establish a relationship. In some population colonies and social groups, we have witnessed this courage and freedom of action from women, which ironically resulted in the formation of stable relationships and marriages.

The women who have taken the first step to get married and have been the proposers have had so much character and freedom that they considered the position of men and women to be completely equal and did not follow their passive state.

It is not clear where the root of this idea is: if a woman goes to a man, it is not compatible with his modesty and modesty? This is despite the fact that if a woman breaks this taboo and wrong idea and proposes marriage to the man she likes more. Above all, he has proven his courage and should be respected more than others and characterized by sobriety.

In criticizing the traditional marriage system, it is enough that if two people decide to be with each other with desire and love, there is enough suitable material for the formation of a relationship. What better if this relationship lasts as long as their lifetime! But if there comes a time when they feel that staying together means bitter experience of unhelpful incompatibilities, there is no reason to continue the relationship.

If the relationship is consolidated in the form of traditional marriage, there is no problem. The problem starts from the fact that the little things and guidelines of the traditional system cause the healthy relationship of the parties to be gradually damaged. Because this traditional system does not respect women's rights and gives men an excuse to fight in the realm of inequality they have created for him.

Love, Sex, Marriage, Free Relationship

Consider a young man and woman who meet at a multi-day conference. Their relatively long relationships lead to the creation of a kind of interest that can be called love or "love." They both like each other. They make a dinner date and finally end up in a hotel room and spend the night together. Both of them are young, single and very likely to get married. But should any kind of relationship like this lead to marriage?

This is a question that religious people have a definite answer to. These two must marry each other and preferably not have sex before marriage. But the problem is that during the acquaintance they have had with each other and according to the experience of sex, they do not think that they are good options for each other as husband and wife.

The way that religion puts in front of these two is that they must marry each other in any case, even at the cost of the fact that after some time, personality heterogeneity and asymmetries are revealed and the capacity of acceptance of both sides is over and they divorce each other. It is quite clear that religion and traditional thinking do not have an intermediate path in similar situations. They love each other now. are ready to have a pleasant relationship; but there are no conditions for marriage in them. The religion's answer is self-restraint, sexual abstinence and abstinence.

Modern human reason has found another solution for this problem. This solution is well established in Western countries and is being developed to Eastern societies. The sex of these two in the hotel can be the starting point and at the same time the ending point of the relationship. A relationship that can have tragic results if it leads to marriage.

Religion and traditional thinking also advises them to avoid contraceptives and any attempt to prevent pregnancy. Therefore, the process of pregnancy is assumed in every sex. The result of this recommendation is clear. A temporary life whose destiny is known from the beginning. Also, the birth of a child who must enter the life cycle without one of the parents and in unstable and unsecured conditions.

The Open West Society proposal is to have an open relationship without children and end this relationship after the end of the conference. These two should search for their ideals in the continuation of their life and possible marriage elsewhere. It is obvious that sexual austerity and negative response to all sensual events that may occur during the life of any human being is not accepted by common sense. Therefore, free relationships have become one of the main options of sexual life in free societies.

The benefits and achievements of free sex of the kind we mentioned in the above example are many. Including:

- Preventing the formation of a disorderly marriage and entering into a troublesome process that disturbs their social priorities and main goals in life.
- Preventing the birth of unwanted and abused children, and as a result, creating social crises and educational disorders and lack of quality control of children.
- Preventing divorce as a social problem by preventing inappropriate marriage.
- Preventing ascetic life and self-inflicted sexual deprivation, which may have unpleasant psychological and social consequences in the long run. If the complications and symptoms of this type of deprivation can be seen well in closed societies.

In our example, a man may believe that he has found his ideal partner and that he can live a pleasant and desirable life with her. But the woman's opinion is something else. She believes that according to the inner moods, interests and character of the man, he is not a suitable option for a long-term life in the form of marriage. The woman is interested in spending a happy night with him and at the end of this period, each of them will go to their destiny.

Sexual attraction is still present. They have had extensive fantasies about having a good night and testing their sexual experiences and skills and getting the pleasure they deserve. Both of them are single, beautiful, sexually active, in need of sexual action, respectable citizens, have weight and social prestige and are experiencing the best time of their lives.

The barrier that religion places between these two people does not follow any rational, social or physiological logic. Religion says that you should not have sexual contact. If you love each other, you should get married. Your sex must lead to the birth of a child. You cannot delay the process of pregnancy (even for a short period of time and you need to plan for the years ahead of your life). A woman should change her way of life and abandon her work and career goals and soon enter the painful period of pregnancy and stay at home.

A woman should give birth to her child after 9 months and start breastfeeding and spend the following years raising the child. From the point of view of religion, the heavy price that a woman has to pay for this interest of a few days and this sex is not important. This is the guidance that religion has for the woman in question and emphasizes on it. The other side of this coin is sexual abstinence, sexual austerity, giving up the pleasures that nature has placed in men and women, and suppressing instincts and natural desires. But why and at what cost? This is a question that the institution of religion does not have an answer for.

A woman can spend a night with a man. They can experience the pleasure that is worthy of their freshness and youth and that fate has provided for them. A woman follows her long-term plan for her life. He achieves his goals and successes. In favorable conditions and time, based on her long-term planning, she marries a person who is suitable for her in every way, becomes a good mother, forms a family and ends her life in a humane and favorable condition.

Religion has more strictures for women. He has no other way. Either she should give up this love and pleasure, or she should marry an undesirable man who is temporarily interested and attracted to her, even with the certainty that it may ruin her married life.

The scenario of religion is similar for men. But he has more notes and points in mind. He can give up this occasional love and sex, but use the gifts of patriarchal society to satisfy his sexual needs with little money or effort.

In Eastern and religious societies, men have even more options. He can have sex workers under the name of "temporary marriage" or "concubine." Even after marriage, he can invite other women to bed besides his wife. Law and custom support him for this sexual diversity.

But in the hypothetical relationship of our scenario, there are blessings for the man that cannot come anywhere else. He has to be patient to find another position and try his luck again, in which case he will face the same impasse again at the critical moment. He should seek sex with other people whose bodies can be bought. But there is no gift of love. Sex without love and without sparks of human feeling and inner waves of a deep desire is an act of polygamy.

Sex for money, which is called prostitution, may be considered a depraved and inhuman act for any decent and sober man. So, if the man we are looking for is a lecherous and characterless person, he can choose the second way; but if he is a dignified man with moral and human qualities, the suggested way of religion and all informal methods will be closed.

For him, this love is the best and most ideal kind of intercourse at this moment, due to the knowledge that has been made and the sincere feeling that has been created. In an emotionless sex, the partner (male or female) will feel that his body is being abused. What the religion refers to as "enjoyment" is exactly the promotion of this emotional unrestrainedness and real prostitution. A man can "sexually exploit" another woman by following the options set before him by religion. But he, who is a man who adheres to morals and is free from vices, cannot accept humiliation and emotional unrestrainedness. Therefore, the proposal that the Western society has reached is still the best solution.

A free relationship with a woman he loves is accompanied by moral blessings and achievements: a great amount of love, mutual belonging, sharing in a natural pleasure that is the right of both parties, and a relationship with honesty and free from moral corruption.

How can society and religion offer another solution to the man and woman in our scenario, who can have love, personality, morals, modesty and not ruin the rest of their lives at the same time? There is no answer except to have a healthy and free relationship based on the demands and standards accepted by both parties.

Regardless of the fact that the relationship between the man and the woman in our scenario does not lead to marriage, they will probably only have a short relationship based on their moral standards, this relationship can be the most appropriate in terms of the macro standards of society and morality and virtue.

We examine the moral differences of this hypothetical relationship with a relationship in the form of a traditional marriage without love, list-wise:

- In such a relationship, the parties are in a completely equal and similar situation. No one has moral or social superiority over the other. There is no giver and taker. Sex is completely cooperative and the parties have the same exploitation of it.

- Sex is accompanied by a considerable amount of spice of love. Both parties heartily desire this relationship based on their physical and emotional needs, and therefore sex can be full of ideal components for a harmonious and sensual experience. Both are in the same situation based on their desires.

- Gender equality and non-dominance of one gender over another is established. All in all, no one can imagine a worse or better situation.

- Fear, blame, moral condemnation or special economic or social requirements do not govern this relationship.

- If the parties have a perfect personality match to make this relationship permanent, this small model can be a clear example of a successful marriage or stable relationship. But it is not.

- External forces such as taboos, religious teachings, assistance or mediation of third parties and generally the interference of external elements have no place in this relationship.

- This relationship is formed spontaneously and based on human needs and instincts, and therefore it is the best type of relationship.

- This relationship does not bring annoying feelings and emotions such as heartbreak, guilt, failure, exploitation, hypocrisy, and abuse, and it will not lead to these issues in the future.

- Pretending to love, lies, rules and contractual affairs have no role in this relationship.
- There is no need for special planning and preparations and delays for this relationship.
- This relationship does not create a burden on the shoulders of the parties, and entering and exiting it can be recorded as an attractive adventure in the life experience of the parties.
- This relationship cannot lead to the feeling of "abandonment" after sex, because the same conditions of the parties and the logic of behavior governing it are normal.
- A favorable sexual experience like this can relieve them from negative emotions and daily fatigue and routine form of life while reducing daily stress. The positive effects of positive sexual experiences have been proven by psychological science to strengthen people's psyche.

The list we mentioned above includes the positive achievements of a healthy romantic sex, which is temporary and transitory due to the impossibility of marriage. In front of these two lists, there is a set of disorders and negative points, which is the second form of this scenario; That is, it follows the suggestion of religion and tradition.

With all this said, it is not clear, based on which logical argument and which long-term achievement, religion continues to go its way and without any flexibility and without adapting its proposed models to the living conditions of the modern era, it continues to insist on an outdated method?

Love and Betrayal: Two Sides of the Same Coin

The fact is that love and betrayal cannot be two sides of the same coin. Betrayal happens in the vacuum of love, not on the other side of it. This does not mean that when there is love, infidelity never happens. Rather, it is precisely telling that if betrayal occurs, it is clearly a sign of the absence of love. Love may have once been present in this place; but not now. So betrayal is not the coin of love; but it is another coin.

The crisis of betrayal becomes colorful when love is present. Until around the 18th century, humanity had not yet included the category of love in the subject of marriage. Marriage was a social and even economic and utilitarian matter. These interests fluctuated from having a suitable roof, having a family and children, supporting and being supported economically, to having the possibility of sex in the family environment, to the external and social aspects of being married. But among all these elements, love was not present.

It seems that in such a situation, it is easy to understand the nature of betrayal and cope with it. There is no agreement indicating inner affection and meeting of soul and feeling and no romantic desire. A link to make life better is closed in the form of marriage. The parties provide services to each other. Marriage is a kind of collaboration to facilitate the flow of life and benefit from its blessings. Better food, better sleep, permanent and exclusive sex, reproduction, social status, etc. are part of this facilitation process.

There is no emotional commitment. Feminine beauty is a commodity that can be bought. Beauty complements the quality of sex. A woman's health guarantees the health of children, the social position of a man and complements the social status of the opposite party. In the absence of activism of love, age cannot be an important criterion. Of course, as long as it does not interfere with other elements such as health, sexual ability and beauty.

With the emergence of the new bourgeois philosophy, in the 18th century, love came to the fore. Among the social classes, love became not only the main reason for marriage, but also an important moral justification for the necessity of marriage and the priorities of mate selection. Among two equal and identical men, a person deserves to marry the desired girl who is more loving and affectionate. Of course, provided that the girl is also in love with him.

Therefore, flirting and creating attraction as an important skill among young people became a tool for romantic competition and supremacy. An issue that could be used in the bourgeoisie and among the nobility as a determining factor in destinies.

In this way, marriage changed from a purely social institution to a romantic situation. That is, the influence of the outside world on the phenomenon of marriage decreased and the inner and emotional worlds played a more colorful role.

With the presence of the element of love and emotion, qualitative factors were also added to this arena. Love must be genuine and real. Demonstrators were hateful and immoral people who sought to deceive girls and fake marriage with absurd and unrealistic feelings.

With the predominance of this current, the bourgeois ethics went toward changes in the educational foundations of children. They had to learn to be sincere and honest in expressing their romantic feelings. In this way, a version of betrayal was manifested that included betrayal of feelings. Playing with a woman's feelings with an expression of love, devoid of originality, was a betrayal that was condemned by the modern bourgeois society. The intensity of this confrontation was so much that it could sometimes lead to the formation of a duel.

In this way, young men and women were getting ready for marriage and courtship by emphasizing this strict and emotional aspect. But the matter did not end here. The issue of authenticity of feeling after marriage remained strong. Men should continuously show their affection and love to their wives in a sincere and real way and in this direction, they should not give up any efforts.

In this way, love became a mixture of originality and at the same time abstinence and austerity. A process that was clearly in conflict with the hormonal changes and emotional changes of humans. Therefore, in Western societies, having a steady girlfriend, without the first wife knowing, became a hidden social behavior. Men tried to adjust their outer life with their inner and family life so as to cause the least damage to their public image and women's human feelings. Especially considering the fate and happiness of children in the form of a family was also important.

This kind of external loyalty, although from the point of view of human internal morality, could involve challenges; but in the end, it worked for the benefit of the family and society. Because loyalty had become a valuable and praiseworthy category that could influence people's status and social respect.

Chapter Six
The History of Male Tyranny

Humans of Every Gender Are Organs of One Body

When it comes to human beings, the differences and distinctions between men and women are definitely not important. But this belief is not institutionalized in the upstream texts. In the upstream texts and fundamental thoughts developed in the pages of these books by intellectual and cultural centers of gravity, men and women are not equal examples of the concept of "human."

What is referred to today as the differences between men and women is a kind of precipitation of patriarchal actions that is not rooted in the nature and essence of human creation. Regardless of the desirable differences that bring the concept of woman and the concept of man to the fore as two complementary qualities, male and female beauties are rooted in these desirable differences.

The problem begins when these differences in some cultures and in the opinion of the supporters of historical patriarchy become an excuse to divide the human race into "weak and submissive sex" and "strong, commanding sex."

Intellectually and culturally influential people of human society are divided into two categories so far, the first group are those who, while being original, are producers of thought, and the second group are those who are promoters of other people's thoughts. Ideas such as the "good submissive and pious woman," according to which a woman should be defined by labels such as submissiveness, piety and goodness, are promoted more by those who are promoters of thought rather than its producers.

According to such thinking, a woman is basically like a shoe for a man, which must be suitable for a man's life to be spent well and happily. In this case, a successful and happy man is one who wears the right shoes. Otherwise: "Being barefoot is better than tight shoes."

Like all the fields of life in the past centuries, the field of thought production has also been in the hands of men. In both types of divisions mentioned, men have had the opportunity for many centuries to place the archetype of the "bad woman" in world culture as the activist of Ma Yasha. The issue is not to not talk about the concept of "bad woman"; rather, the question is why has never been written about the "bad man" and its effects in a woman's life. Otherwise, there is no doubt that according to Saadi:

Benevolent woman is very good
But bad woman, God forbid

There is no doubt that there are differences in the creation of men and women. These differences generally include the exclusive characteristics of each gender compared to other genders and do not include aspects of superiority and differentiation. If we look realistically, there are more exclusive features in the woman's creation, which makes the man have less exclusive features.

One of these traits is a woman's ability to create life. Without women, the cycle of existence will stop at once and human life will come to an end. But the man has tried to ignore these issues in order to cover his weakness and to cover up the physical superiority of the woman, in an obvious confusion. In addition to being natural and meeting public needs, women need men's support in a double way during pregnancy, and men have made the most use of this issue for the benefit of developing the dimensions of their dominance.

The only factor in which men are absolutely superior is muscular strength. Apparently, the logical rule that proves the leadership of a man is as follows: any creature that is stronger is the leader, the man is stronger, so the man is the leader. But there is an error in the structure of this logical argument.

If we say that any creature that is stronger is the boss, then the man is the boss. In the second base of this equation, an intentional error is included. If any creature with stronger muscles can be superior, then dinosaurs must be the undisputed rulers of the earth; but they are extinct.

So, male history is exploiting a logical rule, which basically has problems. But men have been able to rely on this baseless argument, turn women into the second sex and the weak and dependent sex and forget the potentials and superiority of women.

Man has been able to use a major part of women's superior potential as a driving force against him. The capacity for love in women is much higher than in men. Love and even sex in women is a deep action that goes beyond the boundaries of her sexual organs and physical presence and reaches the depths and becomes a spiritual and holy matter.

This problem has caused it to be distasteful for a woman to make love and make love with multiple men, so the female soul is in conflict with multiple sexual partners; At the same time, her body is much more capable of managing relationships with multiple sexual partners than men. But the woman has not used her abilities to create a superior position of sex and diversity.

A man is physically weaker to communicate with multiple sexual partners. However, his sexual adventures are more. The reason for this physical-behavioral conflict is that the woman is generally a more moral being and it is the man who is the symbol of sin and sensuality. This fact is exactly the opposite of what man has been promoting since the beginning of creation, with all his tools.

The advantage that a man has created for himself, in the ups and downs of life, has become a factor for creating rights. A right that has been manifested, for example, in the form of polygamy. So, as we can see, men have been able to continuously realize their weaknesses and women's high capacities and exploit them in line with their interests.

We said that the male society has used many tools and instruments to consolidate these discriminatory equations. Beliefs, religion, superstitions, customs, rituals, traditions, superstitious relations, tribal relations and similar things are among the tools that have been used to oppress women and put her natural rights in line with her and turn her into the second sex.

Polygamy, accepted in various forms in different societies, is supported by some religions. If we look at the phenomenon of polygamy without all its accessories and labels, there is practically no difference between men and women in enjoying polygamy. When two people get married as human beings, there is no difference between being a man or a woman. Loyalty in the form of monogamy is one of the hundreds of commitments that two people make to each other. Now, when the marriage does not succeed and one of the couples goes to a third party, the huge difference between the society's reaction to men and women is because it has considered this right for men to have multiple sexual partners.

In front of all the tools and achievements and excuses that men have had throughout history to overcome women, the women's society has been mostly defenseless. To the extent that men have been able to somehow push the issue of women into their domain and take great steps toward owning women. Polygamy can be interpreted exactly from this point of view. Conventionally, one car cannot have multiple drivers, but one driver (owner) can own multiple cars.

The approach of men in their biological relations with women is completely holistic. This issue has even extended to non-material matters such as love. In addition to being perfectionist, the man's view is materialistic and non-spiritual compared to the woman's. Because when faced with the category of love, a woman pays attention to the inner quality of her lover, and a man pays more attention to the physical and non-spiritual condition.

A man is generally an ugly creature, but a woman loves him. It is difficult to imagine that men can tolerate a creature like him. A man sees a woman as a beautiful being and can love her. He is constantly comparing. Comparison is a characteristic of the transactional and totalitarian mind. Comparing one product with another. But women do not compare. Because if a comparison is to be made, the woman should compare the man with herself or another woman, in this case, the beauty and ugliness of the man will be revealed. But a woman's mind does not compare. A woman's mind is receptive to love (regardless of external beauty) because of her high human dignity.

We see that the woman is closer to the logic and meaning of love and mysticism. For this reason, he is probably closer to the Creator of existence and metaphysics (in its spiritual sense). But the irony of history is that women, with all these dignities and existential capacities, have almost no place in important fields, even intellectual and emotional realms such as religion and mysticism. Religion is a completely male thing. In the puzzle of the Trinity, or for example, among the 124 thousand prophets who have appeared on earth, the name of a woman is not observed.

A woman's mind, at least, does not compare matters related to love and spirituality. It is that it does not claim advantages like polygamy. He is deep in love and his permanence in a relationship has more depth and durability.

Should the Female Soul Be Loved Only?

To talk about the female psyche with its enormous energy and influence, it is not possible to speak from a man's point of view. Because in order to judge the female psyche, we will not go anywhere without removing the historical sediments that have poisoned the human mental space throughout the ages.

When we can talk about the nature, identity and psyche of a woman in a precise and unbiased way and without the interference of destructive factors, that we pass the level of a body and the mind dependent on it and reach the level of knowledge and consciousness.

What was deposited in human nature at the beginning of creation, with an almost majority, has a human nature and not physical and sexual. Phenomena such as human mentality, human body, human knowledge and many similar cases, cannot fit into the conventional male and female divisions. But besides this absolute equality, the female soul has given other forces to life.

What binds men and women regardless of their gender is beyond the limited realms of sex. This force is a transcendental element that is the central core of human creation and the center of gravity of existence and consists of a great and eternal knowledge. When the fountain of human life is connected to such a source, the mystic and the beneficiary of knowledge cannot include transverse and unstable elements such as gender, physical difference, differences and needs in defining the existential nature of a person (whether male or female).

When we are going to talk about women as half of the human species, if we don't wear the veils and masks that keep us away from the aforementioned identity, it will be impossible to talk about the nature of women as human beings.

If we consider human existence as a mechanical machine, the differences and basic differences in the physical creation of men and women are insignificant compared to the similar aspects. However, beyond the general nature of creation, the female spirit is a double component in the dictionary of life whose task is to refine life and advance its grand goals.

In addition to these, in the creation of man and woman, so many factors and symptoms from two different poles are interwoven that it can be said that a relative woman exists in every man and a relative man continues to exist in the foundation of every woman. We refer to this issue in more detail elsewhere in this book.

Poets, mystics, even philosophers and thinkers have made many attempts to express the issue we are discussing. That single form and that "indefinable" quality, which is the center of gravity of human life and the common essence between men and women, has been expressed with different interpretations. Expressions that, for example, in Sohrab Sepehri's mysticism and gaze are expressed with two deep expressions "intelligence" and "look."

Wherever there are higher degrees of understanding, consciousness, intuition, mysticism and celibacy, most definitions and frameworks such as male and female, gender and physicality, lost color and macro-inclusive interpretations;

Such as "consciousness," "intelligence," "truth," "essence," "spirit" and the like are used to express the quality of creation.

If we look at the category of women from this angle, then we will see that many positions and approaches of society regarding women are contradictory. Even the most developed and honest opinions expressed about women fall within the circle of fundamental criticism. In their approach to women, various thinkers have even used phrases that justify the difference between men and women and the exercise of male authority out of good faith and good thinking.

Osho, the Indian philosopher and theoretician, who presented the most advanced sociological and anthropological theories about women, sex, marriage and the like, said in a comment: "A woman should be loved and not understood." This way of thinking is very progressive; but at the same time, it unintentionally carries discrimination. If we accept that the same nature that we speak of as "human intelligence" or "human essence" determines most of the examples and conflicts, then loving a woman because she is simply a woman is a derogatory concept or it is authoritarian.

Therefore, if we are going to talk about love, it is better to say "man and woman, regardless of physicality and gender, should love each other." Loving a woman with the position expressed in the above sentence carries with it the suspicion that she is a commodity. It seems that woman is a different creature from human (man) who needs to be loved by us and is a weak creature who is perfected by our understanding and attention.

He says in another place: "If you want to change a woman's opinion, agree with her! If you want to know what a woman really means, look at her, don't listen to her." Although these attitudes seem benevolent and progressive in nature; but in their hearts, they unwittingly continue the same views that have existed for centuries; Looking from top to bottom and looking at the weaker sex or different sex.

In this context, there is no significant difference between different cultures. Language, subcultures, art, literature and human history indicate this way of thinking.

These are just a few examples of the data that tells us that in a man's history, it is always the woman who may be wrong. Now, in another frequent mistake, some modern feminists use the logic of "a woman should only be loved" to deal with such a situation. While basically this logic is in line with the past situation and not against it.

Suppression of Women, Instead of Competition and Opportunity

It is clear that in the realm of sex, men have not been able to compete with women. On the other hand, the physical ability of the man and the lack of need for deep sex, for reproduction, has often tipped the scales in favor of the man.

The possibilities and levers of power have always been in the hands of men, and he does not see the need to give in to such a competition, rather he tries to shirk his responsibility and make more room for himself by suppressing women and denying her power and supremacy.

The man tries to compensate for the feeling of inferiority caused by his weakness by restricting the woman as much as possible. Therefore, history is full of discrimination and oppression of women. A woman is a high-flying eagle whose wings are continuously arranged so that despite the cruelty and oppression she is subjected to, she remains as a tool of entertainment and a pigeon in the hands of a man in his territory.

By picking the feathers of some of their high-flying pigeons, professional pigeon fanciers try to limit the height and range of their flight and keep them in their territory. This is the behavior that has been done to women in human history. In fact, the man has treated the woman as his pet, which is part of his property and has benefits in terms of making life easier.

To facilitate this acquisition and restriction in various societies, cultures and religions, various documents have been used, of which the above items are only a part.

It has been said that in ancient China, men believed that women did not have an independent soul. Therefore, her life is improvisational and dependent on men. Because of this, a man can even kill her without worrying about the law's intervention or reaction. Honor killings are often based on the philosophy that women are part of a man's property. This behavior, contrary to what some sociologists say, is rooted in this belief system.

It is natural that when a woman is a part of a man's property, she can do any kind of interference with him like her other property. In some cultures, a woman does not have the right to remarry after the death of her husband. In fact, an independent identity has not been defined for women. Her existence is dependent on the existence of men. In Jahili Arab societies, a man could have as many slaves as his finances allowed. When a man owns a woman as a slave, he can sexually exploit her without her consent and without any human rituals. Burying girls alive is part of the philosophy of ownership in Jahili Arab societies. A philosophy according to which, the condition of women, girls, and children was ruled by the authority of the religious family with the center of the man.

Men, in order to deepen as much as possible this proprietary domination, have made a great historical effort by resorting to the tools at their disposal. In this regard, religion has helped to suppress women. In fact, most of the customary and legal rules that are rooted in religion are humiliating toward women and even the literature used in the writing of these rules and regulations is also insulting.

For example, in the ruling on temporary marriage, which is referred to as "muta" (sexual exploitation of women), we see that from the beginning to the end of this jurisprudence, the least respect for women was not respected. The word "Muta" means to benefit and exploit. This expression shows that the purpose of this rule is that a man can exploit a woman for a short period of time.

The main purpose of this rule is sexual pleasure. In the explanation of this rule, it is clearly stated that this agreement is a kind of transaction to buy sexual pleasure and use a woman's body, and human, romantic, social philosophy and the like are never hidden in it. In the description of this ruling, it is said that the obligatory works of Muta are as follows:

- Obliging the man to pay the dowry (sex fee) to the woman during exploitation.
- Establishing a woman's legal ownership of dowry and the right to claim it.
- Obliging the woman to observe the Idaho in the temporary marriage, in case of the expiration or death of the man.
- Obliging the man to register a temporary marriage if the woman becomes pregnant during the marriage. (That is, with the

presence of the child, the woman's identity, which was unimportant, finds a reason for a valuable review.)
- Obliging the woman to obey the man in general and special and obliging the man to pay alimony.

As it was said before, if a woman generally has more knowledge, awareness and general understanding, she will avoid giving into such conditions. An informed woman will recognize how insulting and negating her human identity is. Therefore, he will not only allow himself to be the tool of this male collective collusion, but will also fight against this discrimination and disrespect.

But the man still wants to maintain his one-sided status. Therefore, he always tries to close the doors of awareness to women. He tries to introduce the desired woman as "veiled," "in hijab." A woman who has "never seen the sun and the moon" with zero social experience is a more desirable commodity. This is the same concept that lies in the phrase "to be bound" to describe other goods.

Referring to Persian language, folklore, popular literature and even Persian literature shows how rich these cultural resources are with the above concepts. The effort of the oriental man is so exaggerated that he institutionally equates the issue of "innocence" with the issue of "veil." The combined addition of "Veil of Innocence" is based on this thinking.

I knew about Yusuf's ever-increasing goodness
which will take Zulikha's love out of the curtain of innocence

Consistent cultural data also try to relate the fact that women should be veiled to an eternal and eternal issue and the result of the philosophy of creation:

This was God's decree when he created roses and flowers
The first is a beauty in public view and the second remains behind the curtain

In fact, the Eastern veiled woman has a small share of a distant sky, which the hanging of the veil deprives her of. This is how a man deprives a woman of education and confines her to a fence, curtain and hijab. The fate of Eastern women and girls in Afghanistan is one of the clear examples of the rule of this thinking over women. The man tries not to make the woman financially independent. In this case, her reliance on men will decrease. If a woman is not financially dependent on a man, then in long-term relationships such as marriage, love, along with other factors such as equality, respect and common interests, it will guarantee the survival of a relationship and its stability.

It is no wonder that in Eastern societies, officially and legally, these powers are absolutely granted to men along with powers such as the right to divorce. In fact, some religious and legal laws, which are a bit difficult to interpret, are related to this course that we are talking about. For example, the double inheritance rights of a male child compared to a female child is one of the levers to complete this oppressive architecture that has built a large prison for women throughout history.

In the history of dealing with women, sometimes we come across things that are not easy for a wise person to understand. For example, what has happened to Indian women in the Sati system shows how inhuman the treatment of some societies and religions has been. We already mentioned that in such cases, the term "animal" can never be used according to the existing custom. And we explained that the behavior of animals toward the female sex is progressive and based on nature.

Even regarding respect for women and placing women as the center of gravity of the society and the colony, animals have brought perfect examples to the fore. The matriarchal system in the society and life of bees, ants, elephants, whales, spiders, chimpanzees and the like is a complete manifestation of the authority and management of the female sex in the colony or family.

Anyway, in the system of Sati, which was declared obsolete and illegal nearly 200 years ago, the "lost wife" was required to commit herself to the flames in the ritual of mourning for her husband. Interestingly, this heinous inhumane behavior has been mentioned as "a ritual with cultural and religious importance" in the religious system of the Indian region, and it has been considered as a sign of the wife's loyalty to her husband.

Sometimes in such relationships, the nature of the action is not disputed. Rather, its one strain is being discussed. That is, in the language and social norms that show inequality, the lack of "equal institutions" are completely indicative of the situation. In the following example, let's assume that extreme fidelity between a couple is acceptable. But this loyalty is only a woman's duty and a man has no role in it? Only the woman should commit herself to the flames in mourning for her husband, often a man can go to another woman immediately after the death of his wife.

On the other hand, although apparently this ritual behavior was done voluntarily, due to the social hegemony caused by the dominance of taboos and religious demagoguery, it was almost impossible for a woman not to do this. Interestingly, women, as the second gender, have never been able to gain a special human position beyond what is defined by custom, even if they have a high social status. For this reason, this custom has been implemented in a single way both for ordinary women and for women of the elite class.

Although the religious ritual of Sati was finally abolished two hundred years ago after centuries, unfortunately this anti-feminist thinking has continued in the last two centuries due to the fact that it is powered by the same intellectual background that we have described. Tribal systems, which are the biggest source of power for reactionary thinking in the Middle East and West Asia and the Indian subcontinent, have faced huge tragedies in women's social life.

Tribal beliefs in the remote parts of Iran and the countries of the region are still dynamic and even with the migration of population colonies to the central areas, they have survived in these areas and sometimes bring disastrous results that are not dissimilar to the performance of the Sati system.

A tangible replica of the functioning of this social system and its survival conflict in the face of the wave of modernism can be seen in the movie *Bride of Fire*, which was made in 1378. This film, which is based on one of the tribal traditions, deals with forced family marriage.

Ahlam is an Arab girl from Khuzestan who studied medicine outside her hometown in Ahvaz and is a knowledgeable and educated girl. She tries to convince her illiterate cousin to give up his right to forced family marriage due to educational and cultural differences and most importantly, due to the lack of love between them. It is impossible for her and her cousin to marry. But according to the tradition of the tribe, Farhan considers himself the absolute owner and the future husband of Ahlam and says that in case of "disobedience," according to the old tradition, he considers it his duty to kill Ahlam.

The conflict between tradition and modernity is serious. Clan hegemony is strong and no solution can be found. The two get married; but on the night of the wedding, Farhan cuts his leg with a knife and Ahlam burns in the flames of the house.

This story is a small replica of a huge sociocultural crisis. A crisis that men have created over the centuries by creating and promoting such beliefs to dominate women. The purpose of this crisis is the same as we described: trying to dominate the woman. The reason for this effort is the same as we described: the man's feeling of inferiority in the face of women's potential and sexual supremacy.

The important thing to add here is that these thoughts and rules are so old and used that they are often deposited in the collective unconscious mind of a man and settled in the belly of his social personality. Of course, this sedimentation has many layers, the hardness or weakness of each layer depends on the social system and environment in which the man was raised. These layers range from the strictest religious prejudices and social taboos against women to the more lenient laws that are present at relatively conscious levels of society.

Today's civilized men agree or disagree with women's social activities, permission to leave the country and permission to drive, ride a bicycle, custody of a child, permission to marry, the right to choose clothing and dozens of similar cases, are defined solely within the framework of the anti-woman mechanism. Otherwise, it is possible to ask a relatively educated husband who does not issue permission for his wife to leave the country, what is the philosophy of this opposition, and he will not be able to provide an explanation. But due to the sedimentation of the social system and restrictive rules that have been in force for hundreds of years in the heart of the society, he carries with him a feeling that makes it difficult to give simple human freedoms to his wife.

Based on this rule and philosophical and social system, there is a list of restrictions for women that when a knowledgeable person looks at them from a distance, he will find them difficult to understand. This is the result of sedimentation (in the unconscious and unintentional field) and the attempt to dominate and limit (from a deliberate and purposeful point of view). Limitations like these:

- A woman should not go to the stadium to watch the matches.
- A woman should not ride a bicycle.
- Women should not laugh loudly in public.
- A woman should not leave the country without the permission of a man (husband, father, grandfather or…).
- A woman should not marry without a man's permission.
- A woman should not be a judge.
- A woman inherits half of a man.
- A woman does not have the right to divorce.
- A woman does not have the right to custody of her children.
- A woman should not work without a man's permission.
- A woman should not leave the house without a man's permission.
- A woman must obey a man in any case and has no authority over her own body.
- A man can physically punish his wife.
- A woman should not have a relationship with another man, while a man can easily have several relationships.
- A woman should cover her face and almost all parts of her body.
- A woman has to respond to a man's sexual needs under any circumstances.
- And dozens of cases like these.

All these injustices and oppressions, while most theorists and intellectual-philosophical systems generally agree on the issue that a dynamic and active society, in order to function as a living organism, needs capacities that can only be created. It is possible for women.

Despite the fact that a woman is different from a man; but there is never any indication that she was created unequal to the male sex, and the vital and social mechanisms also well show that she can be a great contribution to the dynamism and vitality of social life.

The talents that women have exclusively are not something without which it is possible to continue life. Capacities such as: the power to create life, the power to create convergence and peace and beauty, and to add capabilities to life, family and society, of which love is one of the most important.

These capacities are so great that the inadequacy and incompatibility of women's abilities in matters such as wealth accumulation, management, physical strength, industrial development and the like will never harm the equal nature of women and men.

It seems that the confusion about the issue of equality or non-equality of men and women was caused by a fundamental misunderstanding about the nature and quality of creation. If we understand humans in general in two genders, male and female, and in the form of two complementary parts, we will see that both sexes belong to a whole unit called humanity, which are completely independent and of course equal, despite the need for each other.

The right to benefit from the blessings of life, the right to individual and social independence, non-dependence and lack of disciple-master relationship are the most important principles that are of great importance in this egalitarian idea.

The fundamental differences of creation, which have been deposited in the existence of men and women, do not mean a conflict or a defect and the superiority of one over the other. Rather, these differences mean that these two components can complete and enrich each other.

In other words, men and women can be a source of inspiration and strengthen each other. The inspiration that is available in the first place through the channel of love and in the following forms appears in the form of shared efforts in life and the use of each one's talents.

These differences are the main factors of attraction and belonging between men and women. For this reason, it is never possible to introduce a trait in a woman or a man as something reprehensible and as a weakness, and at the same time benefit from it.

The Role of Religions in Marginalizing Women

As mentioned, one of the tools of the patriarchal society is all kinds of religious systems and structures. In general, religion is one of the most difficult filters that women have not been able to pass through in order to be present in society. Among the thousands and thousands of prophets who have introduced themselves as messengers of the Creator of the universe to guide mankind, there is not a single woman seriously. Religious colonies, of any kind, are devoid of women. In the areas of politics and judgment and some important areas of decision-making, citing religious teachings or rulings, women are prohibited from participating. Religious or superstitious beliefs about the oppression of women have acted in the same way. Suppression of women, whether based on superstitions and social beliefs or based on religious rules, has had different forms and degrees, ranging from burying girls alive to the impossibility of women's presence in sports halls.

The significant issue is that such restrictions or suppressions operate on the same course and are based on a single logic in terms of their nature and overall philosophy. The same logic based on which women are not able to be present in society and actualize their abilities.

Investigating the role of religions and beliefs in the historical oppression of women is an independent matter with very wide dimensions; but a list-based look at this issue may give you a general idea of this complicated view:

- In Buddhism, although the presence of women in the network of Buddhist monks is accepted; but there are restrictions on them. In general, it can be concluded that the principles of the Buddhist religion systematically marginalized women. From the behavior of "Hai Gautama Buddha," it appears that for him, women were low and inferior beings who did not even have the dignity of being in his presence. The general structure of Buddhist thinking about women is that women are the presence of evil forces; but at the same time, it can achieve angelic glory.

Also, women's religious education must be supervised by a male cleric. In fact, in order to reach the stage of illumination, a woman must first reach the stage of "being a man."
- In Islam (in today's modern era), most of the personal, social and financial rights of women are clearly limited, conditional, bound and subject to the fulfillment of conditions, which are generally not the case for men. Obvious differences in the share of inheritance, dowry, alimony, dowry, polygamy, guardianship, custody, divorce, cover, judgment, jihad and dozens of other cases are examples of obvious differences between men and women.
- Christian, Jewish, Samaritan and other known religious scriptures are all male and devoid of the serious presence of women.
- According to the narrative of the Torah and some other texts, the woman was created from the {left} rib of the man. For this reason, in the oral culture of the Tudeh, it is sometimes despised: "Didn't you get up from the left rib today?"
- Although the sale and purchase of slaves included men, the sale of virgin daughters for paternity is reported in Jewish religious texts. This is the same amount that is exchanged today as dowry between the groom and the girl's father. Depending on his financial ability, a man has the possibility to take possession of women, or buy a slave girl as a sex worker from the market.
- Showing the bloody undergarments of the girls' first cohabitation has been one of the most humiliating ways of facing women in some societies. While such a thing was not necessary only for men, but men have widely benefited from the blessings of multiple sexual partners.
- In the extreme parts, most religions, including Judaism and Islam, educating girls is an unnecessary matter and a method for their moral deviation. According to the guidance of Talmud VI, women are prohibited from studying the Torah. Although reforms were made about forty years ago and women were given the right to read the Torah in synagogues; but this forty-

year possibility is very small compared to several thousand years of Jewish history. This extreme view believes that teaching literacy to girls means teaching them rudeness.
- Women's testimony is worth half as much as men's testimony, or they are completely prohibited from testifying in judicial courts. For example, women are still not allowed to testify in Israel's Supreme Court, and most religious positions are held exclusively by men. Also, the process of obtaining a divorce for women from the labyrinth of the Jewish judicial system (with the aim of requiring the submission of women) is extremely difficult.

The possibility of religious and spiritual life and reaching the worlds of illumination has been taken away from women, while considering the wonderful creation of women and the feeling of "childhood," she is full of surprises. A woman is more pure than a man. A woman is more capable of keeping promises than a man. This ability has been institutionalized in him and his great historical experience has refined and purified him and made him a more reliable being compared to man.

The spiritual worlds and the Alevi world have characteristics and qualities that the female creation clearly matches with. But the anti-feminist tradition that exists in the context of religions and spiritual and mystical practices has not allowed women to experience and challenge in these fields.

In order to reach the upper world, the seeker must first of all achieve the childlike state. This is while the desired innocence and childlikeness is clearly placed in the creation of women. But by limiting women to very specific tasks such as motherhood, housekeeping, cooking and taking care of children, men have denied women the right to move and challenge.

Indian philosopher Osho says somewhere: "Whenever a woman has come to hear my words, she has heard me more deeply, more sincerely and more lovingly. But when a man comes to hear me for the first time, he resists a lot. It is very loud. Afraid to be impressed, annoyed that his knowledge is not supported. Or if he is very cunning, he interprets everything that is said based on his knowledge and will say: I know everything, it was nothing new. It is a means of protecting his imperfection. To protect that hard shell. Until that shell breaks and you find yourself in childlike wonder and childlike wonder, it will never be possible for you to be in the position we have always known as our soul or self."

Evidence shows that women have the capacity to listen and become unique. You can see the light of joy and acceptance in his eyes. Being surprised in her is not a superficial issue, and her feelings are rooted in the depths of her heart, and she has much more courage than a man in facing unknown realities and matters that are somehow related to the spiritual and unknown worlds. While a man avoids asking questions for fear of revealing his ignorance, a woman can ask questions with her spirit of challenge without wearing a mask of false knowledge and give her whole being in hearing the answer.

These traits make a woman's approach and attitude to the surrounding phenomena more pure. She internalizes things far more than men and connects with her soul. His look at phenomena such as love, marriage, children, sex and intimacy and unity is more internal and emotional.

But with all these positive differences and with all these wonderful human natures, women have always suffered from humiliation and captivity in the male ecosystem. His economic dependence is transverse; but he has accepted this arbitrary and imposed thing and has suffered from it. A woman's ability to conceive, which is supposed to be an active and dynamic mechanism for the continuation of life and the extension of the human race, has become a factor for increasing her suffering under the control of patriarchal society and reactionary customary and religious laws.

In the eyes of a society that is governed by anti-feminist reactionary thinking, a woman has become a population-generating machine, who must live with the least gifts and even be deprived of her basic rights in sexual participation, and only act as a population-generating engine.

Multiple and unwanted pregnancies have affected a woman's life. Institutions of power, politics and religion put relentless pressure on her to give up all the pleasures of life and constantly think about pregnancy. Because this is the most important task that these institutions have assigned to him. It is that throughout the history of human life, women have been the reason for the flow of constant suffering.

The Exclusive Advantages of Men and Women

The confusion that exists in these discussions is that some people, out of ignorance, have considered equality between men and women to mean the sameness of men and women. This is despite the fact that according to the rules of creation, such a thing is not possible in principle.

At a glance, you can understand that a man can never be equal to a woman. Because she cannot have the properties of pregnancy, and female organs such as the uterus and the like.

In principle, a woman cannot have a man's muscular strength and other physical and masculine characteristics. Therefore, the equality of the rights of men and women should be considered in the form of "equal rights of women as women against men as men" and nothing more or less than this.

While being a woman, it is necessary for a woman to be interested in things like loving and raising children. Paying attention to these matters does not mean that competition and presence outside the home is being negated. A woman's soft and sensitive nature is institutionalized as a deterrent force against evil.

A look at human history shows that there is no trace of a woman in any bloody and brutal historical event. Men's stubbornness has sufficiently stained human history with all kinds of misfortunes and left a heinous track record for mankind. In the meantime, the woman, as the beautifier of this space, must continue to play her role and at the same time adhere to her feminine identity.

A woman should still be sensitive to her womb as a powerful potential for the survival of human life. This is an ability that men do not have, and it introduces the two sexes as two complementary poles and factors in the evolution of life. This does not mean inequality. Perhaps the absence of factors such as interest in home and family and the loss of the natural feeling for reproductive power has caused complications and abnormalities such as homosexuality to arise in the last century.

Perhaps this complication is due to the fact that at the beginning of her path, in order to create equal rights with men by generalizing a male model to female life, women not only overdid it, but also suffered a deviation from the path.

Exaggerating the hostile view of women can strengthen the complications of the modern age, one of which is homosexuality. When the man is the enemy, then how much better it is for every woman to live with another woman.

The philosophy of creation, which is based on two qualities, female and male, should not be questioned by things like what was said above. In this natural proposition, the creation of women is in such a way that the nature and understanding of the natural and primitive creation is closer. In fact, what is referred to as gifts or signs of civilization in human history is a kind of departure from the basic quality of creation. In the meantime, women, as an important part of creation, have clearly acted in alignment with this slower evolution.

It is possible to pull the brakes on continuous civilization by relying on the power of the heart and feeling. The woman has been able to make this braking and slowing down possible by maintaining her position as a force that is more connected to the essence of being and the mysterious feeling of nature than men.

A look at the functions of modernization and civilization will tell us that the only part of the structure of human creation that has been able to stay away from the sting of these changes is human feeling and heart. This factor has remained largely intact in women. In fact, there is no predetermined prescription to understand the feeling and heart of a woman. No formulas or calculation methods are taught in universities and educational centers for success or failure in this field. This is the only part of the creation that still remains in its primitive and natural form, and the woman in the artificial structure of human life is a representative who must maintain this status in the past.

The man is well aware of this female superiority. He feels a void that he is not able to fill naturally and by relying on the skills he has acquired. This feeling of lack has led to a double feeling of inferiority in the male type. His attempt to humiliate women and create a mechanism of historical domination was actually to escape from this feeling of inferiority. He used one of his most important tools to exercise this dominance. It has taken advantage of its muscular strength and financial and economic superiority. This is the reason for the lack of social and economic presence of women in most historical periods.

This was not the only aspect of women's superiority over men. There are many other reasons that make a man feel less sterile and incomplete compared to a woman. The feminine advantages deposited in his natural constitution made him a complete human being. But the man has tried to show this superiority in the form of deficiency and weakness. The oral culture of the masses is full of expressions and references that originated from this effort.

But all these efforts do not change the existing reality. A man has the muscle superiority factor as the only decisive component of his superiority; but a detailed list of women's abilities can be mentioned against this superiority, the following are part of it:

- Women naturally live longer than men.
- Women are more resistant to all kinds of diseases and
- suffer less from diseases.
- Women are more stable and resistant to mental and emotional disorders.
- The frequency of men suffering from psycho-physical diseases, insanity and complications such as suicide is almost twice.
- Women are generally more beautiful than men.
- Women, having the ability to give birth and the reproductive system, are considered as the center of gravity for the continuation of human life.
- Women have far more relationship capabilities. Non-sexual sex and the power of consecutive ejaculations are only part of these abilities.
- Women are naturally sensitive and benefit from the human and caressing spirit.
- In human history, women have a clean and untainted record in terms of moral vices and crimes. In contrast, there are men who have filled human history with all kinds of crimes and filth.

- Bloody figures, dictators and ugly figures of history are all rough men without feminine souls. On the other hand, most of the justified, peace-loving, guiding and calm historical figures such as Christ, Buddha, Zoroaster and the like have had a distinct spirit and even a feminine appearance.
- Art, literature and beauty created by mankind are full of women's praise. In fact, men have been continuously praising women through art and poetry. But when they are going to judge women directly, they find a biting and reprimanding language. In other words, men whose souls are polished by association with art, poetry, and other beautifying catalysts immediately begin to praise the feminine element. But when a man is completely away from these spaces, he finds a completely different relationship with a woman.
- Whenever the female spirit has penetrated in a particular area, the space is refined. Then it is time to create beauty, glory and splendor. The art-artist-work of the art cycle has always had such a formula. The great artists of the world often have the quality, spirit and dignity of women. They benefit from the special elegance, feeling and softness that exists in a woman.

It is understandable that considering such a prominent position that women have assigned to themselves as a beautiful and beauty-creating part of existence, men cannot be far from historical envy and jealousy.

The miracle of creation is that it is fully aware of this soothing function of the feminine soul. Likewise, the pragmatism of the male spirit has been neglected. Therefore, he has deposited a glimmer of the feminine spirit in men and a moment of the masculine spirit in women. As an uplifting factor, the feminine spirit is an absolute must for men who work in emotional and aesthetic fields. Without the female spirit, it can be said that male art cannot be realized. Likewise, without the male spirit, women cannot be expected to achieve success in advancing social goals and actions.

Now, wherever necessary, these elements can be increased or decreased in the form of adjustable wicks. In fact, creating a logical balance between the two physiological and mental parts of the creation of men and women can keep the mechanism of social life of mankind in a state of balance.

To understand the quality of the peaceful and complementary coexistence of men and women in the biological structure, it is necessary to know that this duality does not mean a paradoxical function. If so, a lot of life energy would be wasted in the friction between these two conflicting forces. But Hayat is more precise and alert than to create such a contradiction by mistake. This situation has an evolutionary function.

Mankind, with the help of this intelligent structure, can create an acceptable interaction between the seemingly opposite phenomena of existence. Interaction between love and economy, poetry and industry, machine and emotion, heart and brain, sex and virtue, lust and spirituality, and…

For this reason, it should be said that thinking based on the creation of a single-sex quality is an obvious departure from the standards of existence and "leading to error." Without understanding this structure, mankind will suffer the same misunderstanding as it has been until now. One gender serves another gender. The superior race against the weaker race, enemy against enemy. Love against hate, master against slave.

A Sign of Women's Freedom in the Process of Sex

When we speak of the freedom of women and the realization of their rights as a natural and intrinsic matter, there is no room for selecting and censoring certain rights or assigning meaning to others. A woman is either free or not based on her own nature. If she is free, all her natural, social, and innate qualities should be respected as an authentic and fundamental matter. Censoring women and attempting to dictate rules that men do not follow is the starting point of discrimination and misogyny. A woman's freedom in the process of intimacy is crucial for her not to feel "restricted" or "dominated." The routine rule that suggests men must always be the active party and take the initiative is in conflict with women's freedom.

This historical issue has always been problematic for women. Men have attempted various ways to subjugate and censor women (especially if the woman is religiously and legally bound to them). When both parties lose control during intimacy, the imposition of dominance and adherence to taboos causes women to be under control and censorship. Achieving the peak of sexual pleasure and orgasm for a woman may only be possible when she doesn't feel compelled to adhere to restrictions. Imposing silence on a woman during intimacy imposes severe emotional and mental restrictions on her.

In the absence of freedom of action and the suppression of feelings, reaching the peak of sexual pleasure and orgasm will not be realized. Orgasm has a direct connection with the female soul. This is unlike the mechanism of orgasm in men. In men, orgasm is limited to a few specific sexual organs and physical acts, whereas in women, orgasm depends on feelings, soul, heart, and the extent of body parts.

The foundation of initiating the feeling process in women may start with a romantic caress on her ankle and sometimes, orgasm can be achieved without the involvement of reproductive organs.

The basic actions that facilitate a woman's orgasm include moans, groans, whispers, cries, and the like, indicating the involvement of all body parts and the entry of the soul into the sexual process. To achieve orgasm, she needs full engagement of all her senses. This matter, while profound, is very fragile and dependent on the environment.

To disrupt this process and stop the arousal, sometimes just a whisper! In a soft tone, it is enough to cause the collapse of the sexual arousal state and remove the foundation of her primary feelings. This whisper acts as a form of censorship; the woman understands this and feels humiliated, imprisoned, a feeling rooted in her vulnerabilities in historical confrontations.

She remembers that throughout history, she has always been secondary and subject to exploitation. Her unconscious collective memory reminds her that her moments of happiness are entirely temporary, and at any moment an external factor could destabilize this situation. A whisper from a man becomes so heavy for a woman that the physical arousal that had brought her to the brink of orgasm, like a flame extinguished by water, subsides, and her arousal returns to the hidden depths of her spirit. She censors herself, shocked by the blow she has received, and retreats into seclusion. The failure of millions of women to reach the peak of sexual pleasure is due to men not adhering to these backgrounds. Of course, this is not a simple task.

To be able to consider such meticulous details, a man must be not only enlightened and progressive beyond what is commonly seen in society but also a visionary. It seems that the number of such men is not high even in advanced societies. For a woman, complete enthusiasm does not differ significantly from madness. If a man can also attain this level of madness, they will be fully immersed in a profound transformation where the woman becomes a genuine actor, as the famous proverb goes, "When a madman sees another madman, he enjoys it." If the initiative lies with the woman, she will manage the battlefield of love in a way that no similar sexual experience or pleasure will be possible for the man elsewhere. This is not something commonly observed in society. Women are accustomed to always being subordinate, passive, self-contained, and to surrender their controlled and colonized bodies to men.

Male control (a common occurrence) causes a woman to transition from a spiritual and passionate state to a physical and neutral state as a sexual partner. The behavior of the man, his cultural level, and his upbringing will determine the experience on either side of this coin. Societal ideologies in past centuries have transformed this shameful pattern of sexual encounter with women into a norm. This phenomenon is strange but true. Men have essentially objectified women and then engaged with them intimately. For a body, intimacy or violation is synonymous. She has accepted her situation and ultimately coped with the pain. However, understanding men who have engaged in intimacy with bodies and repeated this throughout history and different generations is very challenging.

A Window to the Future

Humanity has so far deviated in its encounter with women. To address this issue, it is necessary for individuals to reconsider their conventional and stereotypical thoughts, without regard to conditional patterns.

For women to break free from past constraints, reclaim their human identity and equal rights, they must not only break away from past patterns but also strive to help the opposite gender understand the necessity of women's liberation. While the process of this enlightenment has begun, it is essential to carefully examine past male-dominated societal strategies in the process of empowering women.

In other words, the question arises: how has the male-dominated society managed to maintain its dominance over women for so long, considering that women are intelligent, sensitive beings who are not unaware of their unequal position? The answer lies in the fact that the male-dominated society has deceived women by exploiting their sensitivities and delicate points, to some extent convincing and controlling them.

The slogan of men in most societies is: "You as a woman are much greater than entering into male relationships, so your mission and responsibility is to raise children and give them life." Men have tried to convince women that this duty indirectly means interfering in the fate and quality of future generations. However, as discussed above, it has been shown that ultimately, with the extensive network of educational systems, the children of future generations also believe in the same beliefs that the male-dominated society holds. Therefore, we see that with each generation, there is no difference in the attitude of today's children and the future men regarding the rights and position of women. This means that women have not had an impact on the transformation of the intellectual life of future generations. Because if such effects existed, they could have amended the public perception of the social position and rights of women. Without realizing the nature and form of this great deception, women have allowed the intellectual and practical system based on the exploitation of women to continue in the same context through neutral performance.

With the beginning of a new era, this sequential process was disrupted. A generation of progressive and equality-seeking women endeavored to transform society's intellectual system regarding the perception of women by relying on public awareness. Women were able to remove some of the old constraints and create enlightenment movements by utilizing the resources provided by medical knowledge and the information explosion of the era. However, the massive waves of this enlightenment have not yet been able to deeply penetrate distant parts of the world, including underdeveloped and impoverished countries. Consequently, the primary mission of women and women's liberation movements of extending the reach of the waves of knowledge and illuminating awareness on backward societies remains distant. What women worldwide must understand is that effort is necessary for success. History does not recall anyone voluntarily granting the gift of freedom. To achieve equality and equal rights above all, one must demonstrate eligibility for these rights. Now women must unleash hidden individual and collective capabilities, release immense energies, and utilize them on the path to securing their rights. In fact, what a male-dominated society perceives as a woman's weakness is her strength, and women must utilize their strengths throughout the world to secure their freedom in the coming century. Next, we will delve into some signs and examples related to women's strengths.

One of the strengths of women is their ability to imagine, a power that has been suppressed within the narrow circle of home and responsibilities such as housekeeping and raising children. A woman must expand her realm of knowledge and wisdom by spreading her wings and practicing flight in this infinite space, aligning herself with men. To achieve this, the way a woman perceives things must change so that housekeeping and child-rearing are only a part of her life philosophy, not all of it. A doctor, an engineer, an influential politician, a commander of a space station team, and an impactful scientist, along with thousands of jobs and social opportunities, are just part of the mandatory outlook for women in the modern era.

The presence of Yasmin Moghbeli, a woman of Iranian descent, as the commander of a NASA space mission who went to space in the summer of 2023, is one of many examples of women's abilities coming into fruition parallel to men, and perhaps even surpassing men by far. Maryam Mirzakhani was another example of such successes.

The destiny of influential women like these clearly demonstrates how open societies, which have provided such opportunities for women, can significantly contribute to advancing the status of women worldwide. It is evident that such women could never have achieved such accomplishments in their destination and birth societies. In the discussion of marriage permission and exit permission for women, controlled by men, it is worth mentioning how absurd it is to think that such women do not have the autonomy to make a simple decision about marriage or leaving the country. This is a characteristic of closed societies that do not facilitate the realization of women's capabilities.

The modern era has provided women with the opportunity as half of the human society. Now, women must strive to pursue their idealistic dreams not only through their sons but also through personal experiences. No one can live another person's life. Sons cannot bear the burden of their mothers' aspirations. Ultimately, each human is an independent and unique being with their own specific destiny and life path. Mothers must recognize this individuality and unique life path within themselves as independent human beings with inherent destinies. Yasmin Moghbeli, in a live conversation from the space station, openly acknowledged to Iranian students at Stanford University that with the necessary foundations and platforms for the realization of ideas and aspirations in Eastern women's society, each of them has the potential to reach great heights in any field. The difference in success between women and men lies in the fact that women, despite their success and creation of ideas and values, operate matters and rules in a more humane and optimal manner, given the softness and centrality they possess. Women are significantly softer, kinder, and more balanced than men. This confirms the perspective of some sociologists who say that if the world's management were in the hands of women, the Earth would be a better place to live.

Perhaps it is necessary for women to assert their rights to equality based on the "Burhan Khalf" theory. This means that by realizing certain ideals, as we have mentioned in some examples, they should demonstrate to human society that women are not only deserving of qualities attributed by men but are actually superior to men in practice. Because not only has nature created women to have the maximum qualifications for life, but it has also endowed them with biological advantages that can make them more creative than men. In this context, the only superiority of men is the muscular power summarized in the toughness of their bodies and large bone structure.

This has led men throughout history to exploit women the most in order to rely on them. From the era of cavemen to the pre-modern times, humans have advanced in a way that women, due to their lack of muscular strength against life's challenges and self-defense, have been dependent on men. This rule gradually found its final form within the family structure. In the caveman era, livelihood was also a reason for this. It was the man who could hunt large animals relying on his strong muscles and skills in archery and trapping, providing sustenance for the family and the woman.

This rule became so dominant over successive periods that even in the modern era, where social relations have changed, it still governs the regulation of relationships between men and women.

The modern human no longer relies directly on nature. Any citizen can meet their life needs by paying money. Women are also included in these new conditions. However, men, relying on old rules, strive to keep previous relationships alive and intact. Now that the issue of direct hunting and provision from nature is not relevant, men try to keep women dependent and in pursuit by monopolizing money. Sometimes the situation has been such that the woman has financial independence and is the owner of money, but apparently, due to an old habit, a hidden sense of the necessity of relying on the man has surrounded her. This is why in the oral culture of the masses of women, phrases like "being under the shadow of a man" are frequently heard.

Therefore, one of the educational requirements for reviving an independent female personality and not relying on men is for these hidden data in her social consciousness to gradually disappear. If this happens, a sense of personal and historical independence will emerge, leading to women and men standing on equal footing in all relationships, in a similar situation. In choosing a partner, having an independent identity and self-confidence can create equal conditions for any kind of interaction and even mutual support.

Humiliation of Women in Linguistics

The concept of human thought in the past centuries was based on the idea that woman is the second sex. Due to the dominance of this perception, all areas, even language and subcultures, were filled with contempt for women. A linguistic investigation would reveal that the domain of most common languages on Earth is more poisoned with anti-female cognitive patterns than we might imagine.

In English, the term mansplaining refers to condescendingly explaining something to a woman by a man. This is because it assumes that the listener (as a woman) has limited knowledge and a mistaken understanding of the issue. Conversely, the counterpart term womansplaining means kindly and humbly explaining an issue by a woman to a man. This is based on the assumption that the listener (as a man) has a high and humble understanding of the matter.

In 2008, Rebecca Solnit, an American feminist writer, wrote an article titled "Men Explain Things to Me," where she pointed out that when a man interrupts a woman to explain something further, he is actually explaining a subject that the woman knows more about. Through examining and delving into their native language's culture of vocabulary, everyone can discover to what extent language construction has developed against women. Across many languages, hundreds, if not thousands of words exist that reflect women's incompetence and worthlessness. A linguistics expert can demonstrate gender inequality by compiling words from a language. Studies on "linguistic sexism" reveal how widespread male dominance, patriarchy, and male superiority are in the realm of language.

Although no research has been conducted on this matter, as a linguist, looking at the Persian language suggests that the abundance of vocabulary related to belittling women is significantly greater than in Western languages. If this is the case, it is not surprising. Despite its balanced history of thousands of years in terms of the relative equality of women and men, the Persian language has not been immune to cultural invasions aimed at altering its nature over the centuries. The past millennium has witnessed the dominance of external and invasive cultures over the domain of the Persian language. One of the major identities of these external forces has been the opposition to women, the instrumental and possessive view of women, and the disregard for their social rights. This influence has been so significant that the cultural domain of the Persian language has, in recent centuries, regressed into an area with the highest cultural indicators and anti-female perspectives.

The linguistic domain in terms of the breadth of vocabulary related to disdain and belittlement of women can serve as a thermometer reflecting the cultural status of society. The more the female gender in the field of linguistics is confronted with cultural bitterness, the more this domain is filled with praises for men and an honorable view of the male gender. Most of the time, the "equivalents" related to male authority in language are precisely the opposite equivalents of the same concepts regarding women.

If we compile a glossary of terms related to gender inequality in the Persian language, it will likely consist of over thousands of words. Unless the educational system—the language that begins with a child's first exposure to language and continues in peer groups and society—is not reformed, the bias in this language will not diminish. In a balanced language, phrases like "taking a woman" cannot have a place. In the word "taking," there is no respect or dignity. The verb "taking" is used to express an action or the occurrence of a state that implies an inanimate object or phenomenon. These phrases do not have equivalent suggestions in a masculine context. This is just one example of thousands of linguistic interpretations that can be raised in this area, but due to the lengthening of the pages of this book, we refrain from discussing such topics. Many of the phrases and insults created for women are not directly intended for them. Since women do not have an independent identity and are perceived as possessions and objects of construction for men, they are considered as such. Therefore, in insulting one man to another, a woman is used as the subject of the insult. Terms like "mother whore," "woman whore," "sister whore," or in English, "son of the bitch," and similar words are not insults to women. Instead, they are insults to a man; however, women are openly humiliated and insulted by associating them with men.

In the English expression above, even though the woman is not originally present in the dispute, by attributing the adjective of obscenity to the mother, the attempt is to degrade the son. As mentioned, there is no equivalent entity for such expressions in languages. The equivalent of the entity "mother-prostitution" is the expression "father-prostitution"; however, according to Eastern society, "prostitution" is considered a feminine matter, and men have more freedom in this regard, and generally, these matters do not carry much stigma for men. There are many concepts that apply equally to men and women. However, the predominance of anti-female identity in mass linguistics causes many concepts to have only a feminine aspect. This same expression of prostitution, considering its literal meaning, can be both a feminine and a masculine example. But it is not clear why mass language only uses it in relation to women. The verb "to give," which is used in masculine oral literature and always implies a form of contempt and belittling, indicates that sex in a masculine and backward mindset is an act where the woman gives something to the man. In other words, mass linguistics implicitly acknowledge that in a male-dominated society, sexual misconduct is solely relevant to women.

The acceptance of promiscuity among men in a male-dominated society is not considered ugly. Men not only do not shy away from boasting about their experiences with multiple sexual partners, including lower-class women and prostitutes, but they often proudly recall and consider it a personal success in harmonious gatherings. These differences are very evident in the cultural realm where language reflects the values of society. Language, with all its nuances, is highly sensitive when representing cultural elements. Therefore, by solely examining language data without delving into the public spheres of a society, one can evaluate the status of women in that society.

Mass oral culture and folklore literature contain a significant amount of linguistic quality. These two domains intertwined, serve as a mirror reflecting the extent of degradation and suppression of women in society. This extent, depending on the cultural development of each society, can vary greatly; however, it does not seem to be entirely absent anywhere in the world.

Due to a long-standing cultural habit, desirable and favorable matters are often attributed to the male gender in the structure of language. On the contrary, combining the word 'woman' creates phrases that are antithetical to those preferred concepts. Expressions like 'manliness', 'being a man', 'acting like a man', and similar phrases used in contrast to 'acting like a woman' and similar combinations are observable in almost every language.

The issue is not that chastity is not a sacred and human matter. Rather, history has attempted to control women with various tools (language being one of them) and interpret the issue of chastity to its advantage.

One should question whether the historical narrative of the difference between Mary Magdalene and Mary the mother of Jesus (regardless of the authenticity of these stories) has been entirely honest and accurate. Is it an exaggeration to condemn sinful women in history and highlight the sin of a woman compared to any other man? The reason why historical facts and symbols of sexual sin primarily involve women is because the historical perspective has consistently been anti-women at all times, usually showing a similar leniency toward men.

Most references and signs of historical hermeneutics point to the phenomenon of the "sinful woman" as being gender-biased. If we disregard gender and evaluate other major sins and place the symbols of sin on the table of human life, women suddenly disappear from the scene. Apart from the sin of lust, where all its symbols are condensed in women, in other sins, women's record is clean.

Murder, crime, bloodshed, massacre, plunder, rape, corruption, lies, oppression, slavery, assault, and dozens of other sins are on the judgment table, yet almost no woman is present as a symbol of all this wickedness. However, as soon as we set these aside and place lust on the table, all historical sinners will be women. This illustrates a masculine history that itself is the cause of vices, propagating a great propaganda to depict women as symbols of wickedness and the means of human downfall. Not because of committing thousands of actual crimes across vast historical geographies, but merely due to the illusion of one sin: lust! It is evident that these documents and references are fabricated and outdated, a place of suspicion. Because masculine history has mostly relied on its own propaganda to depict the demonic image of women.

Matters such as the right to divorce, inheritance, testimony, judgment, custody, stoning punishments, and the like, have made the status of women in recent centuries much more critical. In this era, religious texts, clergy, and preachers have constantly been producing content and documentation to demonstrate the superiority of men over women. To the extent that some try to show that in the beginning of creation, Satan only prostrated to Adam and not to Eve. Nevertheless, the trend that has started from the West in recent centuries may well be able to shed light on all hidden aspects of this anti-women history.

With all these circumstances, it must be said that delineating a vision where we do not witness cultural distortions and linguistic patterns overseeing the degradation of women's status is not an easy task.

Male Deception

The man has employed various methods to convince the woman to maintain her previous position and accept him as the authority figure, even if there is no convincing reason for this situation. He has not refrained from both obvious and covert deceptions. For instance, in utmost generosity and charm, he presents paradise to the woman saying, "Paradise lies under the feet of mothers," but surely if paradise had real financial benefits, the man and religion, by monopolizing it, would never give it to the woman.

In practice, the man has not supported the woman's real talents and has made no effort to bring them into fruition. Instead, he has endeavored to suppress these real talents and has offered anything unreal and immaterial in line with that historical deception. The woman is introduced as the queen of the house and the teacher of future generations, someone from whose guidance great men have ascended to the heights of success. However, all these are imaginary scenarios that have cost the man nothing.

This issue, related to the man's pride, is so important to him that the woman has sometimes unintentionally participated in this grand deception to gain the man's cooperation and affection. Sometimes women, to protect masculine pride, have even withdrawn from their talents and abilities, presenting themselves as weak and incapable, perpetuating this flawed cycle to strengthen the foundations of masculine dominance and female dependence.

Examples of this backwardness can be observed in the teachings of traditional societies, even in the Western world. The basis of this idea is that a woman should not be in a superior position in a gathering or assembly where a man is present. The pretense that a woman is in the shadow of a man has been a long-standing principle of education given to young girls waiting for a husband (even among the nobility and elites). For centuries, men have lived their lives under this false and empty pride, bringing women under their control. Therefore, even if women had unparalleled talents and capabilities that could have contributed significantly to the improvement of human society, the male-dominated society has preferred stagnation and backwardness by neglecting the capacities of women. Ultimately, this selfishness is rooted in the history of masculinity.

Literary Texts Are Tools of Male Propaganda

Poetry and literature reflect certain aspects of human philosophical thinking and preserve them as literary products. In these works, as reflections of societal realities, one can observe the main stream of thought. The image that literature and art portray of women can serve as a mirror reflecting the overall status of women in any historical period.

The famous verse "Both woman and dragon in the dust / The world is pure from both impurities" even if attributed as an additional verse to Ferdowsi, actually represents the perspective of Persian literature on women. This perspective ranges from the mocking tone of this verse to softer forms of expression. An important point to mention is that poets and writers are all products of their societies. Societies where over centuries a negative view of women has been promoted and has directly or indirectly influenced the minds of poets and writers, ultimately manifesting in their works.

When Ferdowsi writes this verse, he surely has his reasons and justifications. Whatever these reasons may be, one undeniable fact remains: no thought grows in a vacuum. Therefore, in the third, fourth, and subsequent centuries, the same grand propaganda we mentioned supports this way of thinking.

From a literary critique perspective, Ferdowsi has been completely truthful in the structure of his narrative and has consciously narrated it in the "historical context." The portrayal of women in the Shahnameh, as the most important cultural and historical document of Iran, is not criticized because Ferdowsi desires it. Rather, it is because he is obligated to narrate history without manipulation. Therefore, the image presented of women in the Shahnameh by Ferdowsi is not derogatory or devoid of intelligence. Occasionally, depending on the narrative's spatial and temporal circumstances, we also encounter exceptions like the character of Sindokht Kabul, reflecting specific situations within the overall structure of the Shahnameh.

Prominent Persian literary texts, whether in poetry or prose, are almost entirely free from insults, denigration, and indecency toward women. The language and positioning in these works regarding women are so bitter that perhaps the Shahnameh, alongside the Masnavi Ma'navi, could be considered among the most balanced among Persian poetry and prose works. The primary perspective of Persian literary works on women, in a general evaluation, is almost in line with the hypothetical line drawn in this text. The main aspects of looking at women in Persian literature include these concepts:

- Men have absolute superiority over women. This viewpoint is considered self-evident, and speakers usually do not feel the need to provide evidence or arguments to prove their point. As the saying goes: "The sun itself is evidence of the sun."
- Women are seen as symbols of sin, and as collaborators with the devil in deceiving men and leading them away from knowledge and spirituality, qualities that men should distance themselves from.
- Women are portrayed as fearful, deceitful, suspicious, and weak beings, completely opposite to the masculine qualities and virtues such as wisdom, intelligence, courage, warrior spirit, knowledge, ethics, and magnanimity.
- The identity of a woman is tied to trivial matters and she is always occupied with worthless tasks like spinning thread or

grinding grain, and household chores. Whereas men are always engaged in noble and valuable pursuits.

- A woman is considered the property of a man. However, she is deemed a worthless possession that a man should distance himself from as much as possible. In other words, a woman is likened to a possession, categorized among material goods and worldly pleasures. As expressed in the writings of Shams, where it is stated that a human (meaning a man) should not "chase after the world," emphasizing a connection between money, the world, and women.

Men have absolute superiority over women. This viewpoint is considered self-evident, and speakers usually do not feel the need to provide evidence or arguments to prove their point. As the saying goes: "The sun itself is evidence of the sun."

Women are seen as symbols of sin, and as collaborators with the devil in deceiving men and leading them away from knowledge and spirituality, qualities that men should distance themselves from.

Women are portrayed as fearful, deceitful, suspicious, and weak beings, completely opposite to the masculine qualities and virtues such as wisdom, intelligence, courage, warrior spirit, knowledge, ethics, and magnanimity.

The identity of a woman is tied to trivial matters and she is always occupied with worthless tasks like spinning thread or grinding grain, and household chores. Whereas men are always engaged in noble and valuable pursuits.

A woman is considered the property of a man. However, she is deemed a worthless possession that a man should distance himself from as much as possible. In other words, a woman is likened to a possession, categorized among material goods and worldly pleasures. As expressed in the writings of Shams, where it is stated that a human (meaning a man) should not "chase after the world," emphasizing a connection between money, the world, and women.

When it comes to the identity and image of women in Persian literature and Iranian cultural productions in the post-Islamic millennium, it is necessary to briefly recall three points so that this brief yet essential discussion does not remain vague.

Firstly, the portrayal of women in Persian literature over our millennium remains consistent from the time of Rudaki to around the era of Tahereh Qorrat al-Ayn. However, with the advent of the Iranian Enlightenment era that began with the Constitutional Revolution, changes emerged. The entire millennium is filled with the prevailing notion of demeaning women. Yet gradually in the contemporary period, signs of intellectual transformation become noticeable. In modern literature (especially in modern Persian poetry), the depiction of women has softened significantly, with poets and writers looking at "women" somewhat respectfully and empathetically.

Even this desirable atmosphere paved the way for the emergence of some female poets who, while discussing the "secrets of femininity" in their works, became influential pioneers of the women's equality movement in the contemporary century. Additionally, it should not be overlooked that efforts to improve this situation have been made by non-religious reformers and enlightenment advocates, which have mainly provided comfort and solace rather than being a substitute for the truth. Interestingly, many of these reformers have been men.

Secondly, the image of women in Persian literature is inherently dual-faced. This difference is apparent in a way that it seems we are faced with two different women in our Persian literature. The first woman is the same being we depicted earlier. This woman is often seen in specific literary genres such as epic literature, didactic literature, and mystical literature. This is the same woman who is portrayed as malicious, materialistic, demonic, worthless, and scorned, from whom a complete man should distance himself or restrict his exploitation.

However, the second woman present in Persian literature is in the realm of mystical poetry. The woman in mystical literature is the same as the "beloved." A beloved for whom the most beautiful Persian poems have been composed. For instance, Saadi, who in his educational and social books addresses the extreme oppression of women, suddenly speaks so passionately and almost madly about women as beloved in his poems that it seems this supernatural being is fundamentally not a woman.

In mystical literature, the beloved woman is compelled to compete with the beloved man, who is a beautiful-faced youth in new attire, as observed in Persian "flirting with boys" literature. Part of the beloved in Persian poetry is also mystical and abstract. Regardless of these two beloveds, a considerable portion of being a beloved in Persian poetry is attributed to women. However, this is the same woman who holds no value in other forms of literature. The duty of poets like Sanai Ghaznavi is clear. In *The Garden of Truth*, he likens women to animals and tells numerous indecencies to her, yet in his poems, the intended meaning of the beloved for him is mystical and abstract. Although he also draws upon the beauties of earthly women in his collection of similes and symbols.

But when it comes to Saadi, the matter becomes slightly different. A portion of Saadi's poems entirely focuses on the human and earthly beloved (female gender). In his poems, Saadi praises in an exaggerated manner the same beloved that he portrays as a fearful and worthless being in "Golestan" or "Boostan."

Third point: Considering the profound difference in the portrayal of women in Persian literature in the millennium after Islam, compared to Pahlavi and ancient Persian literature, along with the religious texts of this era, it might be closer to reality to say: Looking at women in Persian literature in the millennium after Islam, more than being a representative of Iranian culture and civilization, she is a representative of Islamic civilization.

In its place, we have repeatedly indicated that the position of women has always been a subject of dispute and scrutiny since the beginning of creation and the presence of Eve on earth. Throughout this millennia-old history, acceptable and even remarkable points are also considerable and identifiable. Some of these prominent points belong to the Iranian-Zoroastrian civilization. Even historical discussions about brief periods of female dominance or matriarchy in history are closer to ancient Iran. Thus, it is observed that the intensity and severity of the degradation of women in Persian literature over a thousand years are a result of the same historical-cultural rupture after the Arab invasion of Iran. Among the few philosophical and social systems that have respected the body of a woman and her overall identity throughout human history, ancient Iranian historical geography has always been at the forefront alongside civilizations like Greece and Rome. The absence of the cultural region of the Arabian Peninsula does not require argumentation in the geography of human culture (from the perspective of women). Nevertheless, how can texts of literature from a thousand years after Islam be considered as cultural evidence of Iran regarding the perception of women? Just as Venus, as the goddess of love, beauty, and fertility, holds a prominent place in Roman myths, Anahita (Aredvi Sura Anahita) in Iranian civilization, as the goddess of the waters of the world, holds significant power in ancient society. She is the guardian of divine knowledge. Her name, meaning purity and cleanliness, oversees the respect and dignity that the feminine spirit and body hold in this culture. Just as texts like the "Tantric" in Hindu culture and myths assign a special place for women as a feminine goddess. With these characteristics, it is natural that the cultural rupture resulting from the Arab invasion of Iran has never given the inhabitants of the cultural region between the Caspian Sea and the Persian Gulf the opportunity to return to their roots. Therefore, the sources and references used for cultural thought production in Persian literature have been more Arabic and Islamic than ancient Iranian cultural documents. In such a situation, producing literature similar to what we described above and looking at women in this literature is a matter that is neither natural nor representative of the Iranian cultural region.

In future centuries, a man begins to face a logical encounter with a woman. However, the encounter is within the same boundaries and standards as before. The man tries to create a more logical mechanism for advancing household affairs through a kind of division of labor and description of duties for himself and the woman. But this does not mean allowing the woman into prohibited territories. All of this is conditional on him not intending to take a step beyond the defined boundaries. If he deviates from this line, society will turn the other side of the coin to him, and he will become a vile demon, the source of all evils and wrongdoings. He will turn into the gateway of hell. A symbol of darkness devoid of any kind of sanctity. He will become a mistake that creation has committed. The same situation that we have depicted a glimpse of in literary texts.

Eastern Burned Mother, Archetype of the Flaming Candle

When the ancient model of the burned Eastern mother governs the relationships between men and women, as mentioned earlier, the man's utmost effort to compensate for the comprehensive loss of the Eastern woman is a scarification on the arm of her young child to express gratitude in this way. This issue encompasses all the features of a great historical and social tragedy.

The Eastern man knows the calamity he has brought upon his wife, mother, and sister. He refrains from speaking about it due to the heavy taboos surrounding the matter. However, his social conscience is troubled by this issue. Therefore, he attempts to show appreciation by creating a sacred halo around the mother-wife-sister relationship. Unaware that this very sacred halo is the curse that has turned the garden of the Eastern woman's existence into scorched earth and deprived her of the fundamental right to life.

In the deeper layers of society, the man has surpassed his desires. While he values the sanctity of family and producing a sufficient number of children, he goes beyond seeking his own diversities, leaving the realm of the household and pursuing other forms of happiness in a society that has provided him with opportunities.

He knows that to reduce his heavy responsibilities as a man, he must pay attention to modern tools such as condoms and various forms of contraception. He seeks happiness that traditional marriage and Eastern family structures do not offer him. However, the woman remains the same woman; accepting, reactive, and suppressing all her suppressed desires that she has learned to adapt to the surrounding conditions through a long historical process of education.

As the man ascends the staircase starting from the initial sexual attractions, passing through a peak of excitement, and reaching the suppression of the woman—the wife of convention by crossing the taboo of sexual relations with relatives, day by day, it deprives him of the possibility of recreating an exciting sexual space with his wife. The functioning of this staircase clearly demonstrates Freud's finding about the diminishing of sexual attraction between man and woman. This staircase leads the man through various stages toward progression or upward movement. In this progression, his sensual feelings are gradually reduced, and his oppressive and "motherly" feelings toward his spouse are intensified.

- Dating and trying to attract the attention of women.
- Proximity and creation of sexual relationships and marriage.
- The peak of the sexual relationship, including the honeymoon and the stages after that.
- A woman's pregnancy and the appearance of signs of the presence of a child.
- Child birth and breastfeeding.
- The intensification of motherhood and the addition of a holy aura around the mother with subsequent children.
- Man moving away from woman and not returning again due to contradictory feelings and repetitive processes.
- The withdrawal of women and drowning in the role of mother.
- Suppression of sensual desires and the end of women.
- The start of the grieving mother.
- The appearance of my grandmother.
- Grandmother's death without benefiting from her natural and biological gifts.

Before the child is born, the factors involved in the coldness of the relationship can be kept at the sidelines. If contributing factors such as libido boosters, youthful exuberance, sexy clothes and props, travel, diversification, sex education and the like have any effect on improving the relationship, there is only so much. But as soon as the sound of the wheels of the baby carriage is heard in the house and the surrounding sidewalks, these factors lose their effectiveness.

The obvious point that attracts attention is the spontaneous action of archetypes and hidden data of the pronoun. In other words, a person may be fully aware of the fact that his wife is not his mother in the field of external wisdom; but he does not notice that he is secretly imprisoned by chains and hidden forces dominate him.

In other words, man, often, does not voluntarily assume such a role for himself or his wife; but it implicitly witnesses the presence of this external factor and this "omniscient." The spirit of blame that is always present; but his existence oscillates like an ethereal being on the border between existence and non-existence.

Observing the signs that indicate the presence of this dominant spirit is not a difficult task. It is enough to pay attention to private conversations and exclusive expressions between men and women. It is not unlikely that a person has called his wife many times as mother or sister or even brother. or has used phrases that refer to these concepts. These concepts can be traced in the literature of private discourse between men and women. Usually, after some time passes between husband and wife, a kind of expressive culture and sincere spoken literature prevails that only they know the meaning of some concepts and words. In the manifestation of this discourse, the inner child also plays a major role.

That is, they are phrases and words that they have made to express certain concepts that are not used in the external and general levels of language; rather, like MERS codes, they require interpretation. Men and women usually create a symbolic or constructed language to express some names, sexual organs, sexual actions, which only has meaning between the two. This linguistic culture is not general. Naming the penis, naming the act of sex, expressing a desire for sex, naming women's underwear, some sexual operations, certain moments such as orgasm, pre-orgasm and many others are among the areas that women and men talk about in literature and language. They invent their own.

In this dictionary, where men or women have invented words to express their closeness or relationship, we can find signs of maternal and paternal tendencies between husband and wife. An obvious example of this language invention that has become popular is the word *Baby*, which has a feeling of love and closeness in it.

The truth is that two spouses have an equal position in terms of establishing a relationship, and although the idea of flirting with a father or mother is disgusting, in practice, they do not face such a risk. But for men and women, it is difficult to consider this obvious and at the same time elusive truth both consciously and unconsciously. When men and women leave long-term stable relationships for new and perhaps younger sexual partners, it is often assumed that this is a pathetic search for lost youth. But Freud and Jung and many other leading psychologists have proven that the reason for seeking a relationship outside the family has to do with unconscious motivation and is much deeper than trying to relive youthful memories.

As mentioned, usually a parent-like ghost surrounds the spouse and makes any sexual intimacy with him impossible, and their goal in leaving the relationship is to escape from that ghost.

The Fundamental Rights of a Natural Sinner

In many societies and according to human beliefs and archetypes, women have been considered as a reproductive tool. In this case, what happens to the woman and her bodily needs after the pregnancy process, there is a deep silence. The woman's nature is manifested in her pregnancy, and the man's nature is manifested in the subsequent exploitation of this pregnancy and ownership of all processes.

In mythological texts and historical documents of the first and second millennia, the identity of the Holy Mary is summarized in her fertility. Summarize the Holy Mary in one sentence: a noble girl who was once conceived and Christ was born from her womb. We have nothing to do with the quality and philosophy of this story. But has another function been defined for Maryam as a woman? He is holy without a wife. As a human being, it does not matter at all in which direction his human needs have flowed in the later periods of his life. There are no stories about other parts of his life.

This statement does not mean doubting the nature of dualities of good and evil, goodness and evil, Ahura and Ahriman, Satan and God, and other dualities. The dualities of good and evil are one of the most important factors in creating balance in the organization of human life. But the point is that the man has tried his best to expand these dualities with the help of sexual power.

Up to this point, there is no problem; but history has embodied the power of evil in the form of a woman, and when lust begins to work as evil, no trace of a man can be seen. This means that sexual acts are not considered evil for a man. It is only the woman who turns into absolute evil with the slightest slip or the slightest expression of carnal desires.

Those who seek to change the traditional equations between men and women in the form of women's equality movements have gone astray. They should base their activities on the above topic. While issues such as women's voting rights, custody rights, divorce rights, or male manifestations and actions and fake resemblance to men, have formed their main priorities. Male similarities are not only a virtue for a woman, but also a defect for her.

The natural quality of the human genetic map suggests that women are superior to men in many cases, but history clearly ignores women in pursuit of monopolistic interests and goals. Religious beliefs have contributed to this problem in all ages. Adam is created and then Eve is given to him as a tool to meet his needs. There, the conspiracy to destroy the woman's identity immediately begins. It is your mind that is guilty. He is the one who eats the forbidden fruit. He is the one who causes humanity to be thrown out of the Garden of Eden and forced to endure earthly suffering. You see! From the very beginning, the conspiracy against the woman has started. In this context, throughout human history, the door has turned on this heel.

Men's history, men's religion, men's philosophy, men's sociology, men's art, men's cinema, men's music, and many other men's fields, where men have tried to make a woman a sinner by nature.

This incessant attack has had a profound effect on women as half of humanity. This widespread promotion has gradually been deposited in the DNA of the world and even women themselves, and the archetype of "sinful woman" has been institutionalized in human nature (even in female nature).

Because of this, women have always been afraid of men and harbored a secret feeling of guilt. For this reason, in other eras, every judgment that was made about him was accepted without protest. At times, she has been half a man. He has won half of the inheritance. He did not have the right to vote. He did not have custody of the children. He did not have the right to leave the country. He did not have the right to judge. He did not have the right to drive. He did not have the right to ride a bicycle. He did not have the right to show his face. and thousands of other rights.

The point is, who should have granted him these rights? Of course he's dead! Therefore, it should be said that a woman did not have the right to have "rights" during her lifetime. Even now that women's demand movements have started in a part of human society, they should demand their rights from men. It means from the one who deprived him of his right!

For centuries, women have been asking men to return at least a part of their rights to her. Just like a thief enters a house and takes most of the property and things in a bag. After a long time, the owner of the house went after the thief and asked him to return at least the most necessary and important items needed in his life. This is the story of a woman in a male society.

Sexual Power Is the Criterion for Evaluating a Woman

An important factor that history has included in its assessment and judgment toward women is how she acts in the face of her sensuality. It is natural that such a factor, even if it is called desirable or acceptable from the perspective of tolerance, is not the case for men.

Men are evaluated with factors such as management, combativeness, authority, intelligence, knowledge, and the like; but women are specifically evaluated by their sexual personality and the way they act and react to this phenomenon. This problem has spread in all aspects of human existence, including in art and literature.

What is the difference between Rabia Qazdari and Rabia Adavieh? In what factor is the difference between Forough Farrokhzad and Parvin Etesami or Parvin Etesami and Mehsti Ganjavi in terms of male perspective? Probably being in "Shahr Ashoob" (society's sexual response to their cities). The one who causes chaos in the city with her different actions, she faces the arrow of criticism because she is a woman. Otherwise, in Persian literature, there are dozens of examples similar to Mehsti, whose being a man has given them the permission to speak any kind of erotic speech far more naked than Mahasti, and their speech is not considered "Shahr Ashoob."

In this way, it is clear that with the way men face the category of gender and the natural needs of women and the identification of men with the opposite sex, even in the field of literature and culture, the criterion for evaluating women has been first of all the sexual aspects and physical differences.

A New Era and the Beginning of New Relationships

While systematic discrimination against women continued in various forms, humanity entered a new era. The modern age and Toffleri's three waves arrived and each of these currents created deep and deep-rooted effects in cultural and social life, the relationships and status of women in society were also affected.

In the new era, the first serious window was opened for women to look at the prospects of equal rights and free life. In the beginning, it was just a window that could show a favorable view in the distance. Women had a difficult task ahead of them to pass through this window and have a sensual and real presence in the midst of that promising landscape. But the dark experience of the past warned them that any kind of procrastination and despair might mean a possible return to the dark past.

The dark past of women is detailed and has its requirements and characteristics in every part of the world. But the nature of this cruel behavior has many commonalities. These aspects of sharing include tying women in line with the customs and tastes of the male society. From this point of view, the burqa and niqab of women in Afghanistan, the compulsory hijab in Iran, and the mutilation of women under the name of "circumcision" from the Nile Delta to the ends of the world, are practically no different. When modern women look back, they remember the dark Victorian era, for example. A period when the behavior of the patriarchal society, including the aristocracy and the bourgeoisie, was exaggeratedly petrifying and cruel toward women, and women were exactly like puppets, captive to misogynistic thoughts, and in practice, there was no way out of this situation for women. did not have. Although the industrial revolution had also arrived during this period; but until the first sparks related to women's liberation movements and the revival of female identity began to shine, it was inevitable to endure this situation.

The agricultural revolution and the industrial revolution, which later created the information and communication revolution. At least in the Western society, it changed the view of women. The women, now informed, sought hard to consolidate the foundations of their social rights. The slogan of "equal rights of men and women" and pragmatisms of the type of feminist movements and even the appendages and self-proclaimed guests of these currents such as "homosexuality" were the product of this revolution and public awareness.

Now the common equations were obsolete and the pioneers of equality thought, who were mainly influential theorists, in various fields such as sociology, philosophy, psychology and law, even biology and biology, revealed great injustices that put women in an unacceptable dark room.

Sigmund Freud and his peers were able to bring the knowledge of sexology and psychological studies related to the differences between men and women into a new field. A new look at the issue of men and women had led to the formation of new ideals and the continuation of fundamental research.

Political, social and economic theories without involving the issue of women in human society had a major shortcoming. The new psychology not only believed that in terms of structural biology and historical sociology, men and women are equal, but any kind of idea and thought or belief that aims to establish male supremacy is inhumane and caused by totality is sexual. A thought that seeks to exploit women has no place in modern society and the new era.

Although Marx's views did not directly address the issue of equality of women's rights (such as workers' rights), later this theory became the basis of one or two feminist movements such as "socialist feminism." According to the philosophy of class discrimination, just as the ruling classes want the workers to be in hardship and they live in euphoria and pleasure, in the same way, men as the ruling class are interested in women's lack of sexual pleasure. While they themselves want extensive sexual pleasure and diverse sexual freedoms. Marxist reform theories have always had a partial look at the women's issue. It may be said that the idea of equality between men and women is more compatible with the "commune" system than with the capitalist system. Because in the commune system, the basis of the thought and structure of the society is without the concept of class and division. Therefore, gender division will also be unnecessary.

In this way, the way was opened for extensive research in neglected areas. The achievements of the research group consisting of William Masters and Virginia Johnson, pioneer researchers of sex science in their 40-year research, showed that before the age of enlightenment, women lived in a dark house of ignorance and male tyranny. It is obvious that a considerable part of this encyclopedia of ignorance was caused by the lack of correct understanding of human beings about the mechanisms of creation, ethics and society. Although this claim is not based on documented scientific research; but it can be said that part of this male tyranny was intentional and due to the totalitarian policies and the desire for ownership that men used in the face of women.

The achievements of scientists, of which the American Masters and Johnson's research is a full-view mirror, in addition to discovering unknowns and historical deviations, led to the invention of various methods and disciplines to optimize the love-emotional-sexual relations between men and women.

Sexology, which was a science based on the research of Masters and Johnson, while examining the interests and sexual behaviors and performance of people, tries to use the findings of psychology, biology, sociology, criminology, medicine, etc., to investigate the complications of human sexual behavior and check his success or failure in a standard relationship.

Many norms and anomalies were examined in the dictionary of this new knowledge, which has been effective in creating a better society and optimizing the position of women in the equation of life. Issues such as: sexual orientation, sexual identity, sexual relations and activities, sexual interests and deviations (both normal and abnormal), as well as issues such as sexual tendencies and actions at different ages and among different strata and inefficiencies of sexual behavior in cases such as erectile dysfunction, anorgasmia and other disabilities and abnormalities were investigated in these studies.

What makes Masters and Johnson's research unique is breaking the taboo in speaking about the realities of the world of sex. A world where human sorrowful homelessness is one of its undeniable manifestations.

During the three revolutions that occurred in recent centuries. An invisible revolution called "Sex Revolution" has been taking shape in the concrete of society. The interweaving of these events was such that when Masters and Johnson's famous book Human Sexual Response was published, critics could hardly determine whether this book was the result of the sexual revolution of the 1960s in Western society or whether it was the cause of such. It has been revolutionary.

This research was trying to answer the questions that some time ago, basically, in society, there was not even the "face of the problem." These questions included the following items:

- What happens to a woman during the sexual process?
- Where does female arousal occur? Does this arousal occur only in the clitoris or does it include the walls of the vagina? In this case, vaginal lubrication through vaginal fluids is the exact result of which interaction?

The importance of Masters and Johnson's research is that; Before they answered these questions, not only did no one in the world community know the answer, but no one knew the question itself.

The above examples were considered as a prelude to bigger conclusions from the researchers. For example, it was discussed that during long centuries, women were cruelly deprived of reaching the peak of sexual pleasure, and it was even determined that men treated women inhumanely during the sex process.

As mentioned earlier, the behavior of men with women is like the behavior of a sex machine. A passive machine that must regulate and even suppress all its sexual behaviors and bodily needs in line with the man's desires and wishes. In this way, the man, in line with maximum pleasure and in line with his comfort, has not allowed the woman to enjoy as well. The man has always been on top. He has taken the initiative and has adjusted and personalized the entire process depending on the timing of his ejaculation. In the meantime, women's desires have no place in the Arabs. Women's potential is ignored and suppressed. The power of repeated ejaculations in a woman (deep sex) and the possibility of spreading sex to all cells (extensive and quality sex) are part of her potential that has been suppressed over the centuries.

With the beginning of the triple revolutions and the beginning of the secret human revolution in the field of sex, Western women began a wide and continuous struggle to achieve their social and sexual rights in both social and sexual spheres. Although these struggles sometimes went astray and sometimes the freed energies were spent on marginal and wrong things; but the fact that the current of enlightenment and rebellion against the old foundations and structures had started was a positive thing in itself.

Parallel to the changes in the West, in another part of human society; That is, in the Middle East, traditional beliefs and mentality continued as before. The oriental woman is so unbelieving about her inherent rights that she doesn't even know about them. Therefore, it is not surprising that according to unofficial statistics, more than 95% of Eastern women are unaware of the peak of sexual pleasure.

In an ideal situation, all the moments of sex are considered as steps that are supposed to bring the man and the woman closer together moment by moment. Perhaps one of the appropriate words used in some cultures to express sex is the word "closeness." Closeness does not mean physical and physical closeness, but rather the closeness of two souls and two feelings during moments that are not unlike the moments of a mystic's journey or the Sufi's experience of discovery and intuition and the experience of a seeker of pure moments of meta-awareness.

In the "nearness" of all forms of communication between the two parties, it is a means to bring two huge realities closer; it means two people. An experience that, although it ends with ejaculation, the energy created guarantees the durability of a deeper relationship. For this reason, social psychologists emphasize the success or failure of the relationship, i.e., the authenticity of closeness, in examining the causes of couples' separation and divorce.

Orgasm is one of the symbols of this closeness, but not all. Therefore, in the pre-divorce survey forms, legal and psychological experts ask couples on the verge of divorce about their success in orgasm. Due to the lack of documented and official research, specific information about the effect of experiencing or not experiencing orgasm or the quality of "closeness" in breakups has not been published. If such data exist, they can be used as a rich source of first-hand information in promoting promotion plans in the field of preventing relationship breakdown. But unfortunately, the importance of this issue is basically ignored.

When we say that sex is something beyond the body and body parts. When it is said that sex in women is a divine and sacred matter that acts beyond the cells of the body, it means that a woman is not only her body in the course of sex, but a woman's body is only a part of the whole, which is the heart, soul, five senses, subconscious mind, lived experiences, etc. are all other parts of this whole.

The woman forgets the body in the semi-mystical and semi-discovery and intuitive moments of sex. His experience is one of oneness, and this oneness would be very perfect if it ended with simultaneous ejaculation.

This is why we said that if the management of the sex process is based on past experiences and with the benefit of specialized training and skill enhancement, in such a way that the woman can have several preliminary ejaculations before the final ejaculation, that is exactly the promised paradise of the relationship.

But the truth is much more distant and bitter than this. Due to the fact that throughout the history of thousands of years, the man has been real powerful and has always been a hasty, selfish and imperfect being, very quickly and selfishly, he destroys the relationship at the very beginning, and it is the woman who must be self-controlled and fulfill all her needs.

A man naturally does not have the inherent ability in his body and creation to be able to bring a woman to paradise; but this is not all. He does not consider it necessary to mix this tact and intelligence together with the management and skill of sex to create such a situation.

The differences between men and women are sometimes natural and sometimes related to creation. There is no choice but to accept this fact; but men's irresponsibility has made the story more complicated. Therefore, despite the fact that nature created man and woman for each other; but it seems that the extreme differences in the creation of the two creatures have made the possibility of mutual understanding impossible. Earlier, we mentioned some differences. In the following, we will try to clarify the difference and differentiation of the issue by setting up a list of these aspects.

- Multiple ejaculations versus single ejaculations.
- Long time to ejaculate vs minutes to ejaculate at best.
- More prevalence of sex-related complications; including erectile dysfunction and premature ejaculation and other cases in men.
- Expanding the process of sexual stimulation in the whole body in contrast to the man being limited to the sexual organs.
- The spiritual nature of sex for women, as opposed to the physical and superficial nature of sex for men.
- A woman's high focus during sex on actions and symbols, in contrast to a man's low focus and his superficiality.
- The high level of purity, elegance, relaxation, relaxation and complete envelopment in the process.
- Longer interval of sex needs in women due to the deeper process compared to the needs of men soon due to the superficiality of the process.
- Dependence and unquestionable love in a woman and not paying attention to other men in contrast to a man's superficial dependence and attention to other women.
- A woman's sexual power is active in certain periods and according to her biological calendar caused by menstruation, this feeling can be programmed and calendared in her. While the male sexual power, unlike many animals and creatures, is continuously active.

Motherhood — Femininity

When a girl transitions into the stages of being a wife and then a mother, significant changes occur in her psychological states and emotional well-being. Sometimes these extensive changes happen in a short period of time, making it challenging for women to quickly adapt to the new realities. As a result, women become one of the primary clients of psychiatric clinics. The reason for mental disorders in women lies in this issue. Women are forced to navigate their unstable relationships on multiple fronts with others. These relationships may become disrupted for various reasons. Relationships with spouses and children are among the most significant relational stressors for women. Additionally, women bear a greater burden of responsibility at all these stages compared to men.

Society assumes that every woman, upon getting married, also has the ability to become a mother. This is not always the case. Women need prerequisites and to go through preliminary stages to become mothers. Otherwise, motherhood may impose an unbearable burden on them. Being a woman is a necessary condition but not a sufficient one for motherhood.

Religion is the most serious institution that believes as soon as a girl reaches the age of thirteen or even nine, she is a complete woman. Needless to say, this misguided perspective indicates how far religious institutions are from modern fields of knowledge such as psychology, sociology, and biology. Directives issued by religious leaders in the void of scientific insight and in their empire of ignorance sometimes hold less importance than an organized crime.

Incorrectly, in some societies (especially in class-based societies), women's bodies are viewed as population-producing machines. This perspective not only creates structural problems in society but also severely impacts the socio-economic conditions of women. Observing impoverished and underdeveloped communities reveals that wherever there is economic and cultural poverty, we encounter highly populated families who mechanically engage in population growth without any clear planning or future outlook.

Seeing television images of displaced and distressed population groups in need of international aid and a piece of bread to alleviate hunger clearly indicates that in underdeveloped societies, family planning and developing a program for regulating births are not prioritized. Parents who, in an unstable situation and without even a short-term vision, reproduce mechanically and instinctively primarily suffer from cultural poverty and lack of awareness.

Most likely, in such societies, mothers lack autonomy and decision-making power regarding their own reproductive choices. While foresight and planning in the realm of action and decision-making belong to men. Mothers should be able to have agency over unwanted pregnancies that bring suffering and hardship, but it does not seem that they have such agency under dominant systems. When women lack the autonomy to decide about their bodies, their self-esteem and most basic rights are jeopardized. The perception of women's bodies as population-producing machines is a strategic belief among class-based ideologies. This situation critically endangers the status of women within these population groups.

Children, Mothers, Fathers and Educational System

When a child is born, the person with the most important responsibility toward them is the mother. After nine months of the challenging and exhausting experience of pregnancy culminating in the pain of childbirth, we are now faced with the presence of a child who is directly and entirely dependent on the mother for several years. While society considers all these difficult processes as the definite duty of the mother, it often sidelines her in legal matters, depriving her of her undeniable rights. In some cultures and societies, custody laws regard the father as having absolute authority (ownership) over the child.

Due to her inherent nurturing and natural disposition, a mother never views supporting and raising her child in the following years as a mere obligation. The presence of a child in a mother's life is like the beginning of a feast full of tenderness. A child is an inspiring gift to her. What prevails in the relationship between a mother and child above all is selflessness, compassion, and love.

Unlike the father, a mother has a lesser sense of ownership over her child. She is not concerned with possessing the child but rather all her joys and sorrows are devoted to their happiness and prosperity. The presence of a child marks a significant event in a mother's life, as with the birth of a child, she too is born as a "mother," and this simultaneous "birth" brings about immense changes in her identity.

The significant difference between a mother and a woman arises from the extensive influences that the birth of a child creates in her. A mother is concerned with the principles of raising her child and therefore tends to take fewer risks and make fewer changes in her parenting methods. This is the pivotal point we referred to regarding parenting principles. With a conscious attitude, a mother can guide the foundations of her child's upbringing in a way that in future generations, men's view of women does not include feelings of ownership and dishonor toward women. However, women have been repeating the same unhealthy upbringing foundation for centuries and passing on what they have learned from their mothers to their children. This behavior stems from the strictness and caution she applies toward her child.

Women can gradually initiate a transformation in the outdated upbringing system and start a kind of educational revolution. Eastern mothers can leave behind their classic and hereditary teachings by joining the enlightening waves of the new era. They must avoid repeating themselves and seek proper and new parenting patterns so that in the future, we witness men who not only do not consider mothers and sisters as their honor but fully believe in their freedom. It is natural that social forces will resist in this area. However, what force can resist the penetrating will of a woman in the years when child-rearing is in her hands?

Mothers need a fresh insight into this training course. The more they are approached from a position of weakness and passivity in this course, the men of tomorrow will have less respect and freedom in their own lives compared to women. Criticisms raised about the lack of romantic resources in couples' lives can be addressed in this important educational context. If a mother teaches love to her child and without creating a limited mental structure, makes them receptive and ready to love, she has taken effective steps toward their successes in later life and emotional encounters with the women in their lives. Not depriving children of their freedom of action can make them advocates of freedom. When a child faces unjustified limitations during this crucial educational period, they will learn that depriving others of freedom is a normal thing.

In other words, the formation of societies with deep beliefs in freedom and democracy is possible during this period. Jean-Jacques Rousseau, in 18th-century France, clearly explained the mistakes that occur in child-rearing. Rousseau believes that pressuring children with moral social concepts and ideas is incorrect. To understand these concepts, children should be allowed to go through sensory stages and then enter the stage of mental reasoning to be sufficiently prepared to confront these concepts. Failure to do so may lead the child to evaluate them hypocritically and avoid them when faced with these concepts and moral teachings.

This is an issue that autocratic systems do not pay attention to and try to create generations in harmony with themselves by dictating their desired moral concepts in the form of a complex educational system. Interestingly, these projects often fail and bring about opposite results.

Perhaps for some, talking about the freedom and independence of young children and the necessity of mothers' attention to this matter may seem like a trivial or even amusing topic. However, it is a grave error that human society has fallen into, resulting in a significant amount of selfishness and opposition to freedom and basic rights of women. What mothers can do is practically instill a spirit of resilience and equality in their children through their behavioral culture.

According to educational psychologists, children more so than written sources and educational principles, emulate our behavioral culture. Therefore, when a mother grants freedom of action to her child, refrains from repeated commands, and removes the sense of confinement from the child with a sense of self-restraint, she effectively transfers a sense of independence and nobility to the child. It is not necessary to cater to a child's high sensitivities and needs in the shortest time possible.

Self-restraint in satisfying unnecessary desires and engaging in reflective behavior promotes the child's patience. When a child overly easily accesses their daily and even unnecessary needs in an exaggerated manner from their mother, in the future, as an adult, they will have similar expectations from women in their lives. Just like their mother, they will quickly demand their physical and even entertainment needs from their life partner. The spirit of assertiveness in men's relationships with women, especially in customary marriages, stems from the upbringing practices during childhood and how mothers respond to boys' general needs.

When a child starts to cry, the mother immediately offers her breast as a soothing option. This action is sometimes unrelated to the child's hunger. Crying often serves as the child's language of communication with the environment. Mothers often misinterpret this response and place their breast in the child's mouth. This issue becomes ingrained in the child's unconscious mind and manifests in adulthood when dealing with a life partner as an urgent demand. Psychologists attribute some mental disorders related to addiction, sex, etc., to the individual's childhood. Just as the mother's breast acted as a sedative for the child, now the expectation is that any restlessness or lack of peace should be alleviated by the sedative of sex. Feelings of ownership, deprivation of women's freedom, superiority complex, disbelief in gender equality, premature masculinity versus feminine patience and resilience, one-sided actions in the sexual process, and many behavioral traits shape the dynamics between men and women in this context.

The Third Type of Mother-Child Relationship

Most of the time, men feel a certain fear and confusion when a child enters the relationship between a husband and wife. It seems as if fathers do not love their children enough. With the arrival of a child, a third person enters the relationship framework, taking a significant share of the wife's attention and emotions. With the presence of the child, the woman is no longer the same woman and wife she was before. She, who had previously abandoned her girlish identity with a significant turn and entered the realm of womanhood, now, with a drastic change, steps into the realm of motherhood.

She has undergone significant changes in her actions and emotions. Now she faces the competition between her husband and child. What factors lead to the wife's attention shifting from the husband to the child? The husband tries to discover these factors and show himself worthy of these conditions. He does not want the love between him and his wife to diminish, so he tries to once again attract his wife's attention in the form of a son. The woman is reborn and appears as a mother. Now it is the husband's turn to be reborn and appear in the form of a son. His effort is not focused on winning the child's affection; rather, he tries to mend the damaged relationship with his wife. However, repairing this relationship is not so simple.

When a mother is born, she has waited for this birth for several months, even years, and prepared herself for fundamental changes. The presence of the child has transformed her significantly. The child is a clear symbol of her life and continuity. For this reason, she feels a deep sense of duty and selflessness toward the child. She has a deep emotional and physical connection with the child. In the early months, the child is constantly in contact with her body. This connection at times causes her relationship with her husband to be strained and even impossible for a while.

The mother is the center of gravity for all family communications. Despite this, traditional institutions have tried to deny this centrality and reduce the importance of the mother solely to the services she can provide to the family.

The husband, like the children, relies emotionally on the woman. A man who has grown up under the dominance and protection of his mother for a long time, seeing the mother figure in all women for a period, now expects to have a place under the emotional support of his wife (similar to children).

This projection and homogeneity as an emotional need, when faced with a decrease in attention from the woman, poses a major challenge for the man. He feels like a little boy whose level of emotional attention has now been reduced with the presence of another figure.

The reason psychologists see many mental disorders or behavioral dysfunctions in men as stemming from the actions of mothers. The educational system centered around the mother has perhaps been one of the most unchanging educational patterns in the world. Throughout men's lives, mothers have always raised the men of the future. This educational system has followed uniform patterns. New educational principles have struggled to penetrate this unique maternal framework. A framework characterized by maximum maternal support, maternal affection and love, and the protective shelter of the mother. These characteristics all draw inspiration from maternal instincts. Because the maternal educational system has always been an instinctive system.

Unconditional love, providing all the necessities of pleasure and leisure, and of course imposing restrictions by the mother, which have all been instinctive and may not necessarily align with proper educational styles, are a set of automatic mechanisms that the male societal mindset must explore within them.

A mother's gaze toward her child goes beyond biological boundaries and necessities. She strives to create all possible facilities for the happiness and well-being of her child. Perhaps this approach stems from a strong sense of responsibility or powerful regret that arises within a mother upon the birth of her child. This is because with the birth of a child, there is always the possibility of their suffering in this world, especially when the child is a defenseless infant who is helpless against the forces around them.

This thought leads to an increase in the mother's efforts to provide maximum support to the child. This support causes the man, when faced with his spouse, to seek to recreate the idealized world of the past. It could be said that this issue is the most significant weakness in men.

It is natural that men will never be able to recreate the romantic conditions between themselves and their mother with their spouse. A mother's love for her child and a spouse's love for their husband are of two different styles. Although love in its essence is the same, at lower levels and in details, there is a significant difference between the two types of love. The act of loving someone purely based on external aspects versus someone with whom there is a deep emotional connection that arises from the depths of the soul is different. A mother's love for her child has noticeable differences from a spouse's love for their husband. Some of these differences are as follows:

- In the love of a mother to her child, sex and sexuality are absent or very little.
- In mother-child love, the element of pleasure is absent, or if we trace a kind of pleasure in the mother-child relationship, the nature of this pleasure is not self-conscious.
- A mother's love for her child is eternal and cannot be separated into tests and grades; but the love between man and woman is demarcated and dependent on external conditions and has history and degrees.
- A mother's love for her child does not have a biological or hormonal origin, and its source is mostly within the mother; However, love for a spouse has a hormonal origin and its degree depends on the conditions.
- A mother's love for her child is not reciprocated and there is no counterpoint for it. For example, a woman's love for a man can be mutual points; such as hatred, ownership, exploitation and exploitation; but a mother's love for her child is not like that.

Considering the above, it is unrealistic for the wife to share the maternal love that is dedicated to the child. But since it is based on nature and is caused by an educational vacuum, it is an existing reality and there is no blame on the man for it.

Family Without a Center of Authority

Alongside the growth of human awareness and significant transformations in human interactions in the modern era, the traditional family system is losing its position. For centuries, the family has played a pivotal role in human relationships and served as the primary social institution in the sociocultural process. However, the failure of this social institution to adapt to modern relationships and its lack of success in nurturing human generations have brought into question the intrinsic value of this institution.

The doubts within human society regarding the nature and function of the family institution have multiple reasons. This outdated institution, with its rigid educational principles and inflexible nature, has hindered the mental growth of children in parallel with the convergent changes in human generations. Nowadays, wherever social issues manifest in human societies, the primary cause can be traced back to the traditional family institution. The population imbalance between wealthy and poor countries, hunger, homelessness, religious fundamentalism, declining life indicators, and numerous other issues directly relate to the inefficient functioning of the family.

Hence, some leading theorists believe that the role of the family in modern sociocultural life has come to an end. Despite its long history and role in the mechanisms of past societies, this social institution no longer aligns sufficiently with the dynamics of the modern era. Despite the religious institution's efforts to maintain the family's position, the global community is rapidly moving toward a form of communal living devoid of centralized authority within the family.

Ushu, a socio-biological theorist, states: "In my view, the family of the future will not have a fixed pattern and will have numerous alternative methods. If a few people still want to live within the framework of the family, they must have the freedom to do so. However, this will constitute a very small percentage. Currently on Earth, there are families that are truly beautiful, truly blessed, where human growth occurs; families where there is no authority, no power games, no domination, and where children are not destroyed, where women do not strive to destroy their husbands, and husbands do not seek to annihilate their wives. A place where love and freedom exist: a place where individuals come together only for happiness—without any other motive. A place where politics does not exist."

"Yes, such families exist and have existed on Earth, but they are very rare, not more than one percent. Such families do not need a change in structure. In the future, individuals can still live in families like this. But for the majority, the family is an ugly thing. You can ask psychologists, and they will tell you that various mental illnesses originate from the family. All kinds of neuroses and psychoses have their roots in the family. The family creates very, very sick individuals."

Some scholars believe that many of today's anxieties stem from family roots. These anxieties, based on superficial thoughts that manifest themselves in intolerance toward others and acts of violence and terrorism, all have their roots in the family system. The new human biological patterns based on global village structures and Marshall McLuhan's theories are completely contradictory to the fixed patterns of life and family upbringing.

Family Incompatibility with Women's Freedom

One of the criticisms directed toward the institution of the family is the deprivation of freedoms and social rights of women and girls within it, along with the systematic gender discrimination that takes place. Throughout the centuries, men have been able to impose a form of systematic oppression on women due to having a tool called the family.

The structure of the family is designed in a way that it contains a center of power known as the man. This center of power can completely impose its own interests and desires (even if unjust and inhumane) on children, especially on women. Within the framework of the family institution, a woman has little autonomy to attend to her personal matters and realize her potentials.

If a modern woman is expected to adhere to all the norms emphasized by the family institution, she will never find the opportunity to focus on herself throughout her life. She cannot travel, paint, read, engage in social activities, seek financial independence, create, write, or be an artist. If the family institution becomes intertwined with religious conservatism, the situation becomes significantly more dismal.

The reason for the inflexibility and lack of updating of the family institution is that this institution is primarily based on the teachings of religions. Almost all religions advocate the strength of the family organization as an indispensable method of social life.

On the other hand, all religions oppose the measures that can to some extent keep women away from the suffering of life. Religions and faiths oppose methods of controlling births and anti-conception products. They oppose abortion. They recommend population growth. Governments (especially in underdeveloped societies) are in favor of these methods. For the rulers, the importance of women lies in the fact that by having children, they become a population-generating machine. Populations that are important only as a unit or a soldier in the armed forces, regardless of their biological indicators, future, and identity. Suitable means for killing and being killed. These governments often ignore issues such as employment and the future of these soldiers and are not responsible in this regard.

To promote such an approach, several initial prerequisites are necessary. Marriage, in any form and under any possible standard, forming a family as a production line of soldiers, in any way and under any conditions.

Only a traditional family can provide these conditions for religious people and rulers. But where is the place of women in such a family? If it is necessary to not use preventive measures and abortion is not allowed, and according to the guidance of religions, a woman must have sex with a man and become pregnant under any circumstances, the clear result of this situation is that a woman must be continuously giving birth throughout her useful life, until around the age of 45 or 50.

It has been stated that in such a situation, a woman of approximately 45 years old would be occupied with pregnancy, breastfeeding, or changing diapers of children. It is implicit what status a woman would have in the dictionary of such a family. The conflict between women's biological standards and the institution of the family has led feminist intellectual movements to primarily seek to criticize these outdated patterns. Patterns that, without breaking them, will not see a woman's gender on happiness. Because in the vocabulary of "a woman is always pregnant," the only thing that cannot be imagined is happiness.

Sex for Reproduction, That's It and Nothing Else

Marriage and religious institutions emphasize several key approaches. First, a woman is expected to conform to the requirements of marriage, even if they contradict her human rights and status. Second, physical relationships should strictly serve the purpose of reproduction. Fulfilling the needs of the man takes priority. Third, a woman's opinion in sexual relations, like social interactions, is deemed unimportant as long as the transmission of sperm, the woman receiving it, and entering pregnancy occur, fulfilling the purpose of marriage and religion.

This approach contradicts social freedoms and women's individual rights. Creative sex and meeting women's needs have no place in this context. A woman should never pursue her inner desires and emotions, and it is natural that her quest for diversity will not be tolerated. On the other hand, a man, while having the possibility of engaging with multiple women, can force a woman into "compliance."

The term "compliance" in customary literature and legal language of marriage institutions is considered anti-women discourse. This is evident because compliance is solely about women. If the assumption is that the institution of marriage seeks to promote loyalty, the authoritarian directive of "compliance" should at least superficially extend to men as well.

Another point is that the institution of marriage does not impose restrictive recommendations on women. It is never suggested, for example, that a woman has the right to decide on further pregnancies after the fourth one. Nor is there any right for her to be requested by a man for intimacy a certain number of times within a specific period.

The repulsiveness of this literature is so high that sometimes one hears from proponents of religious marital principles that a woman must fulfill the sexual needs of a man even during menstruation when she is physically unable, implying that the woman lacks personal and emotional independence and has no share in this mutual relationship. Many such instances, which are quite numerous, are just a part of the extensive range of controlling actions leading to sexual slavery for women. The demeaning nature of empowerment discourse for women is sufficient to empty the concept of sex for women of its human nature and essence. A woman is forced, not empowered, to engage in sex to the extent the man deems appropriate, even when her emotions and feelings do not call for it, and to accept his sperm with the aim of pregnancy.

Osho, whose views have been perceived as revolutionary in recent centuries in terms of social relations between men and women, even takes it a step further by considering sex for procreation as a moral sin that humanity should abstain from. He expresses in part of his views, in light of women's liberation movements, "When I say sex for procreation is a sin, the term 'sin' is not used in a moral sense. I simply say it is a sin because it is unconscious and nonconscious. It is not you who are doing it, but you are compelled by an unconscious force to do so." Perhaps from a social logic perspective and due to societal conditioning, including women's society, the idea that sex, even between husband and wife, is ugly and sinful may not be straightforward. However, if we set aside social hegemonic logic and look at it based on human logic and emotional and spiritual analysis, it is quite obvious that sex as a compulsory behavior solely for procreation is ugly and sinful. This issue is more relevant to women.

A woman who engages in forced sex feels the sinful nature of it deep within herself. Unconsciously, she senses that this act goes against her inner feelings and emotional logic. A voice from within whispers to her that at this moment, she has been emptied of her human dignity and reduced to a mere tool for use. She keenly perceives that this act now carries a mechanical and deliberate nature, while sex is neither mechanical nor deliberate.

The feeling of being used is akin to what a woman experiences after being violated. Though the degrees of this feeling may vary, the essence remains the same. It is an internal and gradual sensation. In a one-sided and imposed relationship, a woman finds herself entirely in a state of "powerlessness." Powerlessness inherently involves a degree of violence that can vary.

The sentiment a slave holds regarding their situation is similar. They feel devoid of independence, human identity, agency, and initiative. They are compelled to perform specific tasks for their owner at specific times. Isn't this feeling akin to what a woman experiences in a coercive sexual process, even if it is for the purpose of procreation?

In reality, the situation of such a woman is not even comparable to a woman in a prostitution situation. In a situation of obscenity, a woman engages in sex of her own will. If she had no will for it, she could prevent it from happening. However, our subject woman, who gives her body for sex within the framework of marriage and based on social coercion and the obligations of the institution of marriage, does not have this freedom of action. The interesting point here is that this will not be the end of it. Reproduction means a woman entering a painful period of pregnancy and the challenging project of raising a child. The idea of a woman in a situation of forced social (overt or covert) marriage engaging in such an act is difficult.

The situation of our subject woman is worse than even animal sex in several ways. Animals engage in sex not purposefully and for reproduction, but simply in response to their instincts and temporary needs, in response to bodily changes. However, a woman under the above conditions is not even benefiting from this instinct. She may, despite her own reluctance and in disgusting circumstances, engage in this act based on the coercive dictates of the institution of marriage.

With these characteristics, the institutions of marriage, religion, and government stand firm in their positions. These forces, regardless of the criticisms raised, still view women as a means to serve two purposes: satisfying men's needs and producing children. They believe that sex (regardless of the woman's position) is moral if it is for reproduction. So in their belief, the more animalistic and devoid of emotional and internal aspects sex is, the more moral it is.

A modern thinker argues that sex is valuable when pursued without awareness and solely for pleasure, under equal conditions. To achieve such an experience, the initial stages are biologically driven, but a touch of romance will enhance and perfect it.

Beautiful sex is free from constraints, plans, or specific goals; it begins with biological sparks and evolves through discovery and sensual experiences. This kind of sex can be a source of inspiration for unlocking immense potentials aimed at optimizing the relationship between man and woman, serving the higher purposes of life. Considering the life plans of individuals and aiming to reduce the stress of potential pregnancy, enhancing the quality of sex, all strategies related to infertility, contraceptive tools, abortion, and the like are entirely ethical and serve the advancement of a loving life. A romantic life that is intrinsic and not a vessel for conforming to political, religious, societal, or similar guidelines.

However, authoritarian societies and traditional institutions governing the intellectual currents of societies are vigorously trying to prevent the promotion of this modern thought. From their perspective, a man, in line with his conformity to society, has the authority to exploit women at the level of tools and even livestock, force her to bear and raise his children. In such a view, a man is a farmer and his wife is considered his field. The woman is the cultivated land, while the husband is the wanderer who sows seeds in this land and exploits it.

It is natural that the field and land have no practical choice in the decisions and actions of the farmer. This is why in the linguistic culture of many countries, the term "husband" is synonymous with expressions such as farmer, gardener, planting, and plowing.

Women Flourish in the Absence of Traditional Relationships

In all respects, it seems essential in the modern era for women to overcome the current crisis and achieve their first human rights, enjoying the gift of freedom and dignity by negating traditional ideas, reforming collective actions, eliminating superstitious beliefs, improving misconceptions, and so on.

In a different space where a woman can live freely and equally with men, the dominance of the institution of marriage as the prevailing option will gradually fade away. By moving beyond the institution of marriage and embracing different ways of organizing pseudo-family situations, many ancient and persistent obligations will be lifted from her shoulders.

Compulsory and unplanned pregnancy, transcending gender stereotypes, disregarding emotional needs and inner desires of women in the modern era will gradually disappear without the traditional institution of marriage and family. New ways of living that humanity has initiated and will witness its expansion in the future will provide an opportunity for women to break free from historical feelings of insecurity and lack of self-confidence, and stand shoulder to shoulder with men in the flourishing of their inner potentials. In such a world, the notion that a woman cannot be a mystic, philosopher, and influential figure in society will vanish.

With the removal of traditional gender stereotypes and moving away from conventional relationships, women will reach the heights of excellence in various fields such as literature, art, economy, knowledge, and philosophy. A woman who is no longer confined in the cycle of consecutive pregnancies can delve into her inner self, chart a clear path, and implement a predetermined plan for her life.

A woman who is not forced to compromise and submit to a demeaning relationship can seek to discover her innate qualities and use sex as a determining factor in her relationships and a source of pleasure and satisfaction. Many scholars believe that women not only lack less talent than men in some social spheres, but will perform significantly better.

In such circumstances, awareness plays a major role in determining the biological relationships between women and men and planning for interaction. Unlike the past, sex will take place in areas abundant in choice and awareness. Reproduction and having children, based on comprehensive awareness, with a precise calculation of its risks and considering the abilities of parents and the society's capacity for the happiness of children, will be achieved consciously.

A woman, outside of a life of imposition and full of physical and mental torture, can witness the blossoming and manifestation within herself. In such a world, unlike the past, we will witness the emergence of social reformers, theorists, economic activists, writers, artists, playwrights, doctors, astronauts, engineers, and other influential figures among women. This is an event that is currently unfolding in the Western world.

In such circumstances, women will enter magnificent realms. Realms of knowledge, contentment, pleasure, humanity, and vital contemplation where their identities are discovered, and their experiences in enduring suffering will come to the forefront. In the absence of masculine exploitation, women will become great sources of inspiration for human life and the development of valuable human components such as peace, empathy, and spirituality.

When the management of the global community is entrusted to women more than ever before, undoubtedly the world will be a better place to live. A glance at the history of human life shows that in all historical gaps and tragedies that humanity has recorded in its resume, almost no woman has been present. Therefore, there is no need to argue that when half of human affairs are in the hands of women, the earth will be a better place to live.

The dominance of sensitivity, grace of character, various aspects of contemplation, and maternal instincts of women can be a measure in itself for optimizing socio-biological indicators. Of course, all of this is contingent on the realization of the first assumption. That is, the liberation of women from the shackles and chains that have tarnished her social life and human identity. Women, unrestricted by imposed limitations, will shape a different world on earth beyond traditional marriage systems and their imposed rules.

Democracy and Women's Revolutionary Movement

When we see the issue revolving around a woman's body, all power structures and forces influencing her destiny strive to exploit her body in various ways, without feeling obliged to fulfill any duty or pay any attention in return. A husband or sexual partner expects to exploit her body as desired, often unilaterally and failing to meet the woman's physical expectations. The religious institution aims to restrict women to the maximum extent possible and keep them veiled and covered. The social institution attempts to severely limit their presence in various ways. The political machine and political power are interested in excluding women from social and economic statistics and charts. Therefore, in many underdeveloped countries, the female population is not taken into account in calculating employment rates and social services.

A man, without participating in a woman's suffering or involving her in sexual exploitation or other pleasures outside the home, only uses her to satisfy his carnal desires. Nonetheless, to the extent possible, a woman remains honest in her words and actions. It appears that expressions like "I love you" and "I am in love with you" are often more sincere when said by a woman compared to the same statements made by a man.

In a woman's existence and creation, the ingredients of tranquility and peace are ingrained, and the long-suffering endured by her has not diminished the form and degree of these qualities. An aware woman, when informed of her historical position (this knowledge and education come through university education and training), will then rebel against all these injustices. The main reason for the opposition of religious fundamentalists and backward and tribal segments to the education of women and girls is precisely this.

An aware woman does not submit to oppression and imposition, and at the same time, she will be sensitive and concerned about the fate and status of other women in society (both her own society and the global society). If the number of women who think and act in this way reaches millions and billions, then no authoritarian system will be able to dictate the fate of women as half of the human society according to its own taste and norms.

The collective awareness of women around the world will be achieved through education and promotion of enlightenment and intellectualism. Institutions benefiting from male domination over the female society seek to prevent this enlightenment in order to maintain the status quo.

An aware and enlightened woman will be angry within herself toward men who harass women in any way. If she is a source of change and knowledge or power, she will definitely take action to improve the status of women worldwide. Achieving the status of an enlightened and powerful woman is possible through education and social activity. An enlightened woman will create a kind of effective social dynamism. The more of these women there are, the greater the power of this dynamism will be.

On the other side of the coin, there are passive and accepting women who have accepted their historical fate as men's tame animals. These will be devoid of such dynamism. The second wife is safe for misogynistic patriarchal systems.

In the interval between the two world wars, which brought the world into a new phase of social life, and following the waves of modernity, a significant change occurred in women's society. It turned out that he not only had a correct inference of his own nature, but was also well aware of the power hidden within him. The modern woman was informed that during the history of passive coexistence with the man, how much bitterness has been done to her and how much her basic rights have been denied. He was informed that the man had been conspiring against the woman continuously throughout his history with the woman.

This awareness led to the launch of several movements all over the world, whose main goal was to liberate the female sex and obtain basic and basic rights for women and create an equal position next to men.

The most important problem was that it was believed that women should "fight" with men to obtain basic rights. This thinking, along with trying to make women as masculine as possible, caused some women to become aggressive toward men.

The fact is that women do not need to be angry and vengeful toward men, nor do they need to make themselves completely like men in order to gain an equal position with men. What, in this case, the woman is empty of her true existence as a genuine woman. The truth is his greatest blessing and superiority over men. When a woman is no longer a woman, she does not have an equal position in front of a man. In order to heal the wounds of the past, it is enough for women, while understanding their situation, to try to revive their identity as a "woman-human" and not just a "woman-mother."

It is enough to forgive the man's mistakes and not make him a historical enemy. Because there is no chance to live with a man as an enemy. But there are many possibilities for living with a forgiven wrongdoer.

Men throughout history have tried to make women their slaves. Obviously, this was a mistake. But if there is a chance that women can turn men into their slaves for a long time, wouldn't this method be wrong? Should we answer an error with an error? Since, due to biological determinism, which is institutionalized in the nature of men and women, they are forced to be together. Is there any value in living with a partner who has been reduced to the level of a slave?

This is a difficult question that men have never put themselves in a position to answer or have avoided answering. The question that a man should ask himself is this: Is it worth living with a passive woman who has been reduced to the level of a sex slave and knows nothing but obedience and acts as a full-fledged house maid and sex machine? Is it honorable to live with such a woman or to live with an intellectual, knowledgeable, independent woman who has the same status as a man and as a complete and respectable human being has the power to act and make decisions in all situations and has high human values?

The answer to this question is clear: the first type of woman is desirable for a man who has the same characteristics, but for a man with human characteristics and moral qualities and a suitable social position and as an educated and knowledgeable person who has his human dignity. considers it important, it is definitely more desirable to live with a woman with the position and status of the second wife. Basically, he will not consider himself worthy of living with the first wife.

Therefore, it is clear that the main keyword in the literature of "equality between men and women" and the realization of women's human rights lies in words such as "awareness" and "knowledge" in a general sense. If a man is educated and intellectual and free from superstitions and blind prejudices, he will look for a woman who is his equal and has the same qualifications. Such a man will act with the same mental and intellectual criteria in dealing with society. Also, if such a situation exists for a woman, she will expect the above conditions when facing a man and will act according to her mental and intellectual criteria in her public actions with other women.

It is necessary to repeat once again that the reason behind the opposition of religious fundamentalism and blind tribal systems to girls' education and their presence in society is this simple and clear equation. For such systems, "awareness" and "knowledge" are like a poison that will eventually disable the organism relying on ignorance of these intellectual systems.

Therefore, women's awareness movements and women's rights activists, in the new era, should focus their attention on the issue of "awareness." Adopting aggressive methods against men, keeping alive a historical memory based on revenge, or trying to pretend to be male and look like men, and any other actions and reactions that are not in the way of promoting and developing the consciousness of the global women's community, are the great forces and potentials of women's movements. The great potential of these movements after centuries of submission, acceptance and desperation is a rich and suitable opportunity for the global women's community to take advantage of the opportunity and free itself from the yoke of history by developing the knowledge and thought of female independence and independent identity.

A woman is not supposed to deviate from her identity and nature for the sake of creating transformation and changing the structure of bio-social spheres. A woman's identity is defined by love, affection, gentleness, kindness, motherhood, femininity, feeling and avoiding violence. Any type of women's social struggle should also be promoted by considering these identity factors.

The past full of misunderstandings, which has defined the relationship between men and women until now, can be the driving engine that brings the stormy ship of female identity to the shore of peace. If we accept that the past is the beacon of the future, then this beacon can be used to illuminate the path and not as a tool to condemn the type of man whose historical error is beyond doubt.

In an ideal society where there is no gender discrimination, men will definitely benefit from freedom and independent identity as much as women. The center of gravity of this society is also the issue of responsible awareness and removing superstitions and false ideas from the minds of the society, which have been injected into its mind and consciousness during long centuries and have caused poisoning.

All the damages and disorders that manifest in the relationship between men and women, from the worst form to a simple disagreement and action in everyday life, are caused by the same two fundamental factors: lack of awareness and the presence of superstitious and poisonous beliefs.

Homogeneous behaviors, from burying girls alive in the Hejaz desert, a few thousand years ago, to a suitor throwing acid on his favorite girl in the streets of Isfahan, are all rooted in these two important factors. Therefore, women's movements of the new age should focus on these issues if they are not going to take the path of deviation.

It seems that the deviant currents that have been created in the path of women's rights movements in the new era are somehow rooted in the activities of men to influence this movement. A man can't accept that a woman in his life is just a factor for fun and happiness and nothing else, that he is now trying to create a different world for himself by reaching a level of awareness in the form of social movements. A world in which a woman is no longer the cause of expansion of a man's mind and a means to make his life better; rather, he is an independent human being who must fully participate in social, civil, economic life and benefit from all the blessings of sex.

Now, women don't just enjoy being labeled with the childish attributes they used to receive from men as encouragement.

Now a woman doesn't just want to be: flower, angel, mother, emotional, lover, and gatekeeper of heaven. In addition to these qualities that he has by nature, he also wants to be human, wise, mature, manager, brave, true and complete partner and have the same rights as a human being.

In fact, the attributes of the first type without the conditions of the second type are nothing more than deception. A historical deception that the man, using them, has tried to control the woman and keep within the framework of his desires, needs and desired status. But the various colonies and groups of women, who have now come together all over the world to raise their knowledge and consciousness and make a better situation for themselves, have created a powerful force in themselves that makes them, in the depth of their womanhood, make changes.

The new and common understanding of the world, which is being formed regarding the issue of women, can undoubtedly change the position of women to an ideal situation in the coming decades as an irreversible force. Provided that this great force is not wasted with issues such as unhealthy competition with men. There is no doubt that heavy and violent sports like wrestling are naturally male-specific. A woman, as a delicate and sensitive being, cannot get a better situation for herself by involving herself with these matters.

This does not mean that women should be banned from these activities altogether. Rather, the artificiality that exists in these issues is to mislead the feminine nature of women's rights. Equality does not mean that women are equal to men in all issues and activities. Equality means that a man as a man and a woman as a woman should enjoy all their rights and benefits, and no gender should do anything to dominate the other gender for false reasons, including religious reasons.

Fortunately, in the new age, we are witnessing changes in the behavioral culture of people, especially in developed societies. The communication revolution caused the formation of women's groups and populations related to women's rights in developing countries. With the activity of these movements, we are witnessing the spread of awareness waves to other parts of the world.

The global women's revolution, regardless of the distortions and deviations that have infiltrated it, seeks to correct, optimize and adjust the relationship between men and women as two equal human beings. The ugly relationship between men and women, over the centuries, made less people experience the feeling of true happiness in sex. Although there have long been extensive efforts to train men to behave appropriately with women, today is the time of accelerated procedures. Women tried to make up for the mistakes of the past and move quickly toward the full equality of men and women.

Is Mankind Doomed to Be Alone?

It seems that man was created alone by nature. A look at the "Journey of Genesis" in the Bible and other narratives and myths of creation shows that Adam was created alone and sometime before the creation of Eve. Then the Creator creates Eve to eliminate her loneliness. Most of the upstream documents of Abrahamic religions and creation myths, both in the West and in the East, have drawn the issue of Eve's creation in such a way that Eve was created as a companion and life partner of Adam for the continuation of life and the survival of the generation and is condemned to obey.

Therefore, human beings are generally born alone. He lives alone and dies alone. Since human birth is associated with loneliness, the birth of twin children is an exception and a violation of habits in human culture and causes surprise and reaction from those around. Therefore, being alone is part of our nature. Maybe because in this loneliness and not isolation, a kind of silence and peace has been granted to mankind.

Although being alone is a part of human identity; but he has been able to develop his social funds over time and save himself from this situation. Other biological characteristics deposited in human creation show that social participation and life with others, as an optional element, has become an important part of human biological rule. For example, no human can make love in solitude, have children in solitude, or form biological colonies.

In fact, man is "free" to choose a wife, have a husband and create a better environment for himself by forming a family. An environment where participants can meet each other's biological and spiritual needs and facilitate the path of life. Despite the fact that "being alone" and solitary life is a part of human nature; but "loneliness" is not defined as a negative quality and biological deficiency.

All the interactive methods that man has invented during his life are to fill this deficiency. All kinds of shared entertainment, games, friendships, gatherings, and rituals, etc., have been created to fill this void. Inventing means of mass communication such as television, radio, social networks and shortening communication paths, by speeding up long journeys and the like, is another part of human effort to remove the quality of loneliness from his life.

Even those who prefer to be alone in general prefer their solitude in the form of a group. Someone who lives in his apartment in a city is not really alone. He is surrounded by people who live in close proximity to him and are potentially accessible at any moment. Otherwise, we should witness plenty of people who live alone in the heart of the mountains and deep in the forests.

Humans generally seek their happiness and excitement in the community, and despite the fact that in their privacy, sometimes, they prefer solitude; but in life as a whole, being in the crowd is an undeniable need. Humans generally believe in collective wisdom and benefit from the gifts of this collective wisdom. The main philosophy of democracies, as the highest social achievement of mankind, is the consequences and results of collective wisdom.

Ballot boxes are actually the crystallization of the collective wisdom that individual people benefit from its results. The highest systems of justice and law are also legitimate and acceptable when they rely on collective wisdom and not on the opinion of an autocratic person or a minority group. In the nature of his creation, man is a solitary being, but in the general dimension, he needs and is interested in community life.

The philosophy that emphasizes the authenticity of collective wisdom is based on the view that one person can make mistakes and suffer from corruption and all kinds of vices and errors; but a group never makes a mistake in the way it takes. According to this philosophy, even if a group makes a mistake in one of its choices, because the seal of approval of the group has been put on it, it will not be considered a mistake anymore.

Man tries to find a middle way for the best form of life by creating a balance and a logical fit between his solitary nature and his social dimension, which is a transverse thing. Because of this; He falls in love, mates, marries, creates a family, and has extensive interactions with society.

Man, despite the fact of his existence alone, tries to interact from the first seconds of being on earth. The baby starts crying after birth. This crying, for whatever reason, is an attempt to connect with the environment. You may say that the child is crying and protesting being taken out of the isolated and alone environment. If this is the case, however, the protest is a kind of raising the issue with the people around. He creates a relationship with the people around him and expresses his protest by crying.

The same child, when he grows up, and even before being among his peers, by taking refuge in dolls and objects, he identifies with them and tries to fill the emptiness of his loneliness. In any environment, his first reaction to the surrounding phenomena is the effort to start a project of intimacy.

When an immigrant enters a room for the first time in a foreign land, his first reaction is to open the window and assess his surroundings. His second reaction is to try to identify the wall-to-wall neighbor. The next step is to say hello to him and introduce yourself as a lonely person who likes to share this loneliness in a simple conversation with a neighbor.

Various factors are effective in this simple communication. One of them is the importance of two-way communication. The second issue is the need for mutual respect and understanding. The motives of assimilation and egalitarianism are also caused by human's escape from loneliness. A person who is not in an equal environment feels alone. The next steps are more complicated. The need to love and be loved is a more evolved need that is rooted in eliminating loneliness and filling the void of being alone.

The human infant, in the first instance, begins to love the mother. Then, it is the turn of the father, brothers and sisters. Loving and being loved brings competition. With the entry of multiple components into the space of relationships, the complexity of the matter increases. In much more complex stages, rules and regulations come into play. Now there should be rules that define the boundaries and loopholes of relationships and categorize people and define the form and framework of all types of relationships.

Humans are not allowed to establish any kind of relationship with anyone regardless of lines and boundaries. The mother's position is different from that of the father, brother, sister, and daughter of the neighbor and the people who are far away. "Likes" are also categorized. Actions after the formation of the relationship also have limits and loopholes. A child can love his mother. As well as your siblings. But he can only fall in love with people outside his family. With some, he can have a romantic relationship and with others, he is not allowed to do so.

Using his personal experiences, he learns love for his wife in the stage of love for his mother and by distinguishing the rules and properties of each of these relationships, he blends with his lover or wife. While in relation to his mother and sister, he always stops behind a certain line. Therefore, it defines the coordinates of all kinds of love and channels and regularizes the consequences of each of the different loves.

It is not clear when mankind created its rules in drawing these bio-social coordinates. But the fact is that these rules are present with all their power and have formulated his life and how to get out of loneliness for him. It is not known whether humans had sex with their mothers and relatives centuries ago. We do not know anything about this. Maybe it was something like that. Also, when it comes to the children of Adam, mathematical logic shows that the children of Adam must have had sex with their brothers and sisters in order to produce the next generations. But it is certain that the world of relationships is, at the same time, the world of rules for man, and he has fully accepted this fact.

Since human life experience on earth includes individual trials and errors, and the lived experience of past generations, a large number of failures and hardships also come to him in the process of establishing a relationship. He sees a woman, he keeps trying and making mistakes to develop a romantic relationship with her. In the end, love works as a spice, gets married. But as soon as marriage takes place, another field of discovering the hidden corners of another's existence is created. Here, homogenous biological experiences, over generations, do not work. Under certain conditions, the two of them should discover and deduce a large number of aligned and non-aligned personality elements.

Most marriages end in failure. Because in the field of discovery and inference and trial and error, generally people become more distant from each other than closer. To improve the situation, love can be the way. The most important potential that nature has placed in human nature is the alchemy of love. Love gives a divine quality to a human being. They say that God is the star of defects. With the help of love, the lover can achieve this godly quality and be a star of flaws toward the beloved. Countless marriages and relationships end in failure. The reason for most of these failures is the lack of sufficient or quality love. When a person achieves sufficient and quality love with the help of love and attains the status of God and becomes free of defects toward his beloved, the factors that cause separation fade away and the relationship lasts.

So we see that the operation of getting out of loneliness is associated with risk and danger for humans. He sometimes decides he prefers being alone. But these days, the model of human loneliness has become more complicated.

Techniques such as meditation, discovery and intuition and deep philosophical contemplation have made the human encounter with his loneliness multifaceted and different. Once upon a time, people used to leave the society and seek refuge in the forest cave to be alone. But today, a person has to build his lonely cave in his home in the same framework of society and at the same time benefiting from social services. However, this form of loneliness is different from pure primitive loneliness that was possible in the past. To compensate for this problem, man tries to discover the authentic server hidden in his existence and reach deeper intuitive states.

When a person can explore their inner potential and their spiritual labyrinth, they can have a more pleasant experience when trying to build a relationship. He is inspired by the positive experiences he has had in the worlds of solitude. Therefore, he will not seek raw and incomplete experiences in haste and out of desperation. When he can achieve the possibility of a deep and beneficial relationship, he can perform more creatively. Because this relationship is no longer from the angle of fear of loneliness and as an added value in life. A value created from the perspective of a two-way partnership and to facilitate the process of life and new experiences. This relationship can be a carrier for the manifestation of all the strengths of the parties.

When the relationship is not based on the fear of loneliness, but based on the understanding of the positive view of loneliness, a person will be happy and happy in the form of a relationship and will have high self-confidence. Because the human identity includes a combination of the talent of loneliness along with the biological and social gifts.

A human child begins his life alone. For nine months, his cells are formed in darkness and solitude. But at the same time, he is surrounded by people around him. He is born in the crowd. He organizes his life based on imitating others. He tries to find the answers to his basic questions that are formed in his solitude with the help of others and studying the collective biological experience and in consultation with fellow humans who have had a similar fate. Based on this definition, it can be concluded that human being alone is a positive and independence-seeking trait, but loneliness and isolation can be a form of collective neurosis and incompatibility.

This contradictory quality is an effective weapon for humans. Relying on the aspect of his aloneness, he builds a base for regulating his spiritual and philosophical affairs and can think about the meaning and truth of great concepts such as the meaning of life, metaphysics, God, love, death and the like.

This is why they say that God is present in human solitude. Experiences like meditation and spiritual trances are possible in solitude and in the absence of others. The deepest devotions are recommended in solitude. Even acts of worship such as congregational prayers are designed in such a way that the worshippers practically do not have the possibility of any kind of communication with each other. The same famous saying: "Present and absent existence" is formed in the spiritual glimpses of man.

In other words, the highest temple of man is built inside him. Seclusion and solitude in mystical rituals are based on this philosophy. Rehru tries to get closer to the innermost core of his existence and understand the joys of this connection. Just like a diamond after long isolation and loneliness, it reaches infinite intrinsic value and originality. When a person gets the valuable and infinite treasures inside, he can, based on it, share the other with the romantic worlds inside him and probably have a reliable companion for the rest of his life. He can also help another's quality of life by giving love. The result of this alignment and partnership is the understanding of peace and contentment in the light of self-confidence and mutual respect.

This process is completely personal and experiential. It is not taught in any university, nor is there any training for it, nor can the lived experiences of others be a guide.

Such an experience, if realized in each and every person of the society, will gradually transform the human society, which is now suffering from communication disorders, into the utopia described by utopian theorists.

Loving one's wife and neighbor, which is one of the main guidelines of Christianity, will be realized in such an environment. When a person does not love himself and his wife, when he is faced with all kinds of misunderstandings caused by not understanding himself, how can he have a relationship without misunderstandings with others? To treat others lovingly, you must first love yourself and your loneliness. Then, he started with his life partner and the people around him and finally expanded the radius of this circle of love.

The flourishing of the garden of social relations depends on the blooming of the flowers of human nature, which are located in the hidden layers of human existence. In this case, it will be possible to communicate with others in an aura of culture, dignity, sobriety, free writing and free thinking.

This is the happiness that mankind is looking for and must reach. Therefore, the missing link of human collective happiness is in the potentials that have been deposited in the existence of each human being and must be realized.

Love is a completely individual thing. By looking inside himself and thinking deeply in solitude, man becomes aware of the existence of love inside him. In order to make love with a third person, a person must have the source of love inside him. In this case, loving and loving behavior will be one of the most important foundations of human life. Love can bring many virtues. The first virtue of love is getting out of loneliness. So, love is the basis and prerequisite for collective action.

In fact, man is strangely the assembly of opposites due to having two elements of loneliness and love. On the one hand, love, because it is an internal matter, has its roots in the loneliness and innermost nature of man. On the other hand, because love is manifested in the face of others, it tends to go outwards. Therefore, love is also a union of opposites. When it is said that man is the most complex manifestation of creation, it is for these reasons.

All this depends on the type of initial upbringing of the person. Primary education sparks human awareness about himself. He is the one who chooses what kind of person to be. In the meantime, a large number of people decide not to make an effort to know inside and outside and do not use their capabilities. Just like a seed that is planted in the ground; but for various reasons, it does not reach the growth stage. All humans have that initial seed; but only a few of them allow themselves to excel. Great and desirable relationships are given to those who try hard enough and have good educational backgrounds provided by their parents. The most important turning point is to get out of the cocoon of loneliness and blossom in the community.

A possible misunderstanding should be answered here: entanglement and assimilation does not mean removing the independence of the other person. When such a place is established in the levels of love, all the aforementioned levels will occur independently. The independence of the lover, like other romantic components, is part of the achievements of the romantic relationship. The lover considers the beloved to be a part of him, and just as he wants an independent identity for himself, he also considers the beloved to be worthy of such an identity. This means that love and unity never means taking away the freedoms and powers of the beloved.

Gibran Khalil Gibran explains this situation in the form of an example. According to him, life partners are like two independent and equal pillars that support a roof that is the "building of life." Both columns have the same task and importance. They are part of the macro identity of a structure; None of them overshadows the other. The two, while being intertwined parts of a whole, are completely separate. All of these work in the form of a single organ that aims to advance a single goal.

But this quality is not always achieved. Currently, millions of humans live communally on Earth, who have been defensive against each other since the beginning. They are the seeds mentioned above, they don't try to move toward the sun. They are standing side by side even holding a roof over their heads; but their roof actually consists of two separate roofs that are temporarily placed next to each other. Their being together is temporary. The two have not reached pure unity. It is enough for a flip or an impulse to happen in life for this roof to crack and its two parts to be separated from each other.

When, as human beings, we explore other existential lands and in this pleasant realm, we discover suitable facilities for happiness, we have to allow ourselves to be discovered by the other party. If the treasure within us is valuable enough, then we will not shy away from being discovered. If so, we will eagerly wait for someone else to share this pristine and valuable treasure.

Nowadays, before marriage, they try to identify biological factors and plan to avoid problems. But perhaps more important than biology are plans to know the inside of people. Perhaps it is better to consider a meditation and exercise program to increase self-esteem and improve thinking for couples. Programs that help manifest the inner potential of people to enter a stable relationship.

A person enters the marriage process without sufficient skills and education. Where the top to the bottom requires trial and error and has many variables. Considering this complicated situation, how can we expect that people without training and skill and personalization of data, just by relying on several routine rules, will advance their relationship without problems. Let's not forget that every human is an independent and complex world. When two people meet and fall in love, it means that two worlds will merge and create a newer and more beautiful world. Just like the galactic marriage and transformation of worlds, stars, black holes and constellations and other celestial phenomena.

When two people meet and fall in love, a huge transformation has happened in their existence. The life of two people is exactly divided into the moment before and after this meeting.

Sometimes a moment can completely change the course of a person's life. What philosophers and religious people put forward regarding the category of "predestination and free will" is intertwined in a strange way with the issue of fate, event, and the issue of time and place. These concepts affect our lives in a surprising way. While people's view of these matters is often superficial and naive.

When a man and a woman meet, the first point of connection is pen on paper. This pen is supposed to draw a genealogy over time that will create a new branch of the generation in the decades and centuries to come. Philosophically and historically, the fate of a large number of people on this planet is determined by the meeting point of a woman and a man at this moment. Therefore, every meeting between a woman and a man is of great importance. It is in this way that the two forces of loneliness and sociability in humans shape the structure of life.

What Is the Problem of Being a Man or a Woman?

When the two concepts of "being a man" and "being a woman" are mentioned, many aspects come to mind to define these two terms. In general, there are two main concepts and components to determine the "hypothetical line" between men and women. Biological and physical components and psychological and mental components.

This is why we use the term "hypothetical line" because the line drawn between a man and a woman is by no means definitive. That is, being a man does not end in one place until being a woman begins.

The findings of Freudian psychology have determined that there is a certain amount of man in every woman and there is a certain amount of woman inside every man. Depending on how much this amount is in each human unit, the human will contain certain personal and exclusive characteristics.

Anima or the female element is the leaven that makes a man, despite institutionalized violence and harshness, to have a kind of feminine softness and gentleness in his belly and to be able to achieve masculine and managerial powers while not being alien to delicate, emotional and feminine affairs. It is this feminine aspect that helps the man in mating. Because by resorting to this intuitive and inner power, he can discover the real feminine qualities in the opposite party and choose a good partner.

Animus or the male or masculine element also has the same property in women and strengthens the masculine and violent aspects in a woman. The balance of these elements in a man or woman can lead to the balance of male and female identity.

Therefore, "being a woman" is as much a physical issue as it is a psychological issue. It means that a person can be physically male and mentally female. The opposite of this problem is also true. Some women have a more aggressive spirit and some men have a very gentle and sensitive spirit. What women ignore in their struggles for equality is the need for balance in this part of female identity. The deviation has been made in such a way that it is thought that the more masculine spirit women have, the easier it is to achieve equal rights with men.

To express this issue and the psychological nature of men and women, Osho mentioned an example and said: "Jean-Darque is not a woman and Christ is a woman. Jean-Darque is psychologically a man. Basically, his approach is aggressive and the spirit of Christ is not aggressive at all. He says if someone slaps you on one side of the face, give him the other side of your face. It's psychologically non-aggressive."

Osho adds that: "Non-aggression is the essence of feminine dignity. This is why "science" is masculine and "religion" is feminine. Science is an attempt to conquer nature; religion is a release and dissolution of oneself in nature. A woman knows how to melt and how to become one, and every seeker of truth must learn how to dissolve in nature, how to become one with nature, how to flow with the flow, without resistance and without fighting. As you become more and more meditative, your energies become non-aggressive. Violence in you disappears, love rises. You are no longer interested in dominance, instead, your interest is more and more in the art of submission. This is what makes a woman's psyche feminine."

It has a distinct expression in the mixing of male and female qualities in the mythology of different lands. In Ferdowsi's Shahnameh, some women have strong masculine aspects.

Even though she is a woman, "Gord Afrid" has the status of a wrestler with all the characteristics of a man. According to Ferdowsi, she who is the daughter of Ghastham is a very beautiful woman and at the same time a brave warrior. When Sohrab attacked Iran, he was able to fight well with him, and even until his hat was removed from his head and his beautiful face and black hair were revealed, Sohrab and Turanian did not know that they were fighting an Iranian woman. Ferdowsi has described him as follows:

He was always very famous and brave during the war
There was a woman like a warrior on a horse
Time has never created a woman like her
The one whose name was "Gord Afrid."

In the mythology of other nations, there are statues and characters who have a mixed temperament of both sexes. In the temple of Gangaikunda Cholapuram, India, there is a statue of Ardhanarishva in the form of half man and half woman, which is a combination of Shiva, the guardian of the sky, and Parvati, the goddess of love. This statue, which expresses the ultimate unity between man and woman, on the right side with beautiful hair, breasts and well-balanced hips represents Parvati, and on the left side with a mustache, broad chest and masculine features, it represents Shiva.

Examples of this balance can be seen in other creatures and other parts of creation. Creation relies on the balance of similarities. If the balance is upset, anywhere, the natural process of life will be disrupted. The mechanism of creating balance in creation has been observed both in the field of biology and body, and in the field of human mind and psyche as a component of stability.

Female mind and male mind

The human mind is a combination of female and male parts. In the 20th century, a lot of scientific research was done on the functioning of the human brain. These researches show that each of the hemispheres of the human brain is responsible for doing certain tasks that can be called male tasks or female tasks. There is no noticeable difference in the size and function of the brain of men and women. The most important difference between men's and women's minds is the ability of each to do certain things. Women's minds are more capable of doing emotional and intuitive tasks. The male mind is also more capable in mathematical, comparative and rational activities.

Here we also encounter the same special intelligence of creation. The physical aspect of the creation of man and woman by combining anima and animus capabilities has ensured the balance of life. Regarding the mind, the combination of male and female abilities has once again made balance possible in life.

The result of the difference between the male and female minds is prosperity and diversity in the mechanism of creation. Based on her nature, a woman has a dignified and beautiful mind, and a man, based on the same nature, has a more efficient and practical mind. The combination of all these apparently contradictory components ultimately brings peace and balance in life.

Dominance of the left hemisphere over the right, or vice versa, disturbs the biological balance. Just as the balance between the anima and animus aspects of man is disturbed, it disturbs the sexual balance of the society. Creation has arranged everything according to its rules so that life can continue in the most ideal way. It is obvious that any kind of effort to establish the superiority of one gender over another will make this rule unequal and make life difficult.

The superiority of women in the right hemisphere of the brain, which is the center of poetry and love, does not mean that women are more poets, but it means that women are more poets by profession and lovers. However, poetry in practice is a brain activity of the type of mathematical activity in which men excel. Converting concepts with words and creating a structure in words is an action that the left part of the brain performs. Just as women perform better in mastery of stress, use of language tools and emotional superiority, men process example problems, math and understanding of dimensions and directions better.

Creation has given women the mission to be the guardian and emotional guardian of mankind. The world of women is the world of hearts. But this does not mean that we should direct the woman to the corners of the houses. Because in this case the world will become a completely masculine place. If a man takes the authority to act in a world without women, he will destroy the beautiful spirit of existence and nature.

When faced with nature, a woman acts with her soul and feelings. Therefore, he does not harm nature, trees and forest.

The reason why the Earth's environment is so vulnerable to destruction is because it is completely in the hands of men. The great intelligence of creation has created women to create balance in life, to prevent the destruction of the environment by injecting a considerable amount of spirituality and emotion into the human biological body. But this has not happened in practice. Has the creation made a mistake or have men, by resorting to trickery, distorted the tracks of the creation to reach the ideal destination?

The intelligence of creation in the creation of men and women is amazing. Understanding the greatness of this part of creation is not less than understanding the greatness of galaxies. Let's consider the issue of draining internal forces. There is no doubt that every human being may be activated within him, and the energy of anger or sadness may accumulate inside him. Women, who are half of the society, cry or talk to release these energies. But men punch, shoot or remain silent.

This balance is practically the rule of existence. If all the people on earth were violent and repressive, the human race would probably be extinct by now. It is said that mankind has ignited more than 5 thousand wars. But there is almost no direct trace of women in igniting and continuing these wars. If the emotional and brain functions of women were exactly like men, according to the mathematical rule, now humanity would have more than 10 thousand wars in its history.

The ugliest sentence, which is said to male children in some societies, is something like this: "Be a wolf so you don't get eaten." Man, as the best of creatures, has another policy for life. The law of struggle for survival, which governs animals, has no precedent for humans. Because human beings have wisdom, tact, management, fairness, justice, kindness, control, and a thousand other traits and skills that do not need to be "wolf" in their shadow.

On the other hand, a woman should try to fill her behavioral shortcomings in order to strengthen her mathematical and reasoning aspects. He must learn that loving is not absolute. In order to love, consciousness and a little mathematical calculation are also necessary. Love is like a huge ocean in which you must have swimming skills. Without swimming skills, it is possible to drown in the ocean of love. Due to the inability to calculate, heavy damages may be caused to the woman. What has happened today is the strengthening of those aspects that exist naturally within men and women. The woman has been pushed inside the house to be away from any kind of calculating and non-emotional atmosphere, and the man has been taught to never cry and to survive, he must become a wolf as much as possible. In order to create an ideal and desirable world, extensive efforts should be made to balance these areas.

Chapter Seven
Free Relationship, Pornography, Homosexuality, and Other Cases

Free Relationship, Why and How?

In other sections, we talked about the priorities of a free relationship between a man and a woman. Including the fact that a free relationship takes place in a natural setting and without the intervention of external forces, it is usually a quality and romantic relationship. Even if this relationship is limited and short, compared to the relationship that exists in the form of marriage requirements, it has better quality.

It was also pointed out that it is better for people to think about what factors were involved during the free relationship before marriage to create attraction and prevent the coldness of the relationship.

Of course, the meaning of open relationship needs a brief explanation. An open relationship is usually referred to as a romantic relationship that leads to sex under equal conditions, due to interest and love, and due to mutual attraction, in a completely natural environment and with the agreement of the parties. In this way, relationships that take place outside of ethics and custom, for example in prostitution or buying sexual services, are not included in the definition of free relationship.

A free relationship is an ethical and unrestricted relationship whose main criteria are the consent of the parties, the absence of coercion and secondary requirements of any kind and based on mutual interest. In prostitution, neither party is interested in the other. Money or a financial phenomenon determines the form of the relationship, and in order to establish it, the prerequisites, including initial familiarity and deepening of emotions, have not been passed to the bed stage.

In terms of moral-religious criteria, a free relationship is also different from the relationship known as wife. However, religion does not involve itself in classifying and framing the types of relationships outside of marriage and calls any type of relationship between a man and a woman outside of marriage as adultery. But referring to adultery as a free relationship is not correct, not in the sense that it shows the opposition of religion, but in the sense that there is ugliness hidden in this word.

Many families in the West are the result of a deep family relationship without marriage, and children have also been the result of this relationship. This relationship is completely customary, ethical and sometimes very desirable and high quality. But the religion, regardless of the internal and moral qualities of such a relationship, believes that such a man and a woman are committing adultery throughout their lives, and their children are also born of adultery according to the religion.

But there is another side to the free relationship that has always been a challenge for the moral and social system of the society. In an open relationship, the parties have all the conditions listed for a moral relationship, except that one or both parties are married and have families and even children.

Modern ethics, although it takes a more cautious stance toward this issue; but it is not as strict as religion. The most severe punishments for sectarian religions in such a relationship; including stoning.

The reason for the strictness of religion is in its internal relations and trying to restore its authority in society. Otherwise, in terms of human ethics and relationships of the new age, when two people reach a dead end in the form of marriage, an emotional divorce has actually occurred. For modern ethics, emotional divorce can be the basis for looking for a mate for each of the parties. Although it is stated again that it is better for the parties to legally separate from each other and look for another suitable pair; but if the relationship of freedom is formed before the separation, there is no punishment similar to what religion suggests.

There is another situation that adds to the complexity of the problem. In this way, the parties do not have much problem with each other; but one party, which mostly includes men, establishes a short-term relationship with the other person because of sexual adventures. Here the foundations of common life are not at stake; but one of the parties has a problem in regulating his sexual behavior.

The reaction of religious religions is completely different. Religion gives a man the right to legally and customarily have sex not only with one woman, but with many women. But he emphasizes to the woman that she should only stick to the relationship with one man and not make any mistakes. Religion gives a man many opportunities to have a free relationship with other women, in the definitions of modern ethics, this is the same free relationship; but religion deprives women of this right with difficulty and violence.

According to modern ethics, in such a situation, the conditions of men and women are equal. They should adjust the relationship and solve the problem with their personal tact and discretion. For men, although there are shortcut and unofficial ways to have a double relationship; but legally and socially, no distinct right has been given. It may be possible for a man to have a free relationship with another woman by chance, in the work environment or while traveling. In the same way, such an event may happen to a woman.

This is where the moral standards and the level of deep loyalty, love and two-way emotions are decisive. There may even be one or two sexual incidents for each; but in the end, the foundation of their relationship is so strong that it guarantees the organization of the family and the continuation of the relationship. They may return to each other with this momentary experience and continue their lives with more love and intimacy.

After all, an open relationship is something that can happen at any moment in a person's life. Sometimes such an event may have destructive effects and sometimes it is forgotten as a low-value issue or filed away with an apology and consolation from the wrongdoer.

In any case, there are not few men and women who consider this behavior reprehensible based on individual moral standards and have no desire to sleep with people other than their spouse.

The problem of opposition to free relationships becomes complicated when moral judgments are not the criterion of action and instead, the authoritarian system of religion intends to interfere in a person's life and prohibits him from having free relationship despite having all the conditions. Such an approach may cause a person's life to become a boring mess. Because it is in conflict with human nature. These limitations destroy the human opportunities to love and enjoy sensual stimuli.

A dogmatic view of free relationship makes life void of the emotional glory associated with sensual attachments. This approach is opposing life and trying to empty life of joyful elements.

When the open relationship is in the privacy of a permanent and family relationship, the concept and view of "betrayal" immediately emerges. Betrayal becomes meaningful in front of loyalty. In a permanent emotional bond, one of the parties has deviated from this rule and agreement for any reason. The criteria for evaluating infidelity, like other components, are different in different societies.

The situation of religious communities and the stance of religion is quite clear. Therefore, without repeating the stances of religion, we examine this issue from the point of view of modern ethics and the principles related to the human nature of men and women as two equal beings.

Infidelity, which becomes objective as a result of the process of free relationship, is reprehensible from the point of view of modern ethics. Failure to adhere to the agreement is a matter for which there is no justification. Of course, there are logical ways to get out of a contractual relationship. Divorce and breaking the agreement is the main way to get out of the dead end of the relationship. But sometimes the condition of the relationship is not so malignant and critical that it leads to breaking up. This is where betrayal is a cross-sectional issue.

Betrayal undoubtedly leads to mental and emotional damage to the victim. In John Stuart Mill's *Philosophy of Liberty*, we observe that the privacy of liberty can be expanded and sacred to the extent that it does not lead to harm to others. In the case of treason, a person's freedom has been invaded and his good and personal interests have been taken away. Therefore, according to the principles of modern ethics and human freedom, treason is inhumane and contrary to the principles and standards of freedom.

Infidelity, if it happens, has a lot of destructive and perhaps irreparable effects on the continuation of the life together. Therefore, the treacherous person has acted against the common interests and in the opposite direction of his own interests and interests. By jeopardizing the health of the common life, he has committed an act that is not compatible with common sense.

Betrayal indicates a kind of romantic vacuum. If the unfaithful man or woman, who in normal circumstances was a claimant of mutual love and affection, proves the opposite of this issue, it means that he has been behaving for a long time which was even more immoral than betrayal. He has been secretly deceiving and hypocrisy, which contradicts all kinds of human principles and moral standards. Modern morality is sensitive to the issue of lying in any possible form. Lying in the matter of emotional and romantic dependence is one of the worst forms of lying. Because it plays with the mind and feelings of the other person in a painful way.

Cheating shows that the person in question does not deserve to be in a family relationship in terms of moral principles and standards. Lies and deceit are two basic factors that show that we are dealing with a person who is not trustworthy. Such a person cannot be competent and reliable in the family environment and in the process of raising children and other family requirements.

In a multifaceted family relationship, a person is supposed to deviate even from some of his desires and attachments in order to advance the collective goals. Infidelity, which is related to a matter of fun and fleeting lust, questions the competence of the cheating person in this field. If the betrayal happened in an atmosphere devoid of love and full of coldness, no logic supports the continuation of the relationship. If the parties of the relationship agree to the continuation of the relationship under the conditions of "curiousness," it is not possible to have confidence in the competences and tact of the parties.

When a person enters into a permanent family relationship, his main goal is to achieve three things. Love, sex and family are the most important goals that must be realized in the shadow of a permanent relationship (whether it is a formal marriage or outside of it). Proper management of this process requires the application of other management in the field of individual and collective demands. When betrayal occurs, almost all of these matters are questioned. In this case, there are two possibilities: either the necessary conditions for establishing a stable relationship did not exist from the beginning and the parties committed hypocrisy, or the conditions disappeared over time.

The family organization is based on different beliefs and beliefs, all of which take place in a certain direction. Loving, flirting, sex and emotional relationships are given and take that involve people in relationships in the field of psychology. When betrayal takes place, it means that one of the parties has gone beyond the defined criteria for this relationship and priorities beyond what is within the family framework have been created for him.

It is obvious that under betrayal, it is not possible to continue the organization of marriage or a stable relationship. For this reason, psychologists in divorce counseling offices usually try to provide a special service to clients in the form of "betrayal counseling," which may be feasible to restore if the foundations of the relationship have not collapsed. But there are always big challenges and complex questions on the table of such consultations. Questions about deception, concealment, fakeness of love, trust, competence, offensiveness of betrayal, self-esteem of the betrayed person, disillusionment, psychological damages and the like. Even if such consultations lead to the continuation of the relationship, it will eventually become an example of the same poem that we mentioned above:

If the thread is broken, it can be closed
But there will always be a knot in the middle

What Is Sexual Fetishism?

When we talked about the peak of uniqueness and departure from the norms of behavior in romantic sex, it was briefly mentioned that irregular behaviors may also introduce external influences into the process. There are different degrees of taking help from different tools for double stimulation.

It may be said that sexual fetishism is an extreme form of "tool-oriented sex." But under normal conditions, the parties can take advantage of the objects and elements they have in their possession to increase sexual imagination and more excitability. Of course, it is clear that sensual "tool worship" can be considered abnormal and classified as a mental illness if it is excessive and centered on the tool. This issue is not the subject of our discussion; but paying attention to objects in the conventional form can include acceptable norms. Choosing certain colors for bedroom curtains, wearing different underwear, wearing masks and leather clothing, having long nails to make small scratches on the lover's body, and dozens of similar cases are some of the early cases of normal sexual fetishism.

Sometimes a person's reliance on fetish materials is so high that he cannot achieve orgasm without resorting to tools. In fact, mechanisms such as body, flirting, conversation, and sensible violence are sometimes necessary. Because without them and without external tools, the body capacity of some people may not be enough for sexual stimulation. In such cases, the person's body, without external tools and devices, has lost the power of imagination and stimulation. Excessive use of tools in such a situation can be an abnormal quality.

Regardless of this issue, it should be said that almost all people, to varying degrees, have fetishistic tendencies. When a man says to his wife, "I really like this dress of yours" in normal conversation, he is actually referring to his fetishistic tendencies. Clothing, in itself, cannot be tempting, unless we look at it from the point of view of sexual fetishism. The list of people's desires in the issue of lust creation tools includes different degrees and different tastes.

Man has often used tools in matters related to his inner self and in relation to the beyond. For example, in carrying out a spirit summoning process, a set of external and physical materials are used, which in fact have nothing to do with the phenomenon of spirit and spirituality. These tools are actually a mediator that can create two spiritual phenomena; That is, to connect the "summoner" or medium, and the summoned one or "spirit." Creating the right environment, such as darkening the space, special lighting, and creating silence and peace, burning incense, lighting candles, and similar tricks, play the same role as the foundation and Chinese introduction to the realization of the matter. However, the phenomenon of meeting with the soul is in itself a completely non-physical, non-material and metaphysical thing.

This rule also applies to sex. The tools that are used to improve the erotic quality have the same mediating and double role. Depending on the person's moods and life experiences, the tools help him release more sensual power and serve a strong relationship by conjuring up meanings and images of sexual milestones and lived experiences of the person.

Perhaps a man's first experience as a young adult is seeing a glimpse of the blue bra of a school teacher, the girl next door, or the wife of a relative. This image, at the beginning of puberty, has left a huge impact on his erotic imagination. This internalized experience may unconsciously create enormous stimulation in the new sexual environment.

Most of the time, the target person may be unaware of the reason for this irritation. But when her sexual partner appears in front of her in the same blue bra, she is indescribably aroused. In this case, it is completely justified to ask him to wear such underwear on special occasions as an effective tool. This factor, which is the origin of his passion, while helping to create an attractive relationship, can soften a part of his hidden inner self, as an inner disturbing force, and free him from the burden of such a force.

Sometimes it may be difficult to understand these preferences and instrumental tendencies; but in fact, its roots go back to our biological experience. The mind of every human being is a huge storehouse of lived experiences. These experiences may be buried under the dust of time, so that it is not possible to summon them to the conscious part of the mind. But in any case, these lived experiences, which are present in our womb, have an effect on our sexual action and motivation.

Sometimes these tendencies are rooted in collective experience. That is, it is present in the hidden layers of the collective unconscious mind. For example, in the dressing culture of today's society, high heels are considered a provocative tool. The red color may also be like that.

These two objects are in clear conflict with the traditional woman, which the moral society tries to present as the symbol of the modest woman. This conflict, which is rooted in our unconscious mind, is revealed when it becomes possible to reveal itself with a fetishistic nature in the form of the above two objects.

These factors can be purposefully personalized. For example, the first experience of a man's sexual arousal goes back to the story of meeting a university library librarian who is wearing a navy coat with simple nursing shoes. He has fantasized about this visual experience for some time. Now these two simple and seemingly non-sexy objects have become a symbol of sensuality and arousal for him. Hence, when, for the first time, he sees his lover in similar guise on a park bench, he finds him very different compared to others.

The range of object-oriented tendencies can be very wide and depending on the biological experience of people, it can include a wide range of objects. From a pair of rubber glasses to a short plaid skirt and pink nail polish and tons of other things.

So more often than not, fetishism involves the use of tools to stimulate erotic fantasies and achieve ideal sex. Therefore, most of the time, instead of being a worrying complication, fetishism is actually a psychological potential that can activate the couple's sexual power.

To better understand this issue, we must refer to a wonderful fact. In the sense that sex is almost the only human action that completely engages all human senses. That is, in addition to the five senses, the secondary understanding of humans, which is referred to as the "sixth sense," is also aligned. The all-round conflict of man has gone even higher and engulfs his other human, animal, moral, evil, innocent and wicked feelings. In fact, the process of sex includes a process that dominates from the most mundane animal feelings to the highest spiritual and holy degrees.

The power of objects in sex starts from the sense of sight and by wandering into the most hidden corners of a person's personality and psyche, it accompanies him with a course that passes through the labyrinth of the mind and returns to the body. The reason that objects may be the best means to reach orgasm in some cases is because of the cooperation of body, soul and mind. Therefore, it is possible to match the tool-oriented tendencies and the object-oriented tendencies with Freudian psychological findings.

One of those who scientifically researched the subject of non-sexual behavior was Richard Van Croft Ebbing. For a long time, Van Croft's theories were considered the scientific reference for the analysis of unconventional sexual behaviors. Until this time, any type of sexual behavior that was performed with a purpose other than reproduction was considered reprehensible, and any non-subversive sexual behavior, fetishism being one of them, was considered deviant.

Therefore, the most important point in fetishism as a model of sexual behavior is that this non-sexual act is formed when sex is not a routine behavior and only for reproduction. If the act of sex is based on traditional principles and as a task for reproduction, then neither a man's old leather watch is important as a tool to increase sexual heat, nor a woman's red high heels are attractive.

Although Kraft-Ebbing does not have independent research in fetishism; but his ideas about the non-transgressive components of sexual behavior initiated the identification of sexual actions beyond traditional behaviors. In fact, what makes the issue of fetishism thematic includes the symbols that appear in pornography products in the new age. The use of accessory tools or paying attention to a special form of clothing and belongings related to men and women, which are referred to as "sexy," can generally be studied under the issue of fetishism.

If we put the model of the staircase of love, which is described in the book of Plato's Banquet by Socrates and quoted by Diotima, about fetishism as the criterion of action, we can conclude that any kind of tool, as the initial steps of an evolutionary process, and as a good tool, is justified. When we are attracted to something through the sense of sight, the visual becomes spiritual and leads us to more sensory horizons.

From this point of view, the hypothesis "the goal justifies the means" arises, based on which the objects and phenomena that can be part of the evolution of the sexual process from the point of view of fetishism will not be reprehensible. Of course, like any other field, moral and customary frameworks in actions and reactions are the criteria of action. Extremism, in general, in any field, can be criticized. In fetishism, even though the goal justifies the means, the means itself cannot be justified as the ultimate goal. Therefore, objects, under certain conditions and requirements, can be the source of good and a vehicle for achieving excellence, where the peak of sexual excitement and pleasure and achieving ideal sex is the desired excellence.

Pornography, Requirements of the Modern Age

As we have mentioned many times, the requirements of the modern age have left a great impact on the relationship of couples. Some of these effects are positive and in the way of improving the relationship and making it more rational, and some are in the way of destroying and weakening it. The moral requirements of the modern era point out that a romantic relationship is a spontaneous act and in equal conditions, and a man has no right to dictate his wishes to a woman, even indirectly.

The modern age has provided the conditions for a man to pursue modern entertainment when relationship gaps are formed. Nightlife, erotic entertainment and pornography with a multitude of products are among the requirements of the modern age that attract men. When the relationship between the husband and wife is in crisis, the man is attracted to pornographic products because of his diversity-seeking and easily deceived nature. Pornography is a situation that occurs in human imagination. Nothing is real.

In real sex, human organs and cells are completely involved in sex, but when the viewer, by watching sensual and seductive images, gradually reaches the moments of orgasm, he goes through stages that are physically and morally contrary to his human nature. It is that the dangers of addiction to porn products are more than one might imagine.

The man in our scenario, when he reaches orgasm, is dealing with both the guilt of leaving his wife and taking refuge in his study, as well as morally collapsing and despairing.

If we use Aristotle's statement in the book *Nicomachean Ethics* as a criterion for judgment, which says: "Valamenshi means the full flourishing of the most human characteristics that correspond to virtue," then resorting to pornography to release the suppressed emotions, questions Valamenshi and leaves man with a crisis. faces because his moral virtues and human identity have collapsed in the core of fleeting sensuality, dependent on pornographic imaginations.

Watching the genitals in the ugliest way possible, in an atmosphere devoid of love and romantic ecstasy, displaying sexual behavior, will be despairing for a man who was raised on a natural bed and has enough restraint. This feeling, combined with the emotional breakdown between husband and wife, releases enough force to finally fire an old relationship.

In such an environment, where there is no support from therapists and no adequate filters to prevent men from accessing porn products, it sometimes seems that religious prohibitions about sex are not reprehensible in themselves. However, the prohibitions of religion limit the natural freedoms of human beings (especially women) to such an extent that even if it has reasonable teachings, it gets lost among extremism.

To show how far pornographic products have pushed back the boundaries of obscenity, it is enough to go back to the past and see which products have been censored as literary obscenity in the fields of fiction writing and even documentary research.

In America, for a while, Vladimir Nabokov's masterpiece *Lolita* was not allowed to be published because it was believed to promote prostitution and sexual debauchery and exploit children. This restriction was still applied in some countries for a long time. While in all the pages of Lolita novel, as one of the masterpieces of 20th century novel writing, not a single erotic sentence is found.

Marquis de Sade was ostracized and even sentenced to death for his tendencies in his writings, including Justin's novel, and of course some of his personal sexual acts.

Osho, the Indian philosopher, was criticized by the most progressive Western societies for promoting sexual freedom and equal rights for women and breaking the taboo of sex, and he even faced problems for his travel to free societies.

Forough Farrokhzad was criticized and condemned by religious institutions for freely expressing her emotional and romantic feelings in some early poems.

Western literature is full of works that were opposed and censored because of erotic themes, the works of such people as James Joyce, DH Lawrence, Henry Miller, Anais Nin and many others were among the above. But it seems that the issue of freedom of speech and the right to choose, which are requirements of modern democracy, has left so much space for the production of pornographic works that the tens of billions of dollars of pornography industry with hundreds of millions of viewers in the world is damaging the moral foundations between women. And they are men.

You don't need to be an expert in literature and art criticism to understand the difference between porn movies and erotic literature. Even the average audience can recognize that by reading the Lolita novel, the audience reaches the level of human feeling and discovers the psychological unknowns of today's lonely man, and how much ugly and negative emotions can be experienced by seeing the brutal sex of three men with a woman by the pool. Contaminate the existence of the viewer.

All this while there are not many mechanisms to prevent men from considering such products, neither from psychology nor from scientific and social authorities.

Fortunately, the achievements and blessings of the modern society and the new democracy are such that the wise man of the new age has to deal with thorns of this kind that have grown in the garden of free, democratic and secular human life.

From the point of view of the secular democracy world, citizens are independent in most of their decisions and can watch any picture or scene they like. Humans just cannot do things that violate the freedoms and rights of others. Therefore, if a man wants to look at a pornographic film for a long time and lose his time, energy and enthusiasm, it is not related to others or even to religion.

John Stuart Mill believes in the book *Inquiry about Liberty* that man can pursue his good and interests in any way he wants; but this effort should not be at the cost of depriving others of their own interests or preventing them from achieving their own good. This view considers every human being as the guardian and guardian of his body and mind. He can make any decision about his physical health or mental and spiritual health. What has been legalized as "euthanasia" in some countries is actually based on this idea that a person can even decide about his life and death.

The foundation of liberal democracy thinking is based on several important points. First, democracy is worth tolerating some anomalies, such as the freedom of action of pornographers and their audiences, to protect the ideals of freedom.

The second foundation is that "man as a perfect and conscious being" as the "noble of creatures" has enough intellectual power to distinguish between good and evil and avoid falling into pits and wells. Therefore, humans do not need guardians and shepherds. This thinking is completely opposite to the thinking from which dictatorship and autocracy come out.

Dictatorship thinking believes that humans are like flocks that need a shepherd to distinguish their interests and good and evil.

The widespread prevalence of referendums in democratic countries, which seek people's opinion for every important social issue, along with the existence of Eastern authoritarian systems (which do not even seek people's opinion for the form of government) is due to the difference in the attitude of these two views toward human beings.

This is where the deep conflict between liberal democracy and most religions lies. The philosophy of liberalism, unlike religion, considers man to be the center of gravity of the universe and its brain. While religion believes that humans have come to this world to perform tasks. Because religion is related to the origin of existence, it has the duty to force him to follow biological programs and a certain moral system in the social and personal sphere, even with violence and coercion.

Therefore, wherever the censorship system is working, with a little care, we will find its obstacles in a religious system. Humans are not free in any area, not even their innermost thoughts. For this reason, in many periods of history, a complex network of inquisition and motivation and examination of opinions was set up, which we see as an example in the Middle Ages of Europe and backward Eastern societies in the present era.

According to some thinkers, this is the Achilles' heel or the weakness of the philosophy of liberal democracy, which has sometimes made it vulnerable in protecting people from evil forces (even in areas such as providing security against violence and terrorism).

complex network of toxic content production; Like pornographic products that are constantly operating and endangering the moral health of society, it is a weakness of liberal democracy that censorship and prohibition in general are at odds with the core of libertarian thought.

If certain religions impose the burqa and hijab on women as a method of coercion, they are actually continuing to try to suppress sexual power. Although hijab deeply contradicts the human dignity of women, it fulfills the purpose of religions. Wearing all parts of the body can give even the first sparks of lust at the root. But because the religion also deeply believes in the succession of generations, it recommends sexual intercourse; but he suggests that men and women should not even see each other before marriage. In this situation, in order to verify the health of the traded goods (i.e. the woman), the people around the man can have a complete examination of the goods being purchased so that the man is not confused in this transaction.

Thus, we are currently facing a bipolar world. On one side is the secular and free world, where people are exposed to millions of hours of pornographic films, which is as easy as buying a pack of cigarettes every hour of the day and night. Man in this world is also exposed to the ever-increasing blessing of modern morality and humanity.

On the other hand, we have the closed world of religious tyranny, where a man does not have the right to look at a woman before marriage, even to choose his permanent life partner. But after marriage, the "commodification" of the woman allows the man to treat her in any way he wants. This world is also one of the negative elements of the Western camp; That is, the achievements of pornography are very beneficial. The deep valley between two intellectual and moral camps has made sex a critical issue in human life.

But the question is, which of these viewpoints are better for providing moral happiness, optimizing morale and repairing human pains in sexual life? Should a woman be bought and sold as a sexual commodity, and in this exchange, her dignity and humanity are completely suppressed and she should be owned as an object? Can he take the initiative in all personal and social relationships and bring proper sexual ethics to men in addition to the cunning market of pornography?

It is said that in the Western camp we are dealing with a type of woman who has practically become a commodity and a product, and her body is the raw material for the production of porn products. But the quantity of this type of woman is not enough to endanger the moralistic society of the West.

The irony is that in the consumption of porn products, we suddenly see a strange equality between the two camps of the East and the West. Some research has shown that the search for the word SEX and its derivatives is much higher in countries like Iran than in Western countries. That is, in the porn industry, the producing countries also meet the consumption needs of the third world well.

It does not seem that the above paradoxical and critical situation will end soon. Because of the principles of aesthetics and biological philosophy of the West, it will suppress the issue of women and sex in the way that exists in the camp of the East by seriously opposing beauty and visual elements and individual freedoms. Nor will the new world philosophy of secular democracy retreat from its beliefs about the basic foundations of freedom.

The only solution that seems possible is that with the growth of awareness and the development of libertarian beliefs, the Eastern Bloc will reach social and political maturity and in the shadow of that, the limits and loopholes dictated by religions and governments will be pushed back. As much as the limits of limitation and coercion are pushed back, the limits of the freedom of the Eastern woman will also increase and the two sides of the world will finally meet and interact at a certain point.

The Relationship Between Pornography and Art

Criticisms on the pornography market are mostly based on the fact that it has violated the moral boundaries and fundamentals of visual and spiritual aesthetics of sex and has entered the field of "sexual obscenity." Today's pornography, which applies new deconstructions every day in the competition of production companies, is so extreme that there is no longer any ethical and aesthetic basis for viewing these images.

When a person encounters recent porn scenes, he must unconsciously doubt his human nature and quality. A normal human being, with reasonable human and noble spirits, does not feel comfortable facing these images even in his deepest loneliness.

The human mind is the field of images and memories. The images of porn products are so soulless and devoid of sensual beauty that when watching them, real people, instead of enjoying the images, think of the artificial stupid dialogues and the state of the exploited actors and their heinous and ugly actions rather than the sexual aspects being shown. Because the human spirit is completely missing in these products and only shows the tragic aspects of a helpless human being in a moral crisis.

If the viewer lasts until the end and his work is done, he will immediately feel disgusted. This is despite the fact that after a romantic sex and orgasm with a lover, a person enters a stage of the best tender feelings and the quality of discovery and intuition, which is far more enjoyable than the sex itself.

The point of view that avant-garde literary and artistic critics such as Susan Sontag propose is that pornography can be considered as a literary and cinematic genre. This literary genre can bring double excitement and sensuality by providing factors in terms of imagination or erotic fantasy, as we saw in Shklovsky's view of defamiliarization.

Increasing erotic imaginations can help to increase sexual power. But who does not know how fine the line between pornography and art is. In other words, it is possible to imagine another type of pornography that, in addition to complying with moral standards, also puts artistic standards on the agenda. The most important red line that this genre of art must follow is not to offend the human virtue of the audience. In fact, the increase of sensual desire in the context of works of art, whether written or visual, should not lead to the weakening of high human values. Maybe this border is in works like the movie *Trance*, starring Hedi Lamarr.

In a macro view, we see that all artistic fields are full of inspiration from the sensual foundations and sexual imaginations of man. This issue can be seen even in the field of church art and the highest art forms. As mentioned in the introduction of this book, sex has such a place as one of the main mental and behavioral concepts of humans that no field has been free of its influence.

The timeless appeal of Mona Lisa's smile consists of a combination of imagination and aesthetic principles that oscillate from her sweet smile to her cleavage. The main issue is to observe the principle of balance. Mona Lisa's cleavage represents the sensual side of human existence and the inner beauty of women. Her smile also represents the tenderness and cheerfulness of a woman. As a woman, her body sends signals to the audience, which ultimately makes her sensual and aesthetic power react.

Church art, in turn, shows that sex is not necessarily the enemy of morality and virtue. Rather, like all phenomena related to the soul and evolution, maintaining balance and not stepping on the lines is the criterion for evaluating good and bad in the field of art.

If sex is well managed and under control, it can be considered an empowering and inspiring factor. This inspiration can be seen even in the images of church altars. Even where the subject is the Holy Mary and physical aesthetic principles are not considered.

Even when we look at an image of Christ, we certainly cannot lose sight of his aesthetic foundations and masculine charms. Because man is generally a combination of all dimensions of his existence, one of which is attractiveness, sensuality, beauty and visual taste.

If the Holy Mary is supposed to represent a woman with all human characteristics, along with elements such as sacrifice, kindness, goodness, holiness, and exaltation, she cannot be devoid of sexual aspects. Now this issue depends on how delicately the painter depicts a combination of all these properties and moods to indirectly include the imaginative aspects in his being. This is the border that determines the border of ugliness and beauty in the work of art.

There are many examples of literary ugliness in Persian literature. One of the most brilliant scenes in Persian poetry is the love scene between Shirin and Khosrow. Nizami Ganjavi, without using even a single sexual or obscene word, without directly referring to any of the sensual states in the relationship, has so skillfully depicted the process of embracing and sensuality of a healthy relationship between Khosrow and Shirin that it can be a great example. be a sensual literary work without obscene aspects.

In such a situation, Poran's artwork can even be considered a valuable work. A place where without harming the audience's aesthetic sensitivities and breaking the standards of visual ethics, it will make the erotic movements move inside him and transform his sexual life. This is how the huge gap between sex and virtue can be filled, as the world is suffering from today.

Products that are produced in accordance with these patterns can create a kind of sexual idealism in which a combination of human sensual nature and noble aspects and moral virtues is made, and in this way, while creating sexual arousal and respecting the aesthetic components of the audience, his sexual desire. stimulates in the service of renewing marital relations.

If the modern world has managed to make sex a destructive monster and cause concern for mankind, families and social reformers, this issue cannot change the old definition of the original nature of sex. The production of ridiculous porn content, which often does not benefit from the inherent beauty of sex, is a kind of deviation and misunderstanding of the nature and function of sex.

Humanity has committed destruction and perversion not only about sex, but in all scientific and practical fields, it has a destructive track record! From the chemistry of materials, it has opened a way to narcotics and psychedelics, and from physics and chemistry, it has opened a door to mass death with biological and mass destruction weapons.

Animals and the Conventional Limits of Sexual Morality

When talking about sexual promiscuity in porn products, people unintentionally talk about the animal act of the actors. But this is a gross error and a verbal slip. Not only do animals not perform heinous and immoral acts in sex, but the act of animals can be a model of normal and correct sexual acts.

Man's sexual behavior has fallen into a terrible abyss that rather than conveying sexual excitement to the viewer, it introduces him to the ugly and boring aspects of sexual act.

These actions have nothing to do with the humane and aesthetic principles of sex.

If the new world has taken sex backward by relying on new tools like the Internet, it has nothing to do with the sacred and spiritual nature of sex. Humans have gone so far in this field that in order to correct their misbehavior, they have to use animals as moral teachers and models of adherence to sensual virtue.

There are many points about the superiority of animals in the act of sex. Animals never use sex as a means of sustenance or economic gain. They never overdo it, but following nature, at certain times and seasons of the year, they hold sex like a primitive and original ritual. The courtship of animals benefits from a kind of holy glory and deep spirituality.

Animals, following their moral laws, never violate the rights of their fellows in the category of sexual intercourse. In the spring, when males and females are prone to mating, usually male cats are looking for suitable mates. In a process that takes one to two weeks, each cat makes its offer to the desired female. He is free to accept or not; but finally, after many attempts, each of them finds their suitable pair and flirts in a corner.

When two couples agree, no one violates their privacy. Many times it has been seen that two pairs are courting, and the male cat, who previously wanted the same female, peacefully watches the mating of his rival without any jealousy or aggression.

Flirting has a limited time. After pregnancy, the maternity period of the female placenta begins, and during this period, the male placenta is not exposed to her. After the birth of the children, he occasionally visits the family; but it does not interfere in their affairs.

The reason why the process of mating and sex and pregnancy and the repetition of this cycle in periods and seasons takes place so simply and without any problems is that no external institution is involved in regulating the behavioral nature and social and individual relationships of animals. The beauty and originality of sex in animals is because they do not follow any religion. Their religion is nature.

Basically, wherever man tries to control or limit the natural course of processes by establishing laws and applying restrictions, problems and disturbances have started. The control of religious institutions over the process of mating and sex has been more damaging and distracting than it has been helpful.

The originality of sexual behavior in animals has caused the anomalies created by man to not exist among them. Mating is not observed in baby animals. Rape is not seen. Polygamy is not seen among animals in the same way as humans. Possession of gender has no meaning. There is no proprietary view of the material. The independence of male and female is more than the researcher. Honor killings caused by jealousy and possessiveness do not exist externally. There is no forced sex in any form. Therefore, it is not an exaggeration when it is said that the moral principles of animals in the realm of sex can be an ideal model for correcting human misbehavior.

Female Homosexuality Is More Logical than Male Homosexuality

Although the nature of men and women is generally in conflict with the category of homosexuality; but in practice, we will see that female homosexuality is more compatible with the creation of women. As mentioned earlier, men have not been able to satisfy women's sexual desires due to their natural weakness and even wrong behavior. But this issue, instead of men trying to fulfill women's wishes, led to the suppression of women's capacities. This repression continues in Eastern societies; but the women of Maghreb tried to overcome this situation.

One of the ways for women to overcome male dominance and men's impotence is manifested in the form of female homosexuality. Women flirt with all their being, and sexual motivation in them is not limited to physical flirting and arousal through sexual organs. For this reason, when sex happens between two women, they find more appropriate ways to reach orgasm while fully knowing their desires and physical abilities.

When a woman's sexual partner is of the same sex, the presence of the body is manifested in a transcendental way in the process. They practically do not need sexual organs, either male or female. Homosexuality gives them the opportunity to achieve a deep sex management and achieve a desirable orgasm in a long and deep process, through the involvement of all body organs.

But when it comes to male homosexuality, this act takes on an incomplete and even abominable nature due to the dysfunction of men. Men who turn to homosexuality by imitating women are actually acting against the natural structures and logic of their creation. A man who has not been able to convince and satisfy a woman naturally will not achieve success with the same sex.

Perhaps it is natural because human society is still morally and conventionally facing women's homosexuality with more gentleness and acceptance, and it has much less disgust compared to male homosexuality.

Regardless of whether homosexuality is feminine or masculine, it must be accepted that this phenomenon has a long history. Whether in terms of social culture and philosophical background or in terms of the aesthetic foundations of sex, homosexuality is not a phenomenon limited to the new age. It is not clear exactly when humans have shown the desire for the same sex. But according to the design of this topic in the philosophical and sociological theories of ancient Greece, it can be concluded that the issue of homosexuality was a concern and a mental issue of the theorists of the ancient era.

In the book of Plato's Banquet, as one of the important ancient documents in the field of love, sex and sexuality, the subject of homosexuality is considered. In the debates of this book, most of the participants consider homosexuality as a deviation from the original approaches of the institution of creation.

In a part of this book, Plato mentions from the language of Aristophanes, who is one of the attendees of the assembly and one of the important speakers, relying on the narratives of the creation myth, that after the creation of humans, because of the insolence that humans did, Zeus divided them into two halves. But people who couldn't live without their second half start protesting and striking.

Seeing the plight of humans, Zeus turned their penis forward so that they could embrace each other and continue their generation. After that, an indescribable friendship and interest was established between the two halves of man.

Here Aristotle lays the foundation of the theory of homosexuality and says: "Women who are half of a woman do not desire men, but rather desire women, and that group of men who are half of a man go after men. That is, they love men as long as they are young. They are happy to hang out with men and have drinks with them, or to hug with them, and that group of men who have more masculine qualities than others are the most excellent young people, and they are the ones who will become our rulers when they grow up. This itself is a proof of their superiority and their nature is inclined toward love and they respond to the call of love."

Of course, this group loves boys when they reach a man, and marriage and reproduction are not for them out of love; rather, it is because the law forces them to do this, and if they are left to themselves, they will not agree to marry. Of course, some people accuse these young people of shamelessness and promiscuity, and this is not shameful in my opinion, but it is because of their courage and bravery that they want to be friends with those who are like them.

According to what was said in Plato's language, it can be said that in today's era, women have temporarily found a way to experience deep and comprehensive sex with the help of their same sex after the bitter experience of unpleasant sex with men. Because apparently, only a woman can help another woman to experience consecutive ejaculations after a long flirtation with the knowledge of her body and the feeling of her own body and that of her same sex.

As we can see, Plato, quoting Aristophanes, considers homosexuality to be a moral basis and based on a rule consistent with the creation myth, and despite the fact that he considers it to be a departure from the norm; but he is not to blame. This view can be found in the opinions of most scientists of the new era. Although the opponents of this theory are not few.

These events were taking place in the West at the beginning of the 20th century, while the women of the East were still getting used to their limited and restrained status and continued to live an imposed life.

The aforementioned differences caused it to spread in many Eastern countries and with the indoctrination and propagation of religion that women in Eastern countries are more dignified than their Western counterparts. But the truth was that the Eastern woman's submission was due to not knowing about the discoveries that women had achieved in the free world.

The oriental woman looks more satisfied because she doesn't even know what she has lost and what kind of hat men and sexual partners have put on her. The Eastern woman was enough to be remembered as a dignified woman, a caring mother and the bright candle of the family. Without anyone ever paying attention to his bodily desires and deep feelings.

The combination of these factors caused the women of the East to lag behind in raising awareness and asserting their sexual rights compared to the women of the West. In many countries of the world, even the thought of liberation and transformation in the field of women's sexual rights has not been created. Eastern women are used to conditioning and captivity in the hands of taboos and routine social processes. Consent and conditioning in the context of poverty, slavery, unquestioning obedience and the state of ownership is a function of other social variables. The state of being "shepherd or sheep" is an accurate description of these macro variables.

There is a direct connection between these issues and other indicators such as democracy and cultural development. Human and individual freedoms and social activism and getting out of the outdated social frameworks and rules depend on the existence of democratic spaces and political and social development. Political institutions and ideological systems make a lot of effort to keep women in the status quo. Because the function of these ideologies in the group is the conservative status and general backwardness of the women's society.

What is promoted under the title of "dignity and sobriety of the Eastern woman" is actually the acceptance of fate and the feeling of acceptance. At the beginning of the 20th century, and for the first time in human history, the Western woman was able to rise up against the taboos and restrictions that were imposed on her over the centuries and to some extent push aside the boundaries. He tried to change his destiny with his own hands and for this change, he made a full-scale revolution against two powerful fronts. The powerful force of men and the reactionary view of the nature of women as human beings.

It is natural that a number of thinkers, philosophers, sociologists and psychologists played a prominent role in this intellectual opening as the intellectual pioneers of transformationism. For example, when Karl Marx was able to theorize his theory on "the influence of individuality on destiny," this thought was able to inspire women. According to Marx's belief, poverty and wealth and many and such as fate have nothing to do with categories such as God and destiny; rather, the social, political and economic structure determines the destiny and economic position of humans.

When humans can change their destiny in a desired way and transform the living conditions, they can affect the political and economic systems of the society. On the other hand, when he mentions the component of sex as one of the main human phenomena, he actually refers to the fact that the women of the society, who do not benefit from the blessing of real sex, are deprived of one of the most important biological gifts.

Through psychological insights, Freud prepares the ground for defending the equality of men and women. He believes that men and women clearly belong to one species of creatures called humans, and no theory, philosophy or ideology can condemn women as the second or weak sex to obey men, and such thoughts are inhumane and superior. It is sexual desire.

Masters and Johnson's research opened a new horizon for the Western woman in terms of theory and practice. This research, which was published and received in the form of written and televised works, introduced some of the potentials and differences of female physiology and correctly showed that throughout history, men have been able to oppress women by suppressing these potentials. That is, the woman has not been allowed to enjoy sex throughout her life, because both she herself did not have sufficient knowledge of her sexual organs and capabilities, and men were unaware of this issue and their duties.

While all these factors caused the Western woman to experience a wide material difference in thought and action, the Eastern women lived in the same way as before and passed away from this world after a dull life. However, with the beginning of the fourth revolution, which was more global than the industrial revolutions and the like, and its radius of action became much longer, the whispers of this reformation started at least in parts of the Eastern societies and among the educated classes.

Legal Violation

In the pre-civilization periods when modern moral rules did not rule, it was easier for men to impose their desires on women either by conventional methods or by crude and subversive methods.

The new social rules emphasize that the sex process should be accompanied by standard behaviors that include gentleness, elegance, equality, fairness and consideration of the inner desires and emotions of the woman. It seems that women have never been guilty in this regard and have never been cruel and one-sided in their treatment of men. Modern moral relations have made them move from their comfort zone and accept new requirements. They are not happy with these changes because the new requirements have made their access to sex and pleasure subject to rules.

Various laws, including: banning sex with underage girls and imposing sex on women, whether in the form of marriage or in a free form, are becoming more complicated every day, and judicial systems have taken a lot of strictness. Public opinion and social hegemony have also become very sensitive to the category of sexual harassment.

The new situation corresponds to the human nature of love and relationship. In the sense that love is not formed in an authoritarian and one-sided atmosphere. When we love someone, we expect him to love us too, and the process of meeting two souls on equal terms will continue. These sensitivities have caused the boundary between the imposed relationship or rape and the morbid relationship of the parties to be subject to legal disputes in the courts and wide-ranging media challenges. This border became narrower when women's rights became prominent, important changes occurred in the moral and legal standards of human society, especially in the West.

The legal prosecution of some Hollywood figures and first-class political figures in the West, following the complaint of protesting women, shows that the issue of imposition or any kind of sexual harassment, whether hidden or overt, is followed with high sensitivities by public opinion. The point is that sexual harassment is not covered by the passage of time and sometimes after decades we see that sexual harassers are suddenly caught in the law.

There is no doubt that in today's era, the boundaries of transgression are much narrower than a hair. As the gap between modern societies and backward countries is filled, the world will soon witness a collective convergence toward the recognition of women's rights and the protection of all forms of violence. Although now in Eastern societies, often, regardless of women's will, a form of rape is imposed under the husband-wife relationship; but the outlook for the future seems bright.

Modern morality was able to bring the discourse of equality into families. Now, it is more difficult to regulate personal relationships, from having a simple conversation to asking for sex and regulating the duties of both parties in the family, and it is included in the example of "a thousand points thinner than a hair." In the modern family, small and unimportant matters have no meaning. Any movement, speech or behavior can be considered as an example of violence against women or a desire to force a relationship.

The civilized part of human society hopes and expects that this change of situation will soon spread to backward societies as well. In line with this goal, human rights organizations and women's liberation movements are monitoring the developments of Eastern societies.

Fortunately, the force that is affecting human behavior has succeeded in spreading the hegemony of modern ethics to human relations with high sensitivity. For this reason, the woman of the new age is aware of her equal human rights and identity, and men can no longer be active in our behavioral relationships. In the shadow of double awareness of women, and the increase of behavioral sensitivities, any behavior and speech can cause damage to bilateral relations.

In an environment where the woman is out of the domination of tyranny and old customary laws and the man is still used to one-sided behavior and requests as in the past, relationship management has become increasingly difficult. But this difficulty is compared to the historical bitterness of women as "the drop and the sea."

This situation may continue for a long time, but over time, civilized behavior based on ethics and new social discourse is institutionalized in men. Until then, a man should learn that flirting is not a one-way affair. The man used to think that sex is a special gift of nature and society for him, which is given to him by a woman in the form of a simple and easy-to-reach gift. But now, such tendencies can cause annoyance and cloudiness of the woman's mind and lead to the social embarrassment of the man.

In the past decades, many books have been written and psychologists and social science experts have tried to provide detailed teachings in order to optimize the relationship between men and women. These guidelines are written based on a new systematization and social ethics regarding respect for gender rights. With all this, in sensitive situations and challenges of husband and wife to regulate personal relationships, they are still alone and self-reliant.

The same social morality that is reconstructing the relationship between men and women based on the awareness of the modern age believes that the private sphere of men and women is completely in their own hands. Therefore, it is difficult to imagine an external observer to regulate this relationship.

If this were not the case, the husband and wife of our scenario, instead of going to sleep every night with annoyance in a quiet environment, would sit on the armchairs of a room so that an expert would examine the background and hindrances of their relationship and adjust the relationship from the beginning. Let them see where this coldness and hostility comes from. Perhaps the issue is related to childhood education and childhood emotional intelligence, which has been neglected during this time.

Female Circumcision, a Brutal Russian Way to Suppress Female Sexuality

We mentioned repeatedly that a man is forced to deal with a woman's sexual eruption for various reasons. He uses various methods to control and suppress and seeks help from various tools to justify his actions.

The historical repressive action of men is sometimes accompanied by reasoning and based on soft methods and sometimes accompanied by the most violent methods. Mutilation of the female sexual organ, which is referred to as "female circumcision," is one of the most brutal methods of the patriarchal society to deal with the female sexual power.

This method, which has been widely used in the historical geography of the world, is so inhumane that even the high-ranking religious texts are silent about it without condemning it.

This tradition, rather than having a religious basis, has an ethnic and tribal origin, to the extent that African countries with the highest frequency are the main centers of female circumcision. From the historical point of view, the banks of the Nile River have been introduced as the possible origin of this method. But this tribal thinking is once again watered by a mediator from the same deep historical viewpoint, based on the sexual oppression of women. Therefore, when we look at believing actions in a macro arena, we practically do not notice a difference in the origin of beliefs. Since the time of Adam Abul Bashar, we are faced with a historical act whose center of gravity is the suppression of women's lust by resorting to any means possible.

The long-standing enmity with women is rooted in the biological weakness of men. One of the methods of dealing with women has been to mutilate her sexual organ so that she cannot have the upper hand in sexual relations by benefiting from her double strength. This is a way to cover up the innate weakness of men, outside of healthy competition with women.

According to this historical logic, there is not much substantive difference between gender oppression in glorious times like the Victorian era, and the practice of circumcision in a remote village in Burkina Faso. The historical logic behind these behaviors cannot be very different in different places and periods.

Considering the extreme importance of mutilating women, with the aim of controlling their sexual power, which is in line with the topics of this article, we will briefly examine this phenomenon.

The Purpose of Female Circumcision

To justify the act of circumcision or female genital mutilation in different parts of the world and at different historical times, several reasons have been mentioned that are almost the same everywhere, including:

Decreased libido: The main reason for female circumcision is to decrease libido. However, research shows that female circumcision does not actually decrease sexual desire, but rather decreases the amount of sexual satisfaction and therefore increases the number of sexual acts in women who have been circumcised.

Following the tradition: Female circumcision has been customary as a religious behavior for a long time, and religious people have combined this belief with religious biases.

Formalizing Puberty: Sometimes the reason for circumcision is to mark girls' transition from girlhood to womanhood. Creating social integration and strengthening family unity are among the reasons for this practice. In countries like Sierra Leone, circumcision is the boundary for girls to enter the circle of adult women. However, in some African countries, this practice is performed at the age of three or four, which contradicts the above argument.

Beauty: There are misconceptions that circumcision improves the health and beauty of a woman's penis.

Social taboos: According to some taboos, an uncircumcised woman is not clean, and sometimes, taking food from the hands of uncircumcised women is considered unpleasant in some villages and urban areas.

Improving health: In some tribes, it is believed that circumcision can increase the fertility of women and increase the health and the risk of survival of the baby.

Religious belief: Sometimes the act of circumcision is considered to be in accordance with religious orders. However, in none of the major religions, there is no specific command to perform circumcision.

Although there is no definite order to prohibit this practice in religious texts.

Superstitions: local beliefs and superstitions and subcultures have been more influential than other factors in the category of female genital mutilation.

Husband's sexual pleasure: In the research conducted, some women, including in the country of Sudan, have said that they have circumcised themselves because of their desire to simulate the state of virginity by making the vagina narrower and increase their sexual attractiveness.

Other Factors Affecting Female Circumcision

In addition to the above, other factors have been seen in the field of circumcision or modification of female genital organs. Sometimes women voluntarily undergo plastic surgery to make their genitals more beautiful. This act is not against civil liberties because it is voluntary. However, in the treatment of the body, its compliance with natural norms and rationality is important.

Female genital mutilation is very complex and extensive. This action, with any origin and motivation, is in conflict with the biological norms and the intelligent system of self-management of nature in the first place. Many studies have been done on the aspects of human rights. What follows are the main cases of female genital mutilation or circumcision, which are listed in a list.

- There is no specific treatment method for the victims of female circumcision. However, recently, with plastic surgery, a small amount of damage can be compensated, which does not include the complete restoration of the cut limb.
- Human rights sources generally consider any kind of forced intrusion into the genital organs of girls and women as a violation of the fundamental rights of girls and a violation of equal opportunities and an example of torture, humiliation and mistreatment of women.
- Several conventions have reacted to this issue, including the Convention on Civil and Political Rights, the Convention on

- Economic, Social and Cultural Rights, the Convention on the Rights of the Child, and the Convention on the Elimination of All Forms of Discrimination Against Women (CEDAW).
- On the initiative of an African committee and with the approval of the United Nations, the sixth day of February has been named in the world calendar as the "International Day of Zero Tolerance for Female Genital Mutilation."
- According to the United Nations Population Foundation, by 2006 between 120 and 140 million women around the world were exposed to some form of genital mutilation.
- Social scientists consider the human tendency to do this act in connection with the same will directed to patriarchy. In patriarchal systems, where family genealogy is regulated based on the sequence of fathers, there is a great sensitivity toward women's chastity.
- In the recent century, with the promotion of public awareness and the expansion of modernism and civility, several laws have been enacted to prevent female genital mutilation, and promotional and enlightening activities have been implemented, which have brought great success.
- Waris Deary is a British model of Somali descent who is a victim of female genital mutilation. He is now working as a United Nations ambassador to stop female circumcision in the world. In the book *Desert Flower*, he has republished his childhood memories and facing this problem. He admits that because of this imperfection, he has never been able to understand sexual pleasure. While describing how women's penises are cut off in Africa, he tells the story of his escape to London.

Menstruation Is Aimed at Creation, Not Opinion

The coordinates of women's liberation movements are mainly in the fact that these movements first of all try to take women out of the previous traditional framework and allow her to raise basic questions about the position of women in society, family and relationship with men. Now it is no longer necessary for a woman to be pregnant and serve a man. The process of birth control, which is the result of medical achievements, has given women, before any other time, the possibility to raise their demands and questions in the field of body authenticity with more freedom.

The result of the expansion of these movements has been manifested first of all in the form of the destruction of the family foundation and the marriage foundation. Now, in free societies, neither marriage nor family is the first and last priority of women. These two problems have an equal presence along with dozens of other problems that a man and a woman face in life. Whenever necessary and whenever the situation demands, a woman can get married, start a family and think about having one or two children.

Along with opening these new paths and reforming social thought regarding the nature and social identity of women, other issues are also being resolved. Social taboos and dark tribal and tribal thinking had shown the topic of women's menstruation as an absolute shame. Now, the modern woman is instilling the belief that women's menstruation is just a biological phenomenon that is directed at her creation.

Modern thought asserts that there is no religious or physical rationale for looking at a woman's menstrual period as it has throughout history. The biased and dark-minded view on the subject of women's menstruation follows the same general view of the nature of women as a sinful and absolute evil that has persisted throughout the centuries. We said that historical male domination has used every tool to control the female body. Menstruation is one of the most prone biological excuses to marginalize women.

In the current situation, it is necessary for a man (at least a Western man) to fully recognize the biological and temperamental requirements of a woman while changing his way of looking at women. He should understand that women have exactly the same gifts and rights as men. The biological differences of the female body are just as debatable as the biological requirements of the male body, if not more so.

The periodic change of the body's biological functions is not limited to women. Now, science has well established that men, like women, have monthly or seasonal periods during which significant hormonal changes occur in the body. During the period of men's menstruation, male testosterone levels increase, which can cause feelings and behavioral differences similar to women. with the difference that male period symptoms are more hidden and not visible. However, the field of language and culture is full of derogatory views on the issue of period in women, which unfortunately is used as a taboo against women even in Western societies.

Menopause, end of work or change in life patterns Just as the life of every human, both male and female, contains important stages and parts, women have such seasons in their lives both biologically and intellectually and behaviorally.

Menopause is one of these important seasons in women's lives. A specific change in the life pattern that brings its own requirements. The end of menstruation makes a woman enter a special and different period of her life. Just as there is a negative and illogical view in the minds of men regarding other differences between men and women, menopause is not understood in a logical way by men, nor is it properly faced.

A woman's body goes through important periods during her life. Around the age of 13 or 14, signs of the ability to have sex appear. But his intellectual maturity has not yet been realized. Therefore, social norms do not recognize sexual maturity in the sense of the ability to marry. Here, too, there is a clear conflict between the views of religious people and modern reason. Religion recognizes women as a commodity with sexual capabilities. Therefore, as soon as he reaches sexual maturity, he considers her ready for marriage. Because it is enough for him to be able to tolerate sex and have a child.

But the modern and humane laws of the new era recognize the approximate age of 18 years as the limit at which a woman can make independent decisions and enter into relationships such as marriage. Most countries have started efforts to raise the legal age of marriage to 18.

The beginning of sexual maturity and the activity of sex hormones is almost equal to the beginning of menstruation. This period, which is the longest biological period of a woman, includes a major part of her life. With the end of this period, menopause comes, which, although it does not mean the end of sexual life, is a warning to start a new chapter in a woman's life.

Psychology has also recognized this phenomenon. According to Freud and his fellow psychologists, this transitional stage means the decline of sex hormones in women. But it is not the end of everything. At this stage, life will become more peaceful. Menopause is a way of entering a better state, which can be a source of peace and satisfaction in the case of psychological management. It is the same in men. Men also have a stage without obvious physical symptoms, which is not dissimilar to menopause.

In this period, the mind seeks to find more valuable concepts in life. Man has reached real maturity and evolution, and sex and sexual power seem like a small thing and a light toy.

How to cope with menopause is different in different societies. Western women who have enjoyed the pleasures of sex when they were young suddenly feel empty. But in Eastern societies, where sex has been introduced as an evil demon and especially young women have been introduced as a symbol of Satan and the deception of men, maybe reaching menopause is accompanied by a kind of happiness and satisfaction.

During this period, the Eastern woman feels that a huge burden has been lifted from her shoulder. He no longer has to provide sex and pregnancy services. In this way, he receives more human respect from the people around him. He has finished the period when evil forces were present inside him and entered the phase of wisdom.

The respect given to old women and men in the East is because these people are devoid of sexual power. Therefore, as neutral and safe people, they are worthy of respect.

But in the West, women have had relatively equal respect with men since the beginning. While having sex hormones, she can dictate her human side to men. Now that he is deprived of sensual and sexual aspects, he will not receive anything new against this lack. Therefore, it will feel more empty. Therefore, being old in the West is not a sign of wisdom in that exaggerated Eastern way. Because a person is either wise or not throughout his life. This trend makes the life of a woman in the West not associated with many bumps and menopause is only prominent in the aspect of lack of physical and sexual aspects and female hormones.

For the Western women, the illusion that sex is almost equal to life has existed in practice. But for the Eastern woman, sex has not been a great issue in life. Apart from the fact that it is a one-sided duty and part of his social services in the form of family or wife. In fact, for the Eastern woman, sex hormones and the ability to get pregnant are a disturbing and troublesome element, and now she can breathe a sigh of relief in the absence of this constant trouble.

The difference in attitudes toward the lack of sexual power naturally leads to different reactions in facing it. Sometimes a woman tries to remain graceful and upright by making changes in her appearance. It tries to control and hide the symptoms of menopause. Instead, resort to medical tools and achievements to look younger and more attractive. Diet for having a proper body, plastic surgery, exercise, various drugs, rejuvenating drugs and increasing physical and sexual powers can be part of these activities.

But as soon as the symptoms of menopause appear, an oriental woman suddenly becomes ten years older, her clothes change. She appears in the role of a mother and even a grandmother. Her social connections have changed, and like retired men whose homogenous social groups have changed, the menopausal woman's homogenous social groups are also slowly changing.

These behavioral manifestations occur very quickly in the oriental woman. To the extent that a menopausal woman considers her life to be over. A woman who before menopause still had the activities and signs of a woman with sexual powers, suddenly the spirit of a great mother dissolves in her. His organs become wider and fatter and he gets a different appearance.

Another difference between the Western woman is her social nature. He can strengthen his other social aspects after sexual retirement. There are many women who think of writing a book about their life or experiences after this course. Some people choose sports activities. A group tends to people's institutions, social institutions and charitable activities. Anyway, everyone is looking for a reason to continue their life and continue their social identity. Because he has had these facilities throughout his life and now it is enough to strengthen them in the vacuum of sexual life.

But the Eastern woman has been deprived of these concepts and social activities since the beginning. The oriental man has given a certain definition to him. Sex (mostly one-way), pregnancy, raising children, and finally taking care of housework. At this point, she has lost two of her most important feminine qualities. Childbearing and sex in the shadow of beauty. Although he can still take care of the house, it is less important now. Since his social life didn't exist from the beginning, he can't deal with developing a strong identity for himself.

It seems that at this stage of life, women are still facing a deep misunderstanding in the world. Both men and women should know that full and deep acceptance of the changes that nature has made in the human body is a logical and human issue. Childhood has its charms. Likewise, adolescence and youth, with all the beauty that a woman enjoys at this stage of life, are considered a part of life just like old age.

Old age, if understood well, can be full of obvious and hidden beauties. These beauties can be the engine of a woman's life so that she can live her life to the end without depression and despair.

Silence and peace, meditation and prayer, philosophizing and thinking, transferring the lived experience to the next generations, increasing the dimensions of knowledge and trying to understand the unknowns of life are only part of the glory of old age, especially for women.

In parts of this book, we talked about the importance of love in the relationship between men and women. Now it's time to use all that powerful potential and human drive that love has stored in the body of life. As hormones and sexual urges disappear, love does not disappear, but becomes more mature and complete.

Love does not rely on biological processes. Although these processes can display the sparks of love with more warmth in physical actions and reactions; but love is deeper than just being based on the body.

Now it's time for men and women to live only with the help of love. This is a gift that every human being deserves and should experience once in their life. Nature gives men and women the opportunity to enter this exciting stage.

Now is the time to deal with higher matters. Meditation is one of these ways. An introspection is something that perhaps every human being has longed for in their hectic lives. In the blind excitement of sex, pregnancy, parenting and household management, there was no time for serious meditation. Now is the safe point and the right opportunity for her to look inside as a woman. Discovering the inner labyrinth is no less enjoyable than discovering the outer worlds.

If the menopause category is not faced and managed, the mind will suddenly fall into silence, which is caused by the removal of physical responsibilities. In this meditative atmosphere, a woman's great enthusiasm may make her prone to become a perfect and sublime human being. He must use the power of this passion. Otherwise, it may decline and never appear again.

When the moment of enlightenment comes, it may not be easy to interact with; but with a little practice and meditation, parallel and different worlds are opened before man. When the light of enlightenment embraces you, forces will be released that will be much greater than physical forces and sexual desire.

The power of attraction and desire gives its place to the power of emotion and passion. These forces are almost from the same cell. But they are all stimulating. For a long time, body and hormones ruled. Now it is your turn to realize the rule of mind and heart so that new gates of thinking and intuition will be opened which will lead to a kind of deep knowledge.

Changing the chemical composition of the body does not always lead to stagnation, it depends on how we face it. New combinations can be just as motivating as old ones.

Chapter Eight
Marriage, Reproduction and the Philosophy of Absurdity

Marriage Is Not the Same as Having Children

A misunderstanding that questions the nature of traditional marriage is that marriage promoters believe that every marriage must lead to pregnancy and reproduction. It seems that this requirement is hidden in marriage. This common belief has become a social taboo and has been institutionalized in society over time. We said that marginal requirements are one of the weak points of marriage. Marriage should be true to nature. Whatever the outcome of marriage should be of secondary importance and optional status. But this is not the case and this issue has become another weakness for traditional marriage.

This issue is so institutionalized that as soon as two people get married, it seems that the mental biological timer of the people around them starts working automatically. They expect pregnancy complications to appear in women after six months. After 9 months or a little more, the first child will be born and the rest of the steps will go through automatically. Deviation from this rule and any kind of deconstruction will bring a wave of curiosity and interference from the surrounding people.

Remote evaluations begin with the health of a man or woman. Then practical questions and curiosities will arrive and this process will not stop until a convincing answer is given to the question of the intrusive and questioning society.

The realistic conclusion from traditional society's expectations of women is that women in traditional marriages are judged by their bodies. Among the organs of the female body, several organs are more important. The reproductive system (centered on the uterus) has the highest value. According to the above scenario, as soon as it is determined that reproductive processes have been disrupted, ethical, legal, medical, and familial processes come into play. If the problem is with the female reproductive system, she will face a huge disaster. These all happen in the absence of love. Now imagine that love has the pulse of affairs in hand; We will see that:

Between my moon and the sky
The difference is from earth to heaven

Women in apparently ideal conditions are also captive to the problem of the uterus. In many cases, it has been seen that the foundation of marriage among young couples who like each other's appearance collapses due to the impossibility of pregnancy in the woman. The exact meaning of this situation is that the young man has established a relationship not with "woman as a human being" but with "woman as a womb." It has rarely been seen that the issue of procreation is so unimportant that a man continues his love life with his wife, despite the woman's inability to conceive, without any change in behavior or disturbing the main rules.

The movie *Leila* directed by Dariush Mehrjui is an example of thousands of events that have been narrated in Eastern societies regarding the impossibility of pregnancy for women and it shows that even in the relatively progressive layers of developing societies, the ultimate value of a woman depends on the quality of her uterus and reproductive system. In such an atmosphere, love will be tragically lonely and unsupported. Because the society with all its hegemonic power supports the belief that a woman should get pregnant. A woman's disinterest in pregnancy as a life choice is unacceptable, just like her biological disability. The front facing the force arising from social taboos is too strong for love (if it exists, of course) to deal with it.

Finally, we see categories like love, oneness and acceptance fade away. In fact, these affairs, which were presented as pure gold by the man to the woman before the beginning of the relationship, are emptied of their nature and removed due to a simple issue called "the possibility of a woman's pregnancy." These are all rusted iron sold in the form of magic called love to women.

Now that an original and valuable element called "having children" has appeared for a man, they have simply shed the surroundings and the nature of the heart of these fake values has been revealed. Along with this revelation of fake phenomena, the fake and rusty nature of Sood Mard's gold is also clearly seen.

But the matter does not end here. Now it's time to reveal the true position of the woman in her colorful prison. It is clear that the logic of the ancient history of male tyranny is completely valid. The man is the talkative, tyrannical and lying man who has applied a glaze of intellectualism, feminism, and transformation to himself, and now his hand is turned against him. The woman is the same woman who surrendered to the historical captivity and accepted her painful fate. "Woman as a womb," "Woman as a second sex," "Woman as a mamluk and servant" and…because of this, he indulges in a great depravity. Accepts male prostitution. It even helps him in this way. It gives a rational gloss to self-deprecation.

The originality of "having children" dictated to him by the horrible beliefs of the society is so institutionalized in his mind that he does not even think about its opposite. He has accepted that women are like a womb. He avoids himself and his feelings. As the famous saying goes, he puts on his "Sharia hat" and accepts the originality of the child as the only logic. Meanwhile, based on this originality, which has completely discredited him as a human being and a lover, a few more mornings when he was out of use in terms of the charms of sex and pleasure, his body was ineffective just like his womb. And it will become worthless and fall out of the circle of this relationship.

The lived experience of society shows that most men are "husbands of Laila" who wear a mask of ridiculous civilized behavior. We relied on lived experience for the reason that there is almost no documented research on this to determine how much a woman's intrinsic value is for a loving wife and a man in the society, against the ability to conceive?

As we can see, traditional marriage is not a guarantee for the continuation of a relationship. Rather, the durability of the relationship relies on the components that all of them must be present in a human framework outside the rule of marriage.

Marriage, a Pattern of Communication Between Men and Women; Buts and Ifs

During human life, one of the most important patterns of romantic and sexual relationship between men and women has been defined and recognized in the form of marriage. In general, the institution of marriage seems appropriate and healthy. Marriage can ensure the survival of the family and the basic upbringing of children. For women, the umbrella should bring economic and livelihood support and define clear boundaries for sexual and personal relationships between men and women. Marriage can provide specific definitions in terms of women's social, biological and even security rights.

All these features have made belief systems, politics and upper documents related to social mechanisms, while recognizing the institution of marriage, introduce it as the main approach to romantic, sexual, legal and human relationships. Law books are full of specific principles and rules that define the relationship between a man and a woman in the dictionary of marriage. But is this powerful institution really the most correct rule for the relationship between men and women? Are the rights of men and women considered equal in the constitution that defines marriage for men and women? Have the compilers and propagandists of marriage presented a correct view of the human relations between men and women?

Based on what we will bring in the rest of this section, it is clear that contrary to what the human society, especially the legal and ideological systems, think, the marriage law (at least in its current form) does not fully conform to the nature and creation of women, nor can it provide equality between men and women and guarantee the equal rights and dignity of women (especially in religious and underdeveloped societies). Therefore, either the legal and structural system of marriage should be changed in general, or its promotion as the only communication approach between men and women should be avoided. If the marriage system is optimized based on the ideas of its critics, it will still not be 100% consistent with the creation of man and woman, but it can eliminate some of the gross errors that currently exist.

According to the nature of creation and according to human biological experiences, men and women are not completely created for marriage. According to Osho, the Indian thinker, what happens in the form of marriage between a man and a woman leads to the formation of "an ugly compromise" between the husband and wife. He questions the mechanisms of marriage with the interpretation that this relationship is ultimately "lust that leads to hatred."

According to Osho, "marriage is the ugliest institution invented by man, invented so that you can monopolize a woman as if she were a piece of land or a piece of paper money." According to his belief, in the form of marriage, a woman is reduced to the level of an object.

Before going into the other things that make marriage an unprofitable institution, it should be noted that in marriage it is not just the woman who is reduced to a tradable commodity; but the man does not benefit from this objectification. It is true that in the institution of marriage, the man often enters the field as a buyer and the object of the transaction is the woman and not the man; but in a general view, the man has also entered his identity and function into the mechanism that, although he is looking for his own interests as one of the participants; but due to the nature of this transaction, the man also reduces his value and dignity in the whole of this structure.

Marriage and to Educate Children

In all the explanations given above, as we have seen, children were absent as one of the pillars of marriage and family and the fruit of romantic relationships between men and women. But like it or not, in the continuation of a natural relationship, whether in the form of marriage or under other titles, children will arrive. In fact, one of the main goals that Sharia and custom seek in the category of marriage is procreation.

The customary and social rules of marriage consider matters such as: pregnancy, reproduction and raising children to be a woman's duty. In general, it does not matter to these powerful social institutions whether the children born from a woman's womb are the fruit of a true love and unity between a man and a woman or the fruit of a physical and emotionless closeness. The institution of marriage does not differentiate between these two situations either philosophically or formally and socially.

Even in legal discussions and explanations, when it comes to children, the rights of being a parent, including custody, decision-making rights, and other matters, are given to men. Of course, significant differences have been created between progressive laws in developed societies and regressive societies.

Fortunately, regarding children, their nature and social belonging is more and deeper compared to the relationship between men and women. But some laws have not only depicted the status of children as highly dependent on the male identity, but also sometimes created a possessive aspect in the relationship between children and fathers. This situation is more complicated for female children. To the extent that in some reactionary and backward societies, to a large extent, the father is the owner of the body and life of the girl child. Some laws have humiliatingly made the decision-making power of girls dependent on the permission and decision of their fathers. This issue is sometimes so complicated that it becomes difficult to understand.

In some countries, permission to leave the country for girls up to the age of 40 depends on the father's decision. The marriage permission of mature and wise girls is still dependent on the decision and permission of the father. Interestingly, even if the father is not alive, these permits must be issued by the grandfather.

Imagine a 38-year-old wise and educated girl who is, for example, a university professor and has written several books in her field and is in important decision-making positions, and a large part of people in the society have benefited from her training and teaching as students. They have arrived perfectly. He has been invited by a world-class university to give his speech at an important conference in the field of sociology and the new world order, and now he has to leave the country. The father of this distinguished sociologist and researcher is not alive; but he has a grandfather who is not blessed with literacy and has been staying at home for many years due to illness.

According to the customary, religious and legal laws of the country, the grandfather must determine whether leaving the country is in the interest of this woman or not. He can give permission to leave the country to our desired sociology professor or not.

Such a person needs to obtain the consent of his grandfather in order to marry someone whom he has chosen with his knowledge and wisdom and who is on the same level as him in terms of science and social status. Because this permission is in his hands. Even if the grandfather is not literate and because of his old age he has no connection with the society and practically cannot be considered a human being with the power of reason and decision-making, still this girl's marriage is subject to the permission of the grandfather and to the specification and emphasis of custom. The grandfather must give permission for the daughter's marriage. This illogical insistence and void of any kind of rationality has a hidden philosophy. In this sense, under any circumstances, Sharia intends to humiliate and degrade the dignity of women, not allowing her to make decisions and vote independently.

This bitter irony is just a small example of the types of discrimination that the legal, religious and customary systems in some societies have allowed against women and female children.

If such a girl wants to implement decisions that are not in her power and act against this ridiculous custom, she will definitely face pressure levers. The levers that appear in the form of court, law, religion, custom, culture, subculture and finally government.

Although religion has many levers of pressure, the false social hegemony that provides the ground for applying this pressure is rooted in the childhood education of society's children. If the educational process of the children is outside the educational tyranny of the parents and the formal education system, they will automatically come to the understanding that girls are no different from boys. In the form of a natural and logical interaction that originates from the biological nature and natural human genome, they will come to the understanding that girls have the same right to benefit from the gift of freedom and equality as boys.

In an open and free educational environment, boys learn to see girls as an immediate partner and a friend of the opposite sex, and not as a weak being to be owned by boys. In this case, the world will be the world of lovers and lovers and not the world of maids and gentlemen and the world of wives and husbands and owners and mamluks or worse: the world of slaves and masters and the world of honor and owners of honor.

In other words, that flawed and perverted mentality that thinks all female members of the family are honorable, is the result of the faulty upbringing of fathers who have learned from their fathers that all female members of the family are honorable and nothing else.

In such a vicious cycle, women accept to be men's honor either by necessity or due to forced assimilation. It goes without saying that if this vicious cycle, which has existed for centuries, does not come out of orbit and break in a historical moment, we cannot hope that the position of women will be better in the future, especially in the Eastern lands.

Marriage, as a broad and long rule that has never undergone conceptual development and has always had long and little growth, has affected the relationship between men and women to such an extent that even deeper concepts such as love have been overshadowed by these misunderstandings. The sedimentation of the thought of subjugation in the context of marriage is so much that even in the category of love, "trap" and "hole" are mentioned as a verbal and cultural habit.

In the English language, it is conventionally said to express the occurrence of love: falling in love, while based on the mystical culture and transcendental enlightenment of the East, love is not only "falling" or "falling" in a situation, but also means transcendence and peak. And in one word, it is "unity" and "connection." Connection is the practical, theoretical and main theme of love, and it means connecting with the real and ancient roots of man. Therefore, human humanity is practically realized in connection, which in turn is dependent on the authenticity of love. Love is not "falling" or "caught." Rather, it means liberation and absolute freedom.

What keeps the submissive function of marriage in real conflict with the category of love is this issue. In marriage, there is no room for love. Because the legislator and founder of marriage is well aware of the fact that love cannot be criticized and cannot be considered as a framework. But the matter does not end there. Love is not only in conflict with submission, but if it is locked in binding frameworks, it will soon lose its freshness and freshness and die.

But these are not the concepts that we share with our children during their upbringing. We teach them to look at the machine systematically. We teach them that the machine, system and program are successful and efficient in all matters of life, even in the field of love, friendship and sex, which is the direct result of marriage and love, we consider the systemic view to be the ruling one.

The fact is that human society has continued to live with these established and static methods for centuries and has viewed and managed all its relationships, both personal and public, from this point of view. The dynamic flow of life is interrupted and stagnated in such conditions. Raising children also includes this topic. Women's lives are the same. When the rules of education prohibit us from thinking about different angles, actually thinking that there can be another way to raise children is considered a deviant move and a radical challenge. In the same way, a woman should never think if she will be able to achieve a happy life full of love without putting up with this man, and with another man?

If the educational system is healthy and adjusted according to human nature, the child will learn from his parents that love is not only slavery and ownership, but also freedom. He will learn that marriage, even though it has an anti-freedom nature; but it doesn't always mean that you can't have a romantic and healthy life in the form of marriage.

The type of performance of men can guarantee the survival of love in the form of marriage. This same performance can destroy the healthiest relationships and most romantic interactions between men and women. Marriage can be effective in speeding up this process.

In a word, in order to restore the relationship between man and woman in the form of traditional marriage, men should forget their selfish dictator traits and correct their behavior patterns. Currently, there are very few examples of this supposed relationship in society. Societies are considered progressive and happy when the frequency of these assumed relationships is high and becomes the dominant pattern.

Love is like a slippery fish that requires a lot of delicacy and sensitivity to hold it. Otherwise, the more the pressure and roughness of the hand, the more he will struggle to escape from the situation and jump. Therefore, creating prerequisites and spaces for the growth and maturity of love is the most important thing to do.

The missing link that has caused the historical destruction of the relationship between men and women is the lack of free thinking in dealing with women as lovers, wives or lovers. Therefore, libertarian thinking should be strengthened in the conscious and unconscious minds of men. If there is love, there will be no meaning in discriminating and rejecting a lover.

So we can conclude that our missing link is love. In its nature, love is free from economic and financial equations and calculations and from environments full of greed, greed, calculation and jealousy. This is the environment that humans have prepared for their lives in the past centuries.

Men can at least keep their personal and family privacy away from these relationships. If the lover is free, the possibility of using this right is less than when he is under domination and subjugation. Because in the first premise, this space leads to the creation of a kind of legalism. Women's rights should be demanded for giving love in a free environment and not, for example, for earning a living in an authoritarian and patriarchal environment. This recognition, in turn, causes the continuation and consolidation of the foundations of mutual love. This cycle of completion and evolution can continue indefinitely.

On the other hand, love is in conflict with all kinds of contradictions and limitations. Therefore, the probability of the collapse of the relationship and marriage in the open space is far less than the probability of its occurrence in the enclosed space and behind the iron bars of tyranny and inequality. In the meantime, the most key point for the continuation of a love, whether in the form of marriage or outside of it, is that love cannot be possessed by nature. As soon as the possessive feeling or thinking enters the privacy and area of love, love itself escapes through another window.

Possessiveness can dry the freshness of love and leave it with an artificial and hypocritical appearance. Because of this, many women betray their men in an imperceptible way. Cheating can be mental and never spread to the privacy of the body. But who does not know that mental betrayal is actually worse than physical betrayal.

In this arena, neither a man, nor a judge, a ruler, nor anyone else can apply an opinion and think of a solution for it. But it is regrettable to say that in many cases, rulers, judges, men, lovers, husbands, etc., are contemptuously indifferent to the state of mental betrayal and prefer not to speak about it, nor to give it any relevance in any way. While mental betrayal is the center of huge corruption that threatens the existence of family and even social relationships.

This is why we say that if love and relationships take place in absolute freedom, all parties can benefit from the consequences of this healthy relationship. Progressive societies exploit freedoms in order to improve the moral health indicators of society. Due to the equality achieved by the women population colonies under the new thinking, these societies are more healthy than religious and closed societies.

The summary of this discussion is that if men and women are together in complete freedom, it is much more possible to live together for the whole life. In other words, if there is freedom, it is much more possible for a man and a woman to be together more and spend their lives with more loyalty.

A mechanical and superficial marriage that can be referred to as a formal marriage is itself a source of divorce. If there is no marriage, there will be no divorce. Perhaps this assumption can be extended to more dimensions and say that marriage in the form that is common now is responsible for a large number of social vices, which, in addition to divorce, can include prostitution, polygamy, street children, and the like. The name of the products of this social rule.

In a mechanical marriage and in the absence of love, both parties can survive for a short time because of the novelty they have toward each other. After a while, a man gets bored with a woman. He is looking for change and variety. He is looking for another woman. Again, he does not get the alchemy of love. He looks for another woman or takes other wives (if the customary laws of the society allow it). In such a situation, all his meetings with women are temporary and overnight or a few hours. Obviously, love does not exist in such spaces.

He tries to be romantic. Artificial behavior comes from him. It pays more to get the excitement and revelation of feeling and reach the depths of people's souls. Experienced adventures. But love is still missing. True love should be discovered next to the spouse and the first lover. Because of his selfishness and trying to dominate the relationship, he has lost this gift and cannot regain it. The demand for prostitutes increases and the society is faced with a crisis called prostitution.

Community managers and political leaders are trying to think of a solution to the problem. They have also gone astray. All problems are caused by wrong mechanisms of marriage. They and religious leaders resist. They do not intend to touch the outdated mechanisms of paper marriages and the society continues in this endless cycle.

Now, if a man intends to define new relationships for himself in such a complex crisis environment, with all seriousness, and adjust his relationship with his wife in an ideal and desirable way, it is necessary to start with himself in the first place. There is no other way. If he loves his wife, he should first of all give her freedom.

Freedom, along with love and friendship, are the only important elements for setting up a lasting relationship. If this is the case, there will be no more common male violence during separation. We will no longer read about honor killings in newspapers.

Because under such a relationship, a woman is not a man's honor. He is a friend and companion. She has enough freedom of action and authority to choose whether or not to stay with the man with her own will and authority.

This is where jealousy will disappear. This is where both man and woman will become so rich and pure that they will not try to control each other. They know how fragile and ineffective the levers of control that men and women exert over each other.

Such couples will not allow love to be destroyed and turned into ashes under marriage. Even if their life is destroyed for a while because of a human error, they will have the ability to build a new building like a phoenix on the ashes of this destruction. A building that will be stronger than the previous building.

In such a relationship, love is never destroyed by marriage. The conscious life and action of both parties can even confiscate the tools and mechanisms in the marriage structure for the benefit of consolidating the romantic relationship. What destroys love is the core of a man's mind. The mechanism of marriage is just a tool that men and women use to suppress love.

Conscious couples who put love at the top of their performance will be critical of society's rituals and beliefs regarding marriage. They probably will not deny and abandon everything altogether, nor will they accept the rules and arrangements common in the mechanism of traditional marriage as an interactive method and a means of regulating their personal relationships as a principle. They know very well how ineffective the customary marriage system is for regulating romantic relationships. Because basically, there is no element of local love for Arabs in this system. Sometimes when this inflexible structure tries to look at elements like love and affection, it still leads to error. A clear example of that is the confrontation of customary marriage with the issue of "doom." Affection, affection, love and such things can never be measured and bought and sold with economic and monetary standards and material values.

Meanwhile, one of the common customs in the form of customary marriage is to determine a certain amount of money from the man to buy the bride's dowry. The custom of "dowry" in a humiliating way tries to value a woman's love with a certain amount of money and make it buyable and sellable. This contemptuous look at a spiritual and emotional phenomenon shows how much the customary marriage system leads to errors regarding spiritual issues and emotional relationships between men and women.

In order to improve his marital behavior, a man should educate and train his thinking in the first place. Then train his body and train him in the path of optimizing relationships. Then he must practice to be in love. Romantic relationships are one of the most complex human behavioral relationships. It is strange that some people think that without the slightest attention and practice, this issue can flow by itself. Love is one of the most sensitive human feelings. A coin with many sides. Moving on the narrow and sensitive edge of a wall that can fall toward the deadly waterholes with the least negligence. Floods such as jealousy, crime, self-esteem, possessiveness, etc.

If we imagine love as a painting. Being in love is like being a painter. It is strangely naive to think that a person can become a skilled painter by having tools such as a brush and canvas.

A man meets a woman. Both express their love for each other. They draw an idea of the future. They are going to paint a future. This idea is very beautiful in their minds; but in their world, this beautiful picture should be painted on the canvas called life. If they don't have enough skills, this scene that finally manifests on the canvas can be so ugly and disgusting that it is impossible to imagine.

So it is clear that to have a healthy and successful romantic relationship, life skills, communication skills, intellectual and cultural skills are necessary. In other words, love is an art in every sense. This is the same category that we see in the title of the book *The Art of Loving* by Eric Fromm. According to what was mentioned above, Eric Fromm is trying to show that love is not just a human feeling that anyone can enter into its process after reaching maturity and benefit from its benefits. The author even mentions that this book is not a guide to love, because love is a sublime art rather than a simple relationship.

The summary of the approach of this book is that if a person does not complete the process of all-round evolution of his personality in order to understand and attract love and cannot reach a transcendental romantic worldview, any effort on his part to love is doomed to failure. According to Fromm, a romantic relationship will be based on two main foundations: deep mutual connection plus happiness. Therefore, any emotional relationship that is called love, if it is devoid of these two elements, is definitely not love.

Of course, it should be noted that neither in the book *The Art of Loving* nor in the book before you, there is ever an attempt to trivialize all kinds of human relationships. Rather, the point is that love can correct most of the human behavioral flaws that lead to various misfortunes, especially in the relationship between men and women.

Another point is that love is only one thing and has a single nature. Now mankind does not make any difference whatever name he puts on it. These nouns may include things such as: affection, friendship, love, feeling, interest, conduct, discovery and intuition and the like. These designations do not make a difference in the unique nature of love. Love either exists or it doesn't. To improve the relationship between men and women, the presence of love is inevitable. Love in any form does not make much difference in the story.

The book *The Art of Loving* begins with the question: "Is love an art? If it is art, does it need knowledge and effort? Is love a pleasant feeling whose understanding depends on a person's luck?" The main content of the book *The Art of Loving* is an attempt to develop the discussion around the same first question. But in the following, he pays attention to the topics that we have discussed in this book and the pages above. Topics such as the decline of love in contemporary society and the issue of practicing love.

The point that Erich Fromm pays attention to is that love has no boundaries. As we mentioned above, the marriage code is full of standards and rules that try to set boundaries for love. This is why we say that marriage in the current style is contrary to love, and the parties should pack these rules and put them in the archive when starting life, even in the form of a conventional marriage, and based on their individual principles and standards, that is: "The art of loving" and "the interweaving of love and freedom" continue on their way.

Until love is transferred to the real realm of life with all earthly needs, it is not considered love in this discussion. What Fromm tries to draw in his book in a practical way, about love as an uplifting factor and the driving engine of life, has nothing to do with fictional and tragic loves. True love is that which is manifested in a real way between two physical human beings and the concrete embodiment of its presence can be observed in interpersonal relationships. Therefore, it can be said that one-sided love has almost no meaning.

As a human being, with all his existential coordinates, if he is aware of his original nature and with the help of the essence of love and the light that shines in his life, he sees the world as it is and interprets it according to his understanding and feelings.

When love and wisdom work together as the main elements of determining the path of human destiny, man can bring his wholeness to the fore together with his life partner. In this case, love is an activating potential for men and women and not a passive, enslaving, jealous and unstable element. The characteristic of true love can alleviate many problems and adversities of human societies.

Being in love does not mean an intense and temporary or transitory feeling that one person wants to make a one-sided decision on the basis of which, and aligns the other with one's personal desires and feelings. First of all, love is a form of judgment. A judgment about the other person who has the ray of love on him. After the stage of judgment and selection, it is time for mutual acceptance, and after that comes commitment and loyalty.

Who does not know that having such reserves, two people can live a life full of peace and happiness with pleasure and comfort. Now, whether this alignment is in the form of a traditional and customary marriage or without it, there will be no difference in the nature of the issue.

Now it's time for training. To continue love and explore its labyrinth moment by moment, man and woman must begin to train themselves and their bodies to adapt to love. True, just as a painter needs constant practice and effort to paint his best creative work. Therefore, there is never any room for reflection and pause in order to achieve the most sublime aspects of the arts (including the art of loving).

Just as a person is not born with perfect art, he is not born with transcendental love either. It is clear that some people are more talented than others in all kinds of arts. But there is no difference in the problem. All human beings are relatively artists and reach unknown horizons and peaks with practice. Love is the same. All human beings are born with the innate talent of love. Now, depending on the educational and educational environment and the way of life and the quality of the people around them, they grow or remain useless. With the remark that the art of love is one of the most delicate and original arts.

All humans have a body with similar characteristics. But some of them can reach the peak of creativity by practicing and training their bodies. For example, among dancers, many degrees and stages of art come to the fore. Love is the same. Depending on how much we challenge and interact with the art of love, we can discover more invisible dimensions of it in our personal lives.

With the difference that women are much more talented in this field. Both in the art of dancing and the art of loving. If we compare life experience and skill to walking. The art of making love is like the movements that dancers or ballerinas perform with great skill.

Now that we are talking about dance, it is better to say that making love is ultimately a two-way and group art. Two-person dances are very dependent on the type of movements and performance techniques of the parties. If one of the parties commits a mistake in the complex and delicate steps of dancing, eventually the totality of the art as a two-way action and the expected harmony that is necessary for the continuation of the beauty process will be damaged.

Love is a more complex art. Because in dance and other two-person arts, the emotional conflict is much less. Body movements and technical posture play a major role in shaping art. But in love, the role of the body is less. In the art of loving, there is a kind of homogeneity and convergence between two different worlds. Two worlds that include both the unknown realms of the soul and the sensual realms of the body. When these two worlds get closer and closer, it becomes possible for the parties to connect with the subtleties and unknowns inside each other and touch each other's insides.

This issue works like a double-edged sword. If all the factors involved in this relationship work well, it can be the meeting point of two huge forces and the factor of convergence and creation of a much stronger force. But if the contradictions appear from within this interweaving of feeling and spirit, then the amount of destruction will be much higher, which can cause great damage to the health of the body, soul and life of the parties. For this reason, psychologists put a lot of emphasis on knowledge and familiarity before marriage. Because in case of progress of convergence, with the discovery of possible incompatibilities, the amount of destruction will be more extensive.

It is obvious that by discovering the inconsistencies inside, the parties should take action to end the relationship as soon as possible so that the amount of damage is less. As the old proverb says: "Whenever you prevent a loss, there is a gain," ending a bad relationship is also preventing more losses. But on the other hand, a different saying, which is an example of emphasizing a wrong idea, says: "A woman should go to the house of fortune in a white wedding dress and come out with a white shroud." This language is one of the examples of human ignorance, especially in the Eastern lands. Ignorance caused by society's tyrannical view of women. A view in which women are not important as a passive and worthless being.

Another important point about the importance of love in human life is that love is a generative, dynamic and reactive element. Love is like a mountain that will answer our voices with a voice. No matter how pure, honest and careless we act in the face of love, the reward he will give is far more than our action. According to Rumi's interpretation in Masnavi Manavi: "This world is a mountain, and our verb is a call—come to us, call the calls." In other words, as much as our encounter with love, as a heavy and mountainous reality, is genuine and honest, the echoes and reactions that come back to us will be more valuable.

The first criterion for the stability of love is that neither party asks for love, the process of love happens spontaneously. Humans behave against such a rule. This means that when they sincerely give their love to others, they expect that love will be returned to them immediately. They have put the concept of "heartbreak" for the void of love in these moments.

Heartbreak happens when a person definitely expects a response. Because he considers this feedback as his inalienable right. What is the significance of this inalienable right? They never think about it. They only know that this feedback is their right. Otherwise, in the most cultured way, they bring up the topic of heartbreak.

We said the most civilized state, because it is mostly the case that instead of heartbreak, we have witnessed inhuman behavior and even violence and murder. Honor killings are one of the reactions to the lack of expected feedback. What they expect from the other party, but they don't get it or for whatever reason they don't get the right feedback.

When a person turns violent in response to unrequited love, they are not following the rules of even the simplest transaction. In normal transactions, when the other party does not like the offered product, usually the trader no longer has any rights and the transaction ends, but autocratic love traders have come to the assumption that the other party is forced to accept the product offered by them, which they think is love. Accept it. Otherwise, it will be faced with their strong mental or physical reaction. This reaction ranges from heartbreak to murder and violence.

Such a belief is created because the lover or the trader does not consider the lover or the second party of the transaction to have the same rights as his own. The other party has no freedom of action to accept or reject. This is because when he did not accept, he faced strong reactions. A person who throws acid on the desired person due to the rejection of love or a request for marriage is so captive of the tyranny demon inside him that he does not think that perhaps his lover or desired as a human being has a simple human right called "choice."

Historical male tyranny and improper childhood upbringing have led him to believe that a woman, as the second sex, is in no position to refuse his request. In his opinion, a girl has become his "honor" right from the moment she caught his attention. This hateful concept, when introduced into the mind of a man with a wrong cultural and educational background, overshadows the wholeness of a woman as an independent human being.

In such a situation, mental dogmatism does not allow him to think to know that there are other people and other people whose moods and feelings may be the same as his and have the same spiritual streams. Therefore, the essence of love should be taken away and sought for a transcendent success in another place. This is what animals do in full culture and sobriety. Humans have to learn many civilized and social behaviors from animals. In this case, they learn from animals not to engage in honor killings, or to commit violence caused by refusing to listen.

No animal kills or even hurts another animal because of a negative response in love and does not speak of its heartbreak. When it's time for animals to mate, they offer their love goods to different people. After a few negative answers, finally one comes along who likes his stuff, and from here a healthy relationship is formed, which results in mating and the continuation of the generation.

The reason that humans are not even as civilized as animals in terms of love is that they have been brought up with very wrong upbringing since childhood. As soon as the child grows up and recognizes his physical and physiological differences with the opposite sex, he starts to exercise tyranny toward the opposite sex.

This behavior is accompanied by the encouragement and even happiness of the parents. A male child is taught that he is superior to his sister. He is allowed and even encouraged to exercise dictatorship over him. He controls his movements and criticizes all his actions and always has an authoritarian, repressive and slanderous tone toward him. In Eastern families, it is very rare that their upbringing patterns are such that male children see themselves in a completely equal position in front of female children.

Boys are taught that girls are their chastity and they have a duty to protect their chastity from external factors, especially from exposure to the opposite sex.

Unfortunately, families do not know how much they share in the bitterness of the fate of their daughters and even sons with this wrong upbringing.

With this upbringing, boys seek to start a family and apply their authoritarian and honor-loving view to their wives and children. After starting a family with this kind of view and wrong upbringing, girls realize that in the general view of society, they have no identity other than the weaker sex and nothing but an honor that is always and everywhere taken care of.

This vicious cycle reaches their children and continues from generation to generation. Unfortunately, this tyrannical view and wrong education has become so institutionalized and internalized that when girls are in the position of raising their children, they parrot the same anti-woman and incorrect educational patterns to their children. With a huge wave of awareness, the women of the society can break this vicious cycle somewhere and prevent the continuation of this destructive virus in the next generations.

Insisting on marriage or continuing a relationship that is not mixed with enough love or is accompanied by resentment and misunderstanding is to make life bitter. When misunderstanding is the main basis of the relationship, when two people meet, they produce more suffering and bitterness.

Every movement and behavior will lead to a wrong interpretation. The displeasure of the two parties when multiplied together creates a double amount of displeasure and eventually it will reach a point where each of the parties will go their own way or one of them will oppress and imprison the other or in the best case it will lead to divorce. will be.

Osho says about the mechanisms of conventional loveless marriage: "As far as I know, 99% of marriages end when the honeymoon is over. But then you are trapped, you have no way to escape. Then if you want to leave your wife or she wants to leave you, the whole society, the law, the court will stand against you. Then all morality, religion, priests will all be against you. In fact, society should create all kinds of obstacles for marriage and not for divorce. Society should not allow people to get married so easily. The court has to create all kinds of obstacles—live with this woman for at least two years, then the court will allow you to marry her."

Even the criterion of marriage should not be the beauty of the husband or wife. Beauty is very impermanent and visual appeal is lost very soon. What guarantees the durability and survival of the relationship is the alchemy of love.

Osho says: "The human woman never looks beautiful. A human husband never looks beautiful. Beauty disappears when you get to know each other." He adds: "Divorces exist because marriages are based on emotional states. A person should not marry a woman or a man out of a poetic mood because life is not just poetry. There comes a time when life turns to prose and eventually you may even be dealing with tragedy. Love, because it is realistic and forgiving, can save and move the train of life from all these situations and even crises."

The love of the feelings that is popularly called puppy love is a fleeting feeling that you can never build the foundation of marriage and life on. When they say that love disappears with marriage, they mean such love. True love is strengthened by marriage. Unless the parties (especially men) have not learned the art of loving. The art of being in love while being free. Loving while forgiving and respecting each other. If the realities of love and life are understood, marriage in any form and rule is the great opportunity for the growth and excellence of the parties. An opportunity to grow and evolve. The same possibility that creation has given to man or woman to bring the evolutionary aspects of life to the fore by finding their lost half.

Genuine love is like diamond pieces. Diamond is never destroyed, never changed shape and never combined with other materials. It does not get confused in the surrounding nature. It remains as authentic and holy as it was in the beginning. The alchemical and diamond-like originality of love is also like this. Love does not disappear with marriage, nor fades with the intervention and efforts of those around, nor does it disappear with the discovery of a woman's womb being defective.

Sexual attraction is a temporary thing and the fire is fleeting. But when this fickle flame is connected to the endless substance of love, its flames will never subside. When the lover and the beloved meet again after decades of life and courtship, they will be fresh and unknown and full of freshness just like the first courtship. This issue is the guarantee of the strange durability of the relationships that started with love and survive with the help of love.

When a man keeps a woman locked up in the house and busy with affairs and knocks on every door in pursuit of sexual diversity, she has never been in love. Marriage of expediency or feeling that connected the two to each other was fundamentally wrong. Sexual attraction is always fresh in the unknown. When there is love, the parties are constantly discovering unknown things in the other. But if not, the charms will disappear with the normalization of the unknown elements.

The sexual attraction in the middle of the night is due to the novelty of familiarity, which lasts only once and for one night.

Because no one will fall in love with his bullshit. If there is no love, the task of sexual relationship between a man and a woman is also clear in this way. But because of the more preparations and delays that the establishment of this relationship had, this relationship goes beyond one night, but it is still unstable.

Marriage and Mental Betrayal

As Rumi states, in the absence of love, evils can grow and develop. This is also the case in the marriage process. When love is not involved, everything depends on the rules. Human life has shown that rules are not very effective in the absence of spiritual components.

A man and a woman who start a family life with each other without love and within the framework of traditional ceremonies and in the form of legal restrictions, after a while they get tired and annoyed with each other. This point is the beginning of external and internal tensions on both sides. What Iraj Mirza humorously mentions about men and women going after their whims in practice determines the fate of many marriages. With the difference that men in different societies, especially in Eastern societies that are governed by religious laws, have the upper hand in sexual adventures and diversity.

Legal polygamy and legal prostitution that takes place in the form of concubines and other processes of receiving sexual services have eliminated the problems of men to achieve their urgent desire. But women have a different situation due to the many strictures around them and due to social taboos. When there is no love, attraction and passion, this thing that has now become a duty, gradually turns into hatred and becomes a mental and internal matter. Mental betrayal is the first achievement of such a situation. This phenomenon can be clearly seen in the following story which is mentioned in different sources:

The man was very sick. He had tried all kinds of treatments, but none of them helped. He went to a hypnotist. The hypnotist gave the man a dhikr. "I am not sick," he had to repeat several times a day. "I am not sick. I am healthy." The man felt better after a few days and after a few weeks he was completely fine. He went to his wife and said: "This treatment was a complete miracle. But now I feel that my sexual power has weakened and maybe it is better to go to a hypnotist to treat this deficiency because our sexual relationship has almost stopped."

The woman, who also felt frustrated, was happy and encouraged the man to go to the hypnotist again. The man went to a hypnotist and received another zikr. But when his wife asked him about the content of the new zikr, she did not get an answer.

However, after a few weeks, the man regained his health and his sexual desire peaked. The woman, who was very surprised, kept asking what the miraculous medicine the hypnotist gave him was. The man was still laughing and did not answer. The woman, who became curious, watched the man and one day when he was repeating his zikr in the bathroom, she heard him say, "This is not my wife. This is not my wife. This is not my wife."

This story is a perfect picture of the flawed relationship that many people continue in the form of conventional marriage. Many of them prefer to endure the hell of a flawed and treacherous relationship and not divorce because of the slander of those around them or the pressure that may be imposed on them by the society. Sometimes the existence of children can be the reason and motivation for such couples not to divorce.

When there is no love, formal relationships begin to decline. Sensual needs and sexual attractions fade and men go out of the house as soon as possible to satisfy their sexual needs. Women are also more likely to commit mental infidelity and, if possible, actual infidelity. There is a line between healthy and unhealthy relationships that is right here. When a person allows the thought to enter his mind that the other person is not his ideal spouse. Betrayal and the collapse of the relationship has begun.

Sometimes it has been seen that couples continue to benefit from the blessings of love in spite of reaching old age. Contrary to some people who think that such relationships may be pretentious. In fact, it is not. Love is not a phenomenon for which age has meaning, nor does the soul know age. Therefore, we see that in the life of loving couples, despite their old age, love is still present and dynamic, just like in the first days of dating.

Love and spirit know no time. It does not lose its freshness; the body ages; but the honeymoon of lovers never ends. Every morning when they open their eyes to another day, they are actually in the first hours of their acquaintance. Everything starts from scratch. Traveling does not leave boredom in their hearts.

But when the relationship is devoid of the element of love, the marriage ends the day after the honeymoon. The short period full of freshness of bodies is over in the blink of an eye. Then, everything goes to silence and oblivion. The nagging begins. The feeling of loss and regret comes. The parties consider the other to be the main cause of problems and tensions. The building that was built a while ago starts to be destroyed and the relationship ends. In the vacuum of love, every movement and behavior is evaluated with curiosity and misunderstanding. The parties are trying to beat each other and every day the tensions are piled on each other and there comes a time when it is practically impossible to tolerate the other. The rooms are separated from each other and later it is time to separate houses and lives.

But when there is love, life is an endless journey. A silent inner current that takes place deep within. Sometimes there is no need to speak at all. Instead of rules, feelings speak. There is no place for domination and ownership. because he has found himself in someone else. No one can seek mastery over himself. No one can seek disrespect and deprivation of their freedoms. The world of love is like the world of meditators. Like the world of those who are interested in yoga, prayer and self-cultivation. In every refinement and trimming that happens in this hierarchy of love, a step toward evolution is taken. Therefore, love is far more effective and efficient than religion for the stages of emotional and even physical development.

People also make other mistakes. It is said that too much love can turn into hate. This is a gross error. A mistake that is a kind of disrespect to the privacy of love. Love never turns into hate. If it is love, the idea of throwing acid on the beloved will never come to mind in response to a proposal.

The feeling of hurting a lover who may not be yours is there because the lover has a misunderstanding. He has a strong sense of ownership. In the presence of love, the beloved is never considered honorable. When you consider your lover to be honorable, you have actually violated his privacy and individual freedoms. A lover can never attack the beloved.

In the story of Laila and Majnoon that we mentioned earlier, when Majnoon faces a negative response to his proposal, not only does he not harbor hatred, but love in an elevated form emanates from him and is given to a captive deer:

> This eye, if not the eyes of the lover
> But it is a reminder of her black eye

Love and nature are two intertwined and inseparable elements. Therefore, the lover behaves much more humanely and gently when dealing with other beings. Therefore, when love is woven into the parts of a person's existence, his whole life becomes a meditative process. When we talk about mental infidelity, we are referring to a situation where love is absent. Otherwise, if love dissolves in the life of the parties, speaking in these cases will be completely useless.

Procreation and the Philosophy of Emptiness

What the anti-natalists argue about the need to prevent births goes far beyond the issues we discussed above. In the societies that we have talked about, the issue of preventing children from the human, economic, cultural aspects and of course from the aspect of women's rights is completely justified, logical and even humane.

The philosophy of Antinatalism looks at the matter much further than this. According to this philosophical point of view, first of all, we should know that life in general is a risky thing, and as a result, bringing a child into this world will be a risky thing again. This idea is proposed with the assumption of the realization of the minimum biological facilities for a child.

When the biological standard indicators are available for the presence of a child in this world and parents can provide favorable conditions for his upbringing and livelihood, we are facing the important question of whether parents have the right to arbitrarily force the fate of another person. Despite the possibility of facing the pains of this world, determine?

In cases where parents proceed to procreate without assessing their situation and without a complete picture of the future, the issue is much more than this. In the second situation, we are dealing with a moral and anti-human category. It is unlikely that a couple does not have an understanding of their living environment and the potential dangers that threaten the livelihood and lives of future children. However, David Benatar, as one of the main theorists of the "anti-natalist" philosophy, states in the book *Never to Be, To Be Born* that even the estimation of the quality of human life is unreliable.

Benatar believes that the parents of every child harm him by giving birth to him, and therefore giving birth to a child in general is a mistake that many parents repeat. According to him, as soon as a child is born, he is in a long-term state of pain and injury in his life process. By raising the issue of the asymmetry of concepts such as pain and pleasure, he assumed that life is a futile effort and struggle to understand pleasure, and he believes that this effort can be avoided simply by following the path of "nothingness." Especially as the generations continue and life becomes more complicated, the conflict between these misfits has become more and more complicated and there is no justification for entering into this complicated process. Therefore, never being is better than being.

The opposition to birth or "not being preferred" has much deeper roots than the thoughts of modern age philosophers and theorists like Benatar. It can be said that for the wandering man on earth, the "myth of nothing" has been one of the deep mythological beliefs. This belief exists in different layers and degrees in the literary and cultural works of different societies. The entire Persian literature is full of the preference of absence over existence. This concept can be seen in the writings of poets and writers of the classical era. Khayyam's intellectual and philosophical manifesto, which was later welcomed by many in the West, is about "preferring nothingness" and "taking advantage" because of the baselessness of existence. "The groundlessness of being" is the core of anti-natalist thinking.

After and before Khayyam, traces of this philosophical theory can be found in great poets like Hafez. This idea, either directly or through an intermediary, is one of the dominant elements and recurring themes in Persian literature. The indirect form of this argumentative structure is as follows: since the world is mortal and the principle is based on nothingness, then life should be managed in such a way that it seems as if we are going to travel from the "current urgent situation" to the "permanent promised land." At this point, the best way to deal with human desperation is the philosophy of "Be happy."

Love is also one of the themes and components that are suggested for a person trapped in a temporary existence. Hafez says:

Don't bother yourself about being or not being inside and be happy
Because ultimately everything that exists is nothingness
To suggest love as a suitable alternative, he writes:
O heart, do not be empty of love and drunkenness
Go as if you are freed from the thought of non-existence and existence

The philosophical principle of "existence or non-existence" has been not in the philosophical thought of the East, but in the entire world, including human heart desires. A thought that ultimately leads to the fact that perhaps the best option for humans is to "stay in nothingness"; it means not being born! It is the same philosophical thought that Jean-Paul Sartre examines its dimensions in the book *Being and Nothingness*. Shakespeare also expresses the same idea in the third act of the first scene of Hamlet in an effective way through the language of the story character (Hamlet).

In this world-famous soliloquy, Hamlet poses his question as follows: "To be or not to be, that is the question." After this sentence, Hamlet raises other basic questions that have always been relevant to mankind and it seems that he has not yet found an answer for it. Hamlet asks: "To be, or not to be, that's the question here! Is it more appropriate to submit to the arrow and whip of fate, or to draw a blade and fight with a sea of suffering and end them?" To die, to sleep—and nothing else.

And in this dream, we find out that the sufferings and thousands of sufferings that this earthly body is suffering have ended. This is the end to which one should eagerly aspire. Dying, falling asleep, falling asleep, and maybe dreaming…ha! This is the problem; because the thought of what kind of dreams arise in this dream of death after being freed from this mortal body makes us hesitate; And it is this expediency that adds misery to life. Otherwise, who is there who can bear all the shame and humiliation of the age, the cruelty of the tyrants, the insults of the braggarts, the sufferings of humiliated love, the shamelessness of the office holders who harvest patient and good people from themselves, while he can save himself with a bare dagger.

Philosophical theories based on the birth of antagonism and nihilism that we talked about follow an intellectual policy. Most of these views are based on the biological contradictions governing the relationships of life on earth as the logical foundations of their philosophy. This dominant view of the world is repeated almost uniformly in the philosophy, literature, art and worldview of the West and the East. What Khayyam says is ultimately in line with what Hafez, Maulana, Sartre, and Shakespeare said. This thought has been formed in the mind of man since the beginning of creation, and as his most important philosophical question, a convincing answer has not yet been found.

The extension of this philosophical thought on the historical trajectory has continued until Adam Abul Bashar. In the third part of Shahriar's Oedipus trilogy, called *Oedipus at Colonus*, the ancient Greek playwright Sophocles presents his own view on the preference of not being born in this way: "Not to be born, man, is the highest and best word. But if you see the light of day, seek to return as quickly as possible to where you came from."

Homer, a Greek poet from the 8th or 7th century BC, had the same idea. Just like the Sufi thoughts of the East, emphasizing the instability of the world, he says: "It is best not to be born, if it does not succeed, it is best to pass through the gates of Hades as quickly as possible."

The grounds of anti-birthism are very broad. There are many developers of this theory throughout history. In the following, we refer to these items in a list-wise manner:

- Believers of this theory say that reproducing and forcibly bringing other people into this world, which is full of poverty, suffering and disease, and the inevitable fate of every person is death, is a wrong thing.
- Many books and treatises have been written throughout the ages, all of them emphasize on proving the immorality of reproduction, regardless of the methods of proof.

- David Benatar believes that almost half of the children in the world are unwanted and few people really think about the moral issues related to giving birth to a child.
- Buddha says that if man realized the suffering he would produce by having children, he would refrain from having children.
- Manichaeans believed that procreation puts the soul in the dark prison of the body, so they considered reproduction as a tool in the hands of the devil that imprisons the divine existence in the body.
- Referring to the fact that the world is full of pain and suffering, Arthur Schopenhauer says: Considering all the issues, it would be better if life did not happen at all and there was no desire to live. If the desire to live is put aside, placing a human being in the world is unnecessary and meaningless and is questionable from a moral point of view.
- Miguel Cabrera, a Spanish sociologist, believes that reproduction is an example of total involvement in the destiny of another person, because the born person has no chance to defend himself and prevent his birth.
- Other intellectual standards of anti-birth theory are as follows:
- We have a moral duty not to create unhappy people, and we have no moral duty to create happy people.
- The possibility that a child will be happy after birth is not a valid reason to give birth to it, but the possibility that the child may suffer after birth is an important moral reason not to give birth to it.
- There is always the possibility that one day we will regret that someone's existence depended on our decision.
- People usually feel sad because some people come to this world and suffer, but usually they don't feel happy because some people come to this world and are happy.
- According to Benatar, by giving birth to a child, parents are not only responsible for his pains, but they are also jointly responsible for the suffering of the next generations, of which that child will be the head of the family. If we assume that each couple has three children, the total number of people born next

from this family will usually reach more than 88 thousand people. This number includes enormous amounts of suffering.
- The world is not a safe place to live because: until the beginning of the 20th century, more than 133 million people have been killed in mass killings. In the first eight decades of the 20th century, between 170 and 360 million people died in incidents such as shooting, torture, stabbing, burning, freezing, hard labor, drowning, execution, bombing, or other methods of killing by governments.
- The inevitable fate of every human being is death, so it is better not to create new humans.
- Damage to the environment, animals and the like is a direct result of reproduction.
- Most parents do not properly study the facts around them and this affects their desire to have a child.

The Solution to Birth Opponents

According to the above, one of the major solutions offered by anti-totalists is adoption. Adoption can increase the quality of the population and reduce the number of deprived children while distributing the living facilities more equitably. There are millions of unaccompanied children around the world. If parents are interested in having a child, it is better to think about taking care of unruly children instead of having children.

According to birth opponents, the factors involved in creating interest in having children are mostly unrealistic and unstudied. If these factors are studied in scientific and real conditions, we will realize that irresponsible factors are involved in the interest in having children, or having children in unfavorable or unwanted conditions. According to the theorists of this school of thought, these factors are as follows:

- One of these factors is nature's inherent tendency to reproduce. Nature is designed in such a way that the increase of births prevents the extinction of the generation.
- Another problem is unwanted births and lack of skill in birth control, which is more pronounced in underdeveloped

countries. A look at the number of starving children in Africa and displaced and homeless children around the world is an example of this.

- The lack of prevention tools and the lack of familiarity and skill in using these tools have a great influence on the increase of unwanted births and childbearing in inappropriate conditions.

- Inappropriate intervention of governments in the process of population growth is another factor that disturbs the natural mechanism of reproduction. The leaders of the societies are fueling this issue following their political and economic ambitions. In underdeveloped societies, mothers are considered as soldier production machines.

- Religions fuel the process of unnatural population growth due to the increase of their geographical followers. If stratified religions are combined with ideological governments, they provide one of the most dangerous grounds for the creation of poor-quality populations and the fall of biological indicators.

- The fundamental foundations of religions have automatically focused on increasing the population and fertility of women. For example, in the book of Genesis, we read: "God blessed them and God said to them: Be fruitful and multiply and fill the earth and subdue it." The performance of other religions is almost the same or more thorough than this.

In any case, our ultimate goal of discussing this issue in this book is just a passing reference to the category of pregnancy and the problems it creates for women in life. Because this discussion is very long and requires an independent topic.

A Child Is Not an Imitation Machine

Regardless of the above, the educational system governing children suffers from other defects and shortcomings. The most important shortcoming in the educational system of children is the creation of a kind of dominance system in shaping the mind and consciousness of children. Religious idealisms, political dogmatism, and the dependence of children's education on the issue of geography and the influence of the family on geographic components, such as dogmatic philosophy and theology, make the world society become certain poles.

Sometimes, it happens that after the child reaches the age of puberty, due to being in the path of global consciousness waves, he questions his educational system in general and uses other models for his life. But the prevailing trend is the same as we said.

A child's mind, at birth, is an unwritten blank slate. In addition to the family, which has a great tendency to write their mental menus on this white board, political systems and religious sects, which are clearly scattered in geographical areas, are very sensitive and interested in the regulation of the content of this white board.

In domination systems and societies that do not benefit from the blessings of democracy, this situation is more complicated. Networks and formal educational and educational organizations prepare targeted (and sometimes biased) programs to pursue long-term goals and specific interests by mentally guiding children in a certain direction.

One of the major damages that the ruling systems of the world inflict on children is the attempt to recruit soldiers in order to consolidate ideological foundations. A child is an innocent and receptive human being and is fully capable of intellectual exploitation. In fact, a child does not have the ability and power to reason and say "no" until he has reached intellectual and physical maturity. He is completely dependent on his family and social groups and formal education systems and disarmed against the forces around him.

Superstitious beliefs and outdated ideologies and false thoughts are among the contents that defenseless children are exposed to. Sometimes the mental content that is imposed on the child's mind in the childhood environment is so poisonous and meaningless that the actions of parents and governments take on an inhuman nature.

Imposing data on the minds and beliefs of children and depriving them of the possibility of any kind of independent voting and searching, causes their ultimate personality in adulthood to be accompanied by a large amount of passivity and acceptance, and their mental creativity is crushed.

Blind prejudices, opposition to awareness and knowledge and prejudice instead of originality of research and wrong judgments are just some of the achievements of such practice in raising children. This is how concepts such as discovery, intuition, and authenticity of truth have become alchemical elements in human society.

Family and systems surrounding children, especially in Eastern societies, are fundamentally in conflict with elements such as skepticism, questioning, civil disobedience, intellectual rebellion, and independence of vote. This is because in closed societies, all children are born the same. It is as if all children, as raw materials of educational systems, are cast in a specific and inflexible mold and pass through a specific production line which is controlled by a single centrality, and finally products with specific characteristics are produced.

This issue is completely against the nature of human creation. Every human child is born with a reliable individuality that, if the necessary prerequisites are fulfilled, can benefit from its enormous intelligence to achieve an exclusive and dynamic personality. But the process of machine and factory education burns and destroys these potentials at the very beginning of childhood.

In an ideal educational system where there is no family or systems of dominance and levers of power, we will witness a confusion of conditioning rules. In such a system, most children have the necessary capacity and talent to become a pious, disruptive and questioning human being. In fact, those who we consider today as prominent human figures on earth and in human history are those who exceptionally managed to escape from this routinely conditioned system or grew up in an environment where these systems of domination, power and sovereignty were limited.

In the biographies of some elders, we have heard stories of people leaving the routine educational systems and running away from school and dropping out or not benefiting from a concentrated family. These show well that the power of creativity of these people was caused by their disobedience to the educational and family domination systems. In other words, getting out of the cycle of imitation that most human children have to go through and reach adulthood is the most important prerequisite for making changes in the educational system and achieving great achievements.

In fact, humanity needs to break this vicious circle in order to create a new social life that is full of elements such as dynamism, breadth of opinion, creativity, leaving the circle of dogmatic thinking and understanding the acceptance of others; A cycle that families and governments have experienced working over the past centuries, and its disadvantages are quite obvious.

This destructive educational system has caused children to have no reliable sources of information in their most sensitive educational period, when they need rich and correct sources of information. It is true that sometimes children during puberty, while returning to their childhood educational foundations, criticize it and even hate its principles and standards; but we should not forget that some teachings and intellectual approaches of childhood are engraved in children's minds and remain unchangeable until the end of their lives.

The human subconscious mind is formed to a great extent during childhood. In other words, the leaven of human nature is the alchemy of human existence that is given to parents during childhood so that they can shape it as they see fit. Now imagine that parents who are devoid of any kind of knowledge and awareness and have suffered from an unhealthy educational process, are supposed to be responsible for educating the next generation of society.

This crisis is one of the most important ruptures and faults of mankind, which should be repaired by dismantling the educational dominance of families or increasing their generational knowledge. If this is not done, human society will never witness the improvement of the situation in important areas such as religious dogmatism, superstitions, religious fundamentalisms, terror networks, racism, intolerance, and the like.

Families with the aforementioned characteristics, in the first place, crush the human structure of the child under the initial pressures and then fill their souls with a large amount of pollution from which they themselves suffer. Due to the fact that the child is surrounded by family and clan members and the social environment, the child does not have any access to other sources of information.

Parents think exactly the same way as uncles and aunts and family children think. The child is caught in the middle of a certain colony with certain rules of thought. There is no way to change the color of the congregation and take the color and smell of the people around.

This is the biggest destruction that the family and tribal education system brings to human society. A destruction that is the product of a one-dimensional, petrified, one-sided and passive person who is completely dependent on the mother or the environment in the field of personal feelings and emotional dependence.